THE MANNER BORN

I am native here and to the manner born. —*Hamlet*, I, iv, 14

THE MANNER BORN

Birth Rites in Cross-Cultural Perspective

EDITED BY
LAUREN DUNDES

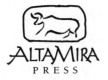

ALTAMIRA PRESS
A Division of Rowman & Littlefield Publishers, Inc.
Walnut Creek • Lanham • New York • Oxford

AltaMira Press
A Division of Rowman & Littlefield Publishers, Inc.
A Member of the Rowman & Littlefield Publishing Group
1630 North Main Street, #367
Walnut Creek, CA 94596
www.altamirapress.com

Rowman & Littlefield Publishers, Inc.
4501 Forbes Boulevard, Suite 200
Lanham, MD 20706

P.O. Box 317
Oxford
OX2 9RU, UK

Copyright © 2003 by AltaMira Press

British Library Cataloguing in Publication Information Available

Library of Congress Cataloging-in-Publication Data

The manner born : birth rites in cross-cultural perspective / edited by
Lauren Dundes.
      p. cm.
Includes bibliographical references and index.
  ISBN 0-7591-0264-3 (cloth : alk. paper) — ISBN 0-7591-0265-1 (pbk. :
alk. paper)
  1. Birth customs—Cross-cultural studies. 2.
Childbirth—Cross-cultural studies. I. Dundes, Lauren, 1962–
   GN482.1 .M36 2003
   392.1'2—dc21

                                                    2002013882

Printed in the United States of America

♾™ The paper used in this publication meets the minimum requirements of American
National Standard for Information Sciences—Permanence of Paper for Printed Library
Materials, ANSI/NISO Z39.48-1992.

CONTENTS

Acknowledgments

I WOULD NOT HAVE ENJOYED the process of editing *The Manner Born* without the assistance of a number of individuals. I am grateful to my editor at AltaMira Press, Rosalie Robertson, for her enthusiasm for the project; to Mary Bearden, who painstakingly copyedited the manuscript; and to Dianne Ewing, my production editor, who facilitated the process of preparing the book for publication. The willingness of long-time friend Kristen Jensen to create the cover art for this book was also much appreciated. Finally, I wish to thank my husband, Mike, and my children, Zachary and Madeline, for encouraging me in my academic pursuits.

Introduction

T
HE ARRAY OF CROSS-CULTURAL CUSTOMS surrounding birth through infancy includes practices that are both fascinating and instructive. One might logically but incorrectly assume that human birth is essentially a "natural" phenomenon, biologically and physiologically determined to a degree that would make the details of parturition more or less universal, meaning virtually identical in all cultural contexts. The theoretical difficulty is that "nature" can never be identified or perceived except through the lens of culture. The visions of nature afforded by diverse cultural spectacles offer a rich panoply of hues and textures. Yet because of ethnocentrism, the idea that the observer's understanding of reality is the "natural" and "correct" one—as opposed to the alternative understandings of the "same" phenomenon articulated by members of other cultures—it is often hard to appreciate the relativity of one's own views. What an individual takes for granted is rarely questioned. In the case of the perinatal custom of circumcision of male infants, for example, many persons outside the United States find this seemingly unnecessary mutilation of the penis (often carried out without any anesthetic given to the hapless subject) to be barbaric, despite many Americans' decision to blindly follow this tradition (for samples of the abundant literature on this topic, see Bryk [1934]; Romberg [1985]; Chebel [1992]). Additionally, Western people might not realize that most births do not take place in hospitals, but rather in homes, that the birth attendant is rarely a male obstetrician, but more commonly a female midwife, and that the optimum birthing position is not a supine position but rather an upright or squatting posture. It turns out that there is considerable cultural variation with respect to almost every aspect of the parturition process. It is my hope that this sampling of the enormous literature available in medical, anthropological, sociological, and public health periodicals and books will convey some of this remarkable diversity. Given the assumption that more rather than less knowledge is a desideratum, the goal of assembling these essays as a whole is to help demystify and elucidate one of the most basic and critical parts of human existence.

Most studies of birthing concentrate on just a single culture or aspect of the process and for this reason it is difficult to get a picture of the full range of variation surrounding this fundamental event. While there are numerous monographs and articles that describe distinct facets of birthing, this book focuses on broad cross-cultural coverage of different birthing issues, rather than on a single dimension. Subjects covered include attitudes and techniques in childbirth, the interaction between human evolutionary form and birthing procedures, the influence of societal factors that differentiate Western from non-Western maternal birthing positions, and the art of midwifery. Also treated are less well-known areas of birthing such as the imagery of birthing, placenta rituals, and popular beliefs about the amniotic membrane called a caul. In addition, the book presents essays that explore humoral medical tradition used in birthing, the possible influence of cultural practices on Sudden Infant Death Syndrome (SIDS), customs and beliefs regarding breastfeeding, weaning, and swaddling, and finally a sociobiological perspective on early infant behavior.

The practices and customs described in the articles, however, cannot represent an entire culture. Nor can these articles discuss every aspect of the puerperal period. Nor can we assume that rituals of birthing remain static over time, especially in light of the increasing worldwide tendency toward globalization. Furthermore, questions of accuracy must be raised whether they result from informants' modesty, their understandable reluctance to share their ways with uninvited guests whom they perceive to be little more than prying, inquiring strangers, or whether they reflect a supposedly objective observer's own unavoidable culture-bound biases (see Freeman [1999] for a detailed if somewhat controversial account of such issues regarding Margaret Mead's work in Samoa). Readers must realize that all data are subject to such lenses.

In a multicultural society, it is imperative that medical practitioners at all levels become at least marginally familiar with the range of traditional behavioral norms likely to be encountered in clinics and hospitals. It is hoped that the diverse essays selected in this volume will aid in demonstrating some of the parameters of parturition as perceived in different cultures. But aside from the important practical reasons why greater awareness of birth customs might be beneficial to both doctor and patient, there is the intellectual rationale aimed at expanding enlightenment regarding one of life's most critical events, the arrival and treatment of neonates.

For much of Western history, infant care was not considered to be particularly significant with respect to the formation of adult personality and character. Often, wealthy individuals would turn over the care of their infants to surrogates, for example, employing wet-nurses to breastfeed these infants. In modern times, with more and more women working outside the home, the number of infant care-providers has increased so that infant care may be left to individuals other than the parents, individuals who may or may not be qualified or really interested in providing such a service. In this context, it behooves parents to be aware of postnatal traditions, especially if the person employed to look after their infant comes from a culture different from that of the parents.

Of course, there are dozens of standard baby books to advise new parents as to what to do with respect to all the questions that arise connected with birth and the period immediately thereafter (cf. Jacobsen, 1995; Hart, 1998). This book is not intended to replace such compendia. Rather it is designed to demonstrate the ethnocentrism inevitably inherent in any one culture. There are indeed many diverse ways of caring for a newborn infant, and it is by no means a certainty that any one of these is necessarily the best or "only" right procedure to follow. Exposure to a selected sample of the world's collective wisdom with respect to birth and postnatal tradition may increase tolerance of alternative customs and in the long run contribute to the betterment of conditions of birth and of infants postnatally.

There is a vast literature devoted to birthing. In one type of article, authors use a narrative style that details aspects of birthing including the parturient's feelings about the event, the family's reaction, customs, beliefs, and specific practices. This personal approach provides the reader with a very compelling understanding of birthing in its cultural context. Authors often provide a composite picture of the birthing experience that gives the reader a more representative picture of the event. Several excellent non-Western examples of this narrative genre include Gideon's (1962) account of a baby born in the Punjab, Barnes's (1949) description of the birth of a child in Zimbabwe, Hanks's (1963) work about the birth of a child in Bang Chan, Thailand, Laderman's (1982) description of a birth in a Malay village, a varied anthology of ancient texts, songs, and birth stories (Meltzer, 1981) and Scaletta's (1986) case history from West New Britain, Papua New Guinea. One of the more unique Western accounts was written by anthropologist Alma Gottlieb (1995) who vividly describes her own experience giving birth while doing fieldwork among the Beng people of the Ivory Coast. An especially detailed account of birthing can be found in Hilma Granqvist's (1947) classic *Birth and Childhood among the Arabs*. In the book's nearly 300 pages, Granqvist includes some narrative-style accounts of birth as well as pre- and postnatal customs in Palestine.

Certain books include a description of birth that is part of an entire life story (see e.g., Shostak's [1981] celebrated portrayal of a !Kung woman, or Delaney's [1991] work on Turkish village society). Still other books (e.g., Turner, 1978) include fictionalized narratives of birth experiences.

The wealth of information surrounding birth is prodigious including the period prior to birth (e.g., rules regarding maternal eating, working, and behavior), predictive techniques, the birth itself, and actions of the midwife. Listova (1991) offers a guide for the collection of material on the customs and rituals surrounding childbirth. Others simply enumerate the birthing customs of a culture. In cases where the information is overwhelmingly voluminous, authors have been known to simply list birthing customs (e.g., Pass [1938] who enumerates 251 birthing customs of inhabitants of Ingria, located on the present border between Estonia and Russia).

Among the copious descriptions of birthing, several include extensive detail, for example, Rombandeeva's (1968) account of the customs of the Mansi (in Siberia), Gaer's (1992) work on the Nanai of Eurasia, Brindley's (1985) paper on the Zulu,

Foll's (1959) research in Burma, and Jensen's (1966–67) study of Iban birth in Borneo, Malaysia.

Other valuable works include Mary Smith's (1981) description of the ritual of childbirth among the Muslim Hausa in northern Nigeria. Smith's extensive interviewing of an elderly woman in a Hausa tribe resulted in a chapter that provides a detailed depiction of birth. Likewise, Rigoberta Menchu (1984) provides an account of birthing among the Quiche Indians in Guatemala, facilitated by the fact that her mother served as a midwife from the age of sixteen until her death at age forty-three. Mary Kawena Pukui (1942) assisted her midwife aunt, who like several other close relatives were experts in delivering babies. Her firsthand experience contributed to her complete description of birthing in traditional Hawaii. Readers interested in the specifics of childbirth in a single culture would profit from consulting these and other similar sources (cf. Diulio, 1986).

In an effort to reproduce the essays in this volume in a form as close as possible to their original design, the chapters will vary in format. The thirteen essays included in this volume were written at different times, the earliest in 1949, and the latest in 1996. One may well wonder at the wisdom of reprinting older papers, but the fact is that the insights contained in Ruth Benedict's 1949 classic comparison of swaddling motivations in Eastern Europe or the fascinating data presented in Thomas Forbes's erudite 1953 survey of beliefs connected with the caul are no less stimulating in the twenty-first century. No one essay could possibly do justice to the complexities of birthing. However, taken as a whole, it is my hope that the sum total of the thirteen essays brought together from a great variety of published sources will provide a unique comparative view of the nature of childbirth as it is found in cultures throughout the world.

References

Barnes, H. F. 1949. "The Birth of a Ngoni Child." *Man* 49: 87–89.

Brindley, M. 1985. "Old Women in Zulu Culture: The Old Woman and Childbirth." *South African Journal of Ethnology* 8: 98–108.

Bryk, F. 1934. *Circumcision in Man and Woman: Its History, Psychology and Ethnology.* New York: American Ethnological Press.

Chebel, M. 1992. *Histoire de la Circoncision: des origines à nos jours* (History of Circumcision: From its origins to the present day). Paris: Editions Ballard.

Delaney, C. 1991. *The Seed and the Soil: Gender and Cosmology in Turkish Village Society.* Berkeley: University of California Press.

Diulio, R. C. 1986. *Childbirth: An Annotated Bibliography and Guide.* New York: Garland.

Foll, C. V. 1959. "Some Beliefs and Superstitions about Pregnancy, Parturition and Infant Health in Burma." *Journal of Tropical Pediatrics* 5: 51–58.

Freeman, D. 1999. *The Fateful Hoaxing of Margaret Mead: A Historical Analysis of Her Samoan Research.* Boulder, Colo.: Westview Press.

Gaer, E. A. 1992. "Traditional Customs and Rituals of the Nanai in the Late Nineteenth and Early Twentieth Centuries." *Anthropology and Archeology of Eurasia* 31: 40–66.

Gideon, H. 1962. "A Baby Is Born in the Punjab." *American Anthropologist* 64: 1220–1234.

Gottlieb, A. 1995. "The Anthropologist As Mother: Reflections on Childbirth Observed and Childbirth Experienced." *Anthropology Today* 11: 10–14.

Granqvist, H. 1947. *Birth and Childhood among the Arabs: Studies in a Muhammadan Village in Palestine.* Helsingfors: Söderström.

Hanks, J. R. 1963. "The Birth of a Child in Bang Chan, Thailand." In *Maternity and Its Rituals in Bang Chan,* edited by J. R. Hanks (pp. 41–57). Cornell Thailand Project Interim Reports Series 6. Ithaca: Department of Asian Studies, Cornell University.

Hart, D. 1998. "'How-To' Literature: A Comparison of Some Texts on Childbirth." In *The Virtues of Language,* edited by D. Stein (pp. 213–228). Amsterdam: Benjamins.

Jacobsen, C. R. 1995. "Lifting the Curse of Eve: Women Writers and Advice Literature on Childbirth." *Women's Studies in Communication* 18: 135–151.

Jensen, E. 1966–67. "Iban Birth." *Folk* (8–9): 165–178.

Laderman, C. 1982. "Giving Birth in a Malay Village." In *Anthropology of Human Birth,* edited by M. A. Kay. Philadelphia: F. A. Davis.

Listova, T. A. 1991. "A Program for the Collection of Material on the Customs and Rituals Associated with Childbirth." *Soviet Anthropology and Archeology* 30: 53–66.

Meltzer, D., ed. 1981. *Birth: An Anthology of Ancient Texts, Songs, Prayers and Stories.* San Francisco: North Point Press.

Menchu, R. 1984. "Birth Ceremonies of the Quiche Indians of Guatemala." In *I, Rigoberta Menchu: An Indian Woman in Guatemala* (pp. 7–17). London: Verso.

Pass, E. 1938. "About the Customs at Childbirth among the Ingers and the Votes." *Opetatud Eesti Seltsi Toimetused* 30: 538–564.

Pukui, M. K. 1942. "Hawaiian Beliefs and Customs during Birth, Infancy, and Childhood." *Occasional Papers of Bernice P. Bishop Museum* 16: 357–381.

Rombandeeva, E. I. 1968. "Some Observances and Customs of the Mansi (Voguls) in Connection with Childbirth." In *Popular Beliefs and Folklore Tradition in Siberia,* edited by V. Dioszegi (pp. 77–83). The Hague: Mouton.

Romberg, R. 1985. *Circumcision. The Painful Dilemma.* South Hadley, Mass.: Bergin and Garvey.

Scaletta, N. M. 1986. "Childbirth: A Case History from West New Britain, Papua New Guinea." *Oceania* 57: 33–52.

Shostak, M. 1981. *Nisa, the Life and Words of a !Kung Woman.* Cambridge, Mass.: Harvard University Press.

Smith, M. F. 1981. *The Ritual of Childbirth among the Muslim Hausa of Nigeria.* New Haven, Conn.: Yale University Press.

Turner, A. W. 1978. *Rituals of Birth: From Prehistory to the Present.* New York: David McKay.

Editor's Introduction

I

Childbirth in Cross-Cultural Perspective

NILES NEWTON AND MICHAEL NEWTON

ONE OF THE PIONEERING FIGURES in the cross-cultural study of birthing is Niles Newton, who was a professor of behavioral sciences at Northwestern University Medical School. For this reason, it is quite appropriate to begin this volume with a comprehensive overview by Niles Newton and her husband Michael Newton, who was a clinical professor in the Department of Obstetrics and Gynecology at the Pritzker School of Medicine at the University of Chicago. They highlight weaknesses in the American way of birth in novel fashion. First, they describe traditional non-Western birthing practices and then contrast them with the analogous American medical model. This format provides an effective means of offering a fresh perspective on generally accepted Western birthing traditions. Earlier, Niles Newton had teamed up with famed anthropologist Margaret Mead in a groundbreaking call for systematic studies of practices surrounding childbirth in diverse cultures. (See M. Mead and N. Newton, "Cultural Patterning of Prenatal Behavior," in *Childbearing, Its Social and Psychological Aspects*, edited by S. Richardson and A. F. Guttmacher [pp. 142–244] [Baltimore: Williams and Wilkins, 1967].)

For later surveys, see C. McClain, "Toward a Comparative Framework for the Study of Childbirth: A Review of the Literature," in *Anthropology of Human Birth*, edited by M. A. Kay (pp. 25–59) (Philadelphia: F. A. Davis Company, 1982); B. Lozoff, B. Jordan, and S. Malone, "Childbirth in Cross-Cultural Perspective," *Marriage and Family Review* 12 (1988): 35–60; L. L. Wall, "The Anthropologist As Obstetrician: Childbirth Observed and Childbirth Experienced," *Anthropology Today* 11 (1995): 6, 12–15; C. D. Laughlin, "Pre- and Perinatal Anthropology II: The Puerperium in Cross-Cultural Perspective," *Pre and Perinatal Psychology Journal* 7 (1992): 23–60; and C. D. Laughlin, "Pre- and Perinatal Anthropology III: Birth Control, Infanticide and Abortion in Cross-Cultural Perspective," *Pre and Perinatal Psychology Journal* 9 (1994): 85–102.

See also Niles Newton's brief essay, "Birth Rituals in Cross-Cultural Perspective: Some Practical Applications," in *Being Female: Reproduction, Power and Change*, edited by D. Raphael (pp. 37–41) (The Hague: Mouton Publishers, 1975).

This essay was originally published in John G. Howells, ed., *Modern Perspectives in Psycho-Obstetrics* (New York: Brunner/Mazel, 1972), pp. 150–171.

Childbirth in Cross-Cultural Perspective   I

NILES NEWTON AND MICHAEL NEWTON

Introduction

ALL KNOWN HUMAN SOCIETIES pattern the behavior of human beings involved in the process of reproduction.[65] Beliefs concerning appropriate behavior in pregnancy, during labor, and in the puerperium appear to be characteristic of all cultures. This review will concentrate on patterns of behavior during and surrounding birth. Special attention will be paid to the primitive and traditional cultures, but examples from modern industrial cultures will also be used. Major trends and contrasts in patterns will be emphasized, particularly in so far as they may have applicability to current clinical issues.

First, attitudes surrounding birth will be discussed: the importance placed on birth, privacy and sexual implications of birth, birth seen in terms of achievement or atonement, birth as dirty or defiling or close to the super-natural, and birth as a painful illness or a normal physiological process.

Then social variations in the management of labor will be discussed, particularly in regard to practices which differ markedly from one society to another, resulting in different types of birth experience for mother and baby. These variations include differences in biochemical management, rules about activity and relaxation, sensory stimulation, emotional support and companionship, and delivery position.

Finally, the effect of social attitudes and beliefs surrounding birth on birth behavior will be discussed, as well as other questions raised by the review.

Limitations on Available Information

Both medical and anthropological literature was searched for information on the patterns of culture in the area of birth. Particularly helpful were the Human Relations Area Files (HRAF), which, at the time the search was made, contained 222 cultures coded in such a way that materials on childbirth could be located rapidly. Medical literature through the years has also concerned itself with certain aspects of patterns of childbirth and was therefore also searched.

Although both medical and anthropological literatures contain considerable information about certain patterns of obstetrical behavior, information is frequently lacking in regard to areas of behavior most relevant to this review. For example, Teit's[96] record of birth among the Nahane Indians of northern Canada devotes more than 450 words to describing the handling of the umbilical cord and to the beliefs concerning it and fewer than 150 words to the other behavior of the attendants and mother during labor. It was not until the 1920s, when the impact of psychoanalysis began to be felt, that ethnologists turned their attention to variations in emotion and personality and began to make more detailed records in this area.

One of the greatest handicaps in the recording of birth patterning among preliterate peoples is the fact that most primitive peoples exclude men from witnessing normal delivery. Although husbands are sometimes permitted to witness their children born, and medicine men may be called in the case of abnormality, other men are excluded from witnessing birth in many of the preliterate societies that have been studied.

Physicians contributing to medical literature are also handicapped, since they tend to see only the cases of extremely abnormal childbirth. Often modern medical advice is asked only when the primitive woman is on the verge of death. Normal childbirth as it takes place regularly in the tribal community is usually out of bounds for the physician as well as the anthropologist.

Implicit in most historical and anthropological writing and medical case reports is the assumption that relatively few observations of behavior in a culture can be generalized into statements about the whole. Due to the extreme paucity of studies done on broad samples collected with controls for observer bias, the limited data available have been used of necessity.

Nature of Conclusions

The nature of the data available at the present time makes it impossible to draw any precise conclusions. What the data can do is to suggest the many variations in the ways in which human beings handle birth. They can suggest certain aspects that have been muted in industrialized cultures and that are more fully developed in other cultures, thus opening new areas of understanding. They can also give perspective, by raising for question implicit assumptions held within our culture, and by exploring various ways in which behavioral issues in our culture are dealt with in other cultures.

A final word of caution is in order in regard to data gleaned from records of so-called primitive cultures. The word "*primitive*" is used only in the anthropological sense, meaning peoples without written language. It is likely that the behavior of most peoples mentioned may often be different from that described in the text, due to rapid changes in culture occurring in most parts of the world. The older accounts are often especially valuable for a study of this nature, since they may record relatively intact societies not yet overwhelmed by excessive contact with industrial culture. Despite the biased and fragmentary records produced by the early ethnographers and other early records, the scholarly world of today owes these men and women a deep debt of gratitude; for they recorded unique patterns of human behavior before they irretrievably disappeared.

Attitudes Surrounding Birth

Birth is an event that is treated with importance. Much cultural patterning surrounds birth as well as other aspects of reproduction. Despite widespread cultural interest in birth, the nature of attitudes toward birth vary greatly. For some it is an open sociable event, while others surround it with secrecy. The sexual implications of birth are developed in some cultures and strictly taboo in others. Various peoples see birth in terms of pay or praise, dirt, defilement, and/or supernatural involvement; or as normal physiology; or painful illness.

Importance Placed on Birth

Among primitive groups and traditional village culture groups, as well as in modern industrial cultures, childbirth is an event of consequence that changes the behavior not only of the mother but of other people in the social group. In primitive culture, by far the most usual pattern is for the laboring woman to have two or more attendants for labor and delivery. Often special huts are built for delivery, and elaborate postnatal patterns have developed. Even among some primitive people, whose life depends on following the food supply, the group will stop migration if possible when delivery approaches, or leave a helper with the woman who must stay behind.

The intense interest in childbirth is reflected in the high degree of knowledge acquired. Thus some non-industrialized peoples have developed the use of oxytocic drugs,[7,73,99] cesarean sections,[105] and operations enlarging the birth passages.[37] Complex cultures have developed sophisticated systems of obstetrics. The medicine that developed in ancient India,[1,80] Chinese medicine of the thirteenth century,[59] and Roman medicine of the early second century in some ways matches or surpasses the obstetrical knowledge of western Europe of only one hundred years ago.

Privacy Surrounding Birth

Although all cultures seem to emphasize in one way or the other the importance of childbirth, there are wide variations in specific aspects. One of these variations is in the area of secrecy with which they surround birth.

The frank open approach of some cultures to childbirth is indicated by the frequency with which they portray childbirth in their art. The Egyptian hieroglyphic for "to give birth to" depicts a squatting woman with the fetal head emerging from the perineum.[49] The ancient Mexican civilizations produced figures of women in the birth position with emerging infants.[99]

Many peoples pattern birth as a social event openly accepted by the community. Thus the Navaho of the south-western United States were reported to show "a great interest in birth. The hogan is open when a baby is being born. . . . Anyone who comes and lends moral support is invited to stay and partake of what food is available."[51]

In some cultures, the games of children reflect the frankness with which birth is regarded. For example, it is reported that a favorite game of Pukapuka preadolescents was to play at childbirth, immature coconuts being used to represent babies. "After a pretended cohabitation, the girl mother stuffed the coconut inside her dress and realistically gave birth to her child, imitating labor pains and letting the nut fall at the proper moment."[6]

In contrast to such open attitudes, other peoples feel extreme secrecy or the need for privacy about birth. Among the Cuna of Panama, children were kept in ignorance of birth as long as possible. They were not permitted to see dogs, cats, or pigs giving birth. Ideally they were not told until the last stage of the marriage ceremony about the existence of the sex act and childbirth.[94] Childbirth was called "to catch the deer": children were told that babies are found in the forest between deer horns or put on the beach by a dolphin.[44] The Chagga likewise surrounded birth with secrecy. Children were told that an animal brings babies or that they came from a beehive in the forest or steppe. In 1926 Gutmann reported: "In former years, the whole country was disgraced when a married man in conversation with minors replied to their questions as to the origin of man: *wandu veketsesau*—man happens to be born."[37]

In contemporary industrial cultures childbirth may also be cloaked with privacy. Seeing birth is often considered appropriate only for medical personnel. An illustration of this was the problem of an American obstetrician who bought a sculpture of a Mexican goddess in the act of giving birth. The fetus was half emerged. He tried putting it in his office, but his nurse and patients objected. He brought it home, but his wife felt it was improper to exhibit it in any part of the house.

Secrecy feelings may be so strong that they tend to persist despite administrative attempts to change them. For example, at St. Mary's Hospital in Evansville, Indiana, fathers are encouraged to participate in the childbearing experience. Fathers attend prenatal classes with their wives and usually sit with them during the first stage of labor. Yet when asked whether fathers should be in the delivery room, 59.4% of 267 fathers said that they did not feel husbands belong there.[25]

However, a protest against the taboo on open childbirth may be developing in the United States. Not only is there a strong minority agitating for permission for husbands to be permitted to witness birth of their babies, but the hippies in communes of northern California are patterning birth as a social home event when it's nice to have one's friends around.[72]

Sexual Implications of Birth

Closely allied to feelings about secrecy are feelings about the sexual implications of birth. Niles Newton[77] has pointed out that there are similarities in the level of physiologically based behavior between undrugged childbirth as observed by Dick Read and the female sexual excitement documented by Kinsey et al.[46] The following aspects of behavior are similar: (1) type of breathing; (2) type of sounds made and facial expression during second stage labor and orgasm; (3) rhythmic contractions of the upper segment of the uterus; (4) periodic contractions of the abdominal muscles; (5) inhibitions and psychic blockages frequently relieved; (6) unusual muscular strength; (7) increased insensitivity to pain and restricted sensory perception at height of reaction; (8) sudden return of awareness at completion; (9) forceful emotional reaction of satisfaction at completion.

These physiological similarities between birth and sexual excitement are developed and recognized in some cultures and muted in others. A 1901 account of Laotian labor states that relatives, friends, or more often young men, hold the woman up and try to divert her with extremely licentious remarks. Some of the young men bring musical instruments and others bring phalli, to which they address such witty approaches that the patient, despite her pain, responds with an outburst of laughter.[83] A Lepcha man of the Himalayan States in Asia told of peeking at a woman in labor when he was eight or nine years old: "I only went because I was very interested to see how a baby was born and because I wanted to see what a woman's vulva was like. I could not now watch this sort of thing as it would have too exciting an effect on me."[75]

In contrast, other peoples have reacted to the sexual implications of birth by concern over modesty. The following remarks by Chippewa Indians of Ontario, Canada, illustrate this problem.[40]

> Some of the fullbloods don't want men around, not even doctors. I, myself, think it is a disgrace the way women submit themselves to strangers today when their babies are born, especially to those doctors. . . . In the old days not even women looked at anyone more than necessary; a big piece of buckskin was placed over the mother to protect her modesty.

The current patterning of the second stage of labor in the United States is in keeping with the tendency to mute any recognition of the relationship between birth and other inter-personal reproductive acts. When delivery seems imminent, the American woman is transported from her bed, wheeled into a room with brilliant lights and medical instruments. She is then put on a special table that has equipment for tying her hands and her feet, and her buttocks are so adjusted that she pushes her baby out into space with no mattress to break its fall should the doctor fail to catch it. Labor is then quite usually artificially shortened by cutting the woman's perineum.[77]

Achievement and Atonement at Birth

In some cultures birth is patterned as representing achievement or an event to be paid for. However, there are marked variations as to who gets the credit and who does the paying. Atlee[2] has pointed out that modern women may derive very little prestige or satisfaction from childbirth. Instead, the feelings of achievement at birth may center around the actions of the obstetrician.

American parlance reflects this feeling. The obstetrician says, "I delivered Mrs. Jones," using the active voice. Mrs. Jones is likely to say, "Dr. Smith delivered me," using the passive voice. The husband and family are more likely to thank the obstetrician for the delivery of the baby than to thank the wife for giving birth.

In contrast to this, the Ila of Northern Rhodesia consider that birth is an achievement for the mother. "Women attending at birth were observed to shout praises of the woman who had had a baby. They all thanked her, saying, 'I give much thanks to you today that you have given birth to a child.'" After the birth, the Ila mother's husband may come in to see her and congratulate her. "Her male relations may also enter the hut, clasp their hand to hers and give her bracelets or leglets by way of congratulation."[88] This feeling of "personal achievement" about labor is so important to some South African tribes that the husband and father may refuse to get medical assistance for a woman in labor on the grounds that she would be better off dead than unable to bring forth a live child by herself.[56]

Perhaps allied with this feeling that birth is an achievement is the attitude that birth must be "paid for." Among the Goajiro of Colombia the father "pays" the relatives of the mother for the suffering and discomfort she experiences in childbirth.[11] The Araucanians of South America may feel that children should be made to "appreciate" their mothers' suffering. Said one informant, "[I] have often thought that when children grow up they need to be told how much their mothers suffered giving them birth."[41] However, the Laotians felt that the mother herself should "pay" for the birth. After delivery she underwent sitz baths and hot body effusions which are part of the custom known as "You Kam"—"to submit to penitence."[21]

Birth As Dirty or Defiling

Ordinary birth was frequently regarded as dirty or defiling. Among the Arapesh of New Guinea, "birth must take place over the edge of the village, which is situated on a hilltop, in the 'bad place' also reserved for excretion, menstrual huts, and foraging pigs."[62] Postpartum purification ceremonies were also reported from such widely scattered peoples as the Hottentots of South Africa,[42] the Jordan village peoples of the Middle East,[32] and the Caucasian region of Russia.[55] Hebrew-Christian tradition has firmly imbedded in it the feeling that birth is unclean. The ancient Hebrews felt so strongly about the defiling nature of birth that the whole of Leviticus Chapter 12 is devoted to the ritual purification of women following childbirth,[49] and even today the Catholic church has a special ritual for women after childbirth, although this is falling into disuse.

The "dirty" view of birth was especially strongly held in some parts of Asia. When labor started, the woman of Kadu Gollas of India was required to move into the jungle hut built for the purpose. She was considered impure for three months after delivery. Anyone touching her during labor "caught" the contamination and was isolated as well. Mother and child could not re-enter the house until they got permission from their deity.[92] Some women in India are reported to be considered unclean and "untouchable" during childbirth and for ten days thereafter.[93] The Vietnamese considered birth so contaminating that, although the village father did all he could during and after birth, he could not enter his wife's room but could speak to her only from the door. In order not to bring bad luck to others, Vietnamese mothers avoided going out for 30 to 100 days after delivery.[17]

Birth As Close to Supernatural

Many peoples see birth as a time of particular vulnerability, when death may be near and supernatural forces are at work. This was expressed very clearly in the Jordan village culture, where the midwife admonished: "The mother is in God's hands and she hovers between life and death. . . . Angels go up and down to record what happens . . . and the mother, after safe delivery of a boy, may be congratulated, 'God be thanked that thou hast risen unhurt.'"[33] The seventeenth-century diary of Samuel Sewall suggests this same sense of vulnerability and closeness to God in colonial New England culture. A 1690 entry reads: "At last my wife bade me call Mrs. Ellis, then Mother Hull, and the Midwife, and throw the Goodness of God was brought to Bed of a Daughter between three and four o'clock."[87] The Moravian village people of Czechoslovakia of the last century are reported to have had strong feelings about vulnerability immediately after birth, when the lying-in woman was susceptible to demoniacal forces, which were particularly strong between sunset and 6 A.M. and again for three hours at mid-day. To avoid their influences, the lying-in woman was supposed to stay in bed and thus obtained some extra postpartum rest.[4]

Death of the laboring woman is widely looked upon as particularly horrifying. Posthumous removal of the fetus was a common pattern occurring not only in the Pacific Islands[61] but also in Africa[13] and Burma.[53] In Samoa the child was cut out of the dead woman since otherwise, it was believed, it would become an avenging ghost.[61] In some areas of West Africa it was considered a disgrace to die in labor. The body of the woman was "treated with contumely" and was burned, as was everything else belonging to her![105] The deep fears stirred by death during pregnancy or labor were particularly prominent in the report of what happened among the Bambara of Africa. The entire female population of the village was upset, marking the event with an elaborate ceremony.[38]

Birth As Painful Illness or Normal Physiology

Is normal birth really a normal phenomenon or one to be treated as a painful illness? This basic question is viewed in different ways by different people. Many peoples in many parts of the world regard childbirth as a normal function. Du Bois,[23] observing the people of Alor, of the Lesser Sundas Islands, states: "One gathers the impression that birth is considered an easy and casual procedure. . . . This does not mean that difficulties never occur, but it does indicate that the society has not emphasized such difficulties." The Jarara woman of South America[36] gave birth in a passageway or shelter "in full view of everyone, even her small children. There was no concern at all over this matter; childbirth was considered a normal phenomenon." From the Pacific Islands it was reported: "Extremely realistic attitudes toward childbirth are held by the Pukapukans. No sense of mystery surrounds the event. It is considered of interest to the whole community as natural as any other fact of life."[5]

Indeed, the sensation of normal labor in some cultures may not be thought of as "pain." For instance, the Navaho have two words for labor—one means pain of labor and the other means labor alone. Thus the vocabulary of the Navaho, which embodies the cultural expectation, encourages the Navaho woman to feel that it is possible to have labor sensations without interpreting them as painful. McCammon, after personally attending more than 400 Indian women who were delivered at the Navaho Medical Center, states: "Many appear to suffer severe pain for many hours. These women do not hesitate to request analgesics and anesthetics. . . . However, I am convinced that not a few go through labor and delivery without pain."[60]

One of the most detailed accounts of primitive labor is of the Aranda, an extremely primitive people of central Australia. The observer, de Vidas, reports that the Aranda recognize the onset of labor by strong contractions which are "painful."[20] However, during labor "little fuss" is made by the woman if the labor is normal.

Nor does excessive pain appear to be part of the usual pattern of the people of Alor of the Lesser Sundas Islands. Du Bois writes: "In the half-dozen births I witnessed, the mothers at no time showed signs of pain beyond acute discomfort. They groaned softly and perspired freely but seemed on the whole to give birth with little difficulty."[23]

In other cultures pain may be quite definite even among people who have had little contact with Western industrial culture. For instance, de Lery[19] writes of the Tupinamba of the Brazilian coastal area he observed in 1557–1558, presumably before there was much contact with European culture. He and another Frenchman were lodging in a village when about midnight they heard a great outcry from a woman. Thinking she had been surprised by a jaguar, they ran to her. They found her in labor with her husband acting as midwife. He caught the baby in his arms and cut the cord with his teeth. A Kurtatchi woman of the Solomon Islands described labor in her culture with these words: "Now it hurts, its mother cries out, now we cut some leaves we make her drink. Now the child is about to be born. Now she is afraid because the child hurts her. She cries out because of the child."[9] Labor pain has puzzled the Ila of Northern Rhodesia so much that they have developed an elaborate theory concerning its origin as being the result of *mupuka* reluctant to let go of a woman.[90]

A number of primitive peoples do have cultural patterns of stoicism that prohibit women from showing the pain they may feel. In Samoa "convention dictates that mothers should neither writhe or cry out."[63] In some cultures, where the expectation of pain is intense the culture uses extreme fear to keep screaming under control. The Chagga are told from childhood that it is man's nature to groan like a goat, but women suffer silently like sheep.[81] Clitoridectomy scars may interfere with delivery and increase pain. Yet the laboring woman believes she will kill her baby if she screams and that her husband may divorce her if, through lack of self control, "the child is killed."[81] She also knows that screams would shame her mother and make her mother-in-law critical of her. Thus most Chagga women are stoic during labor, suppressing loud cries.[81]

American culture has not developed such strong sanctions against expressing pain but birth customs are patterned around the expectation of pain in labor. Uterine contractions of labor are called "pains" not "contractions," and instead of having separate birth attendants specializing in normal birth, the differences between normal and abnormal are so muted that it is considered desirable for a specialist in obstetrical disease to deliver every woman. Atlee[2] described the attitudes of his North American colleagues as follows:

> We obstetricians seem to think and act as if pregnancy and labor constitute a pathology rather than a physiologic process. . . . Our entire basic medical education is so obsessed with pathology that it is practically impossible for us to think of any woman who comes to us as other than sick.

When there is belief that labor is extremely painful, there may be a kind of resignation about the pain and willingness to add to the inevitable; whereas when pain is not considered "normal" extra care may be taken to avoid placing the parturient in extra discomfort. For instance, in the U.S.S.R., where psychological methods of pain control are widely practised,[14] there is a belief that labor is not necessarily painful. Enemas, often used in American labor upon admission to the hospital, are avoided in the U.S.S.R. as "painful stimuli."[67]

Obstetrical Techniques: A Cross-Cultural View

Since patterning of behavior may be particularly elaborated or particularly rigid when events have emotional impact, it is not surprising to find a large variety of well-developed behavior patterns elicited by birth. Differences in management of labor occur in at least five different dimensions, including biochemical management, relaxation and activity, sensory stimulation, emotional support, and delivery position.

Biochemical Management

The culture largely determines the woman's biochemical status during labor. Not only does each society regulate the availability and type of medication, but also determines the availability and type of nutritional support during labor, which in turn influences the parturient's biochemical status.

Non-industrialized peoples have developed the same variety of patterns in regard to biochemical support in labor as have those of Western culture. Some years ago, the first act of the Ukranian midwife was to give the mother a generous dose of whisky to ease her pains.[47] The Amhara of Ethiopia[70] gave a drink of mashed linseed to "relax the birth tract" and to "lessen the pain." On the other side of the world, in Muskrat, North America, a Crow Indian midwife[53] was reported to know of two plants that eased the suffering at birth. The Ojibwa[45] had also developed a pharmacological pattern. They had standard medicines for easing childbirth and others to be taken after normal delivery.

Nutritional regulation was also found frequently in primitive labor. For instance, the African Hottentots[86] fed soups to laboring women to "strengthen them." The Yumans[91] and the Pawnee,[22] both of North America, on the other hand, had developed a strong prohibition against drinking water in labor; it must cease with the first labor pain. Maternal death was ascribed to the breaking of this taboo. The Bahaya of Africa permitted drinking during labor but prohibited eating.[74]

Currently the nutritional approach to labor is so muted in the United States that the idea that food and beverage may play a role in labor may be startling to Americans. American patterns sometimes emphasize the fear that liquid and food given during labor will predispose to the aspiration of vomitus during anticipated anesthesia. A usual pattern is for all food and beverage, and often even water, intake to be prohibited during labor. If labor continues for many hours, dehydration and low blood sugar are combated with intravenous fluids containing glucose. At the same time, a variety of pharmacological supportive measures are administered. The great interest in the United States in the medicinal rather than the nutritional aspect of biochemical support is indicated by the fact that *Williams' Obstetrics*[24] cites 99 references in the chapter on "analgesia and anesthesia," but only 27 references in the chapter on the "conduct of normal labor," none of which deals specifically with the problem of nutritional support.

This is a relatively new American pattern. An early-nineteenth-century obstetrical text[69] urges nutritional supplementation in labor but warns against alcohol, an analgesic drug, as follows: "She should be supplied from time to time with mild bland nourishment in moderate quantities. Tea, coffee, gruel, barley water, milk and water, broths, etc., may safely be allowed. Beer, wine or spirits undiluted or diluted should be forbidden. . . ."

Current European medicine does not seem to mute the nutritional aspect of labor to the same extent as modern American. For instance, a recent British text[79] states: "The labouring woman requires a certain amount of nourishment . . . her own appetite should be a certain guide to what she wishes to eat or drink." The text goes on to suggest that a patient in "trial labour" who may later need a cesarean section be encouraged to eat and drink such foods as eggs, milk, and glucose drinks. In the late 1940s two papers appeared in the U.S.S.R. concerning the oxytocic and analgesic effects of Vitamin B_I in a series of labors. Europeans, whose cultural orientation included some interest in nutrition in labor, picked up the idea and papers were published in Germany, Italy, Hungary, Bulgaria, Yugoslavia, Austria, France, and Greece.[66] Notably absent in a search of literature were American papers, in keeping with their general tendency to mute the nutritional aspects of birth management in this culture.

Relaxation and Activity Implementation

Many cultures feel the need for regulating activity during labor. Patterns involving restriction or augmentation of activity are common.

Preliterate peoples have tended to pattern types of desirable movement during labor although from birth descriptions it is difficult to tell how far labor has progressed before regulations on movement are invoked. The inactive approach to labor, in which much movement is scarcely possible, is described by Schultze[86] in his study of the Hottentots: "Once I saw six women squatting around in one hut scarcely 3 meters in width. . . . It was difficult to recognize which woman was the cause of this gathering who lay on the floor in the background covered with skins."

Other peoples, however, felt that vigorous exercise was beneficial. Among the Tuareg, a nomadic tribe of the Sahara, the young mother followed the advice of her aunt or mother. She walked up and down small hills from the first labor pain onward, in order "to allow the infant to get well placed." She returned to the tent for delivery in the kneeling position.[10] In another group in the same cultural area women not only walked up and down but "pound grain in mortar to provoke the final labour pains."[29]

In the United States activity in labor is usually strictly patterned only after the parturient arrives at the hospital, regardless of the stage of labor. Upon admission, she is put in a wheelchair and pushed to the labor floor. There she is placed supine in bed. Frequently bedpans may be substituted for walks to the toilet. Labor-room attendants may tell the laboring woman to "relax," but only in hospitals where there is interest in psychological methods of pain control may actual coaching in methods of relaxation be given. Relaxation instruction may aim to relieve muscular tension, focus attention away from the pain, or put the patient in a more suggestible state, depending on theoretical orientations,[15] but in all cases inactivity of the major muscles is required.

Patterned inactivity is a relatively new development in American culture, contrasting with previous beliefs that exercise in labor was desirable. An 1816 obstetric text encourages movement:[69] "During the first and second stages (the second stage was defined as terminating before delivery), the patient may be allowed to sit, stand, kneel or walk out as her inclination may prompt her; if fatigued, she should repose occasionally upon the bed or couch, but it is not expedient during these two stages that she should remain very long at a time in a recumbent posture."

As late as 1894 an obstetrical text[54] warns: "The patient should be encouraged not to take to bed at the outset of labor. In the upright or sitting posture gravity aids in the fixation of the head and promotes passive hyperaemia and dilation of the cervix." However, by this time undressing and lying down are recommended as the end of the first stage approaches.

Sensory Stimulation

In quite a number of primitive cultures, sensory stimulation of many sorts plays a prominent part in the management of labor. Music in labor was used by widely separated groups: the Laotians in Indochina,[83] the Navaho of North America,[3] and the Cuna of Panama.[95] Conversation also involves an element of pure sound stimulation and was used by primitive groups who patterned labor as a social event.

Heat is sometimes applied to women in labor in various ways. The Tübatulabel[101] dug a trench inside or outside of the house, depending on the weather, in which a fire was built. The fire was covered with slabs of stone and layers of earth and tule mats were added. The laboring woman lay on top of all this. The North American Comanche[102] simplified the procedure by putting hot rocks on the back of the laboring woman. Farther south, the Tewa[84] fumigated the laboring woman by wrapping her in a blanket and had her stand over hot coals upon which medication was placed.

A common form of sensory stimulation is abdominal stimulation. A tedious labor among the Kurtatchi was treated by an older woman attendant who chewed special roots and vegetation:[9] "She spat the resulting red saliva on to her hand and rubbed Manev's abdomen with it, with a circular motion, all round the edge of the tumid belly. . . . Once in a while the woman kneeling behind moved her clasping hands from the top of the protuberant abdomen to the bottom and shook it violently."

This pattern of abdominal stimulation appears in other widely separated primitive peoples, suggesting independent invention of the technique. The Yahgan midwife of Tierra del Fuego, at the southern tip of South America, made circular strokes on the abdomen with the flat of her hand to stimulate birth.[35] The Navaho sprinkled pollen over the stomach area to make birth easy.[3] The Punjab midwife rubbed melted butter on the abdomen.[30]

Firm pressure applied to parts other than the abdomen was also used in primitive cultures. Among the Pukapuka, the *tangata wakawanau* (medicine man specializing in obstetrics) helped a woman in delivery by pushing with the heel or palm of the hand on the small of her back.[5] The Kurtatchi[9] and the Kazakhs of Kazakhstan in Asia[34] used knee pressure of the attendant holding the woman from the rear. The Punjab village midwife applied strong steady pressure with her feet on either side of the birth canal in the second stage of labor, a measure which was reported "to feel good."[30]

Many primitive peoples provide for skin stimulation by having the woman held in the labor position by others. The contact of body to body, skin to skin, may involve considerably more sensation than the support of an inanimate object. Ford[27] lists twenty-five primitive cultures in which women are supported from behind. Abdominal pressure is often applied as well.

Interest in sensory stimulation is muted in the management of labor in the United States today, except for occasional interest among groups that use psycho-physical methods of pain control. The woman using the Lamaze method of preparation for delivery is often instructed to stimulate her abdomen during labor in the manner similar to that used by various preliterate people. A natural childbirth mother may have a warm water bottle placed on her lower abdomen and have her husband put firm pressure on her sore back. Music may be piped into the delivery room and television viewing may be encouraged during labor. However, this use of sensory stimulation in labor, as a diversionary technique to reduce the sensation of pain, is an atypical rather than a typical pattern.

Companionship and Emotional Support

Birth in most societies is patterned not as an unaided solo act but as a social one in which others help in some way. The emotional impact of the labor attendants is a key variable in the patterning of labor.

Curiously, there is a widespread belief that primitive labors are casual unattended affairs, but records indicate otherwise. Unattended birth does occur in many cultures, but it is a rare event to be gossiped about in the same manner as an American birth taking place in a taxi-cab. Granqvist[33] comments, after giving an account of an unusual unattended delivery: "The peasant women move about outside so carefree although they are already in the last stage of pregnancy . . . their hard life full of heavy work does not allow them to spare themselves. Considering this, it is rather surprising that cases of birth in the open air are not much more numerous." Hilger[41] tells of the resentment felt by the South American Araucanian mother who went into labor when no one except her little boy was at home, so that she could not send for help. In the mountains of Yugoslavia it was reported to be "not unusual" for women to give birth in a field or on the mountain,[98] and in a Bulgarian village[85] an "exceptional" woman was reported to prefer to deliver alone. But in neither case is this the "usual way." A most atypical account is that of the South American Talamanca which states: "When the time of parturition approaches, the father goes into the woods and builds a little shed at a safe distance from the house. To this the woman retires as soon as she feels the labor pain coming on. Here, alone and unassisted, she brings forth her young."[28] However, it is to be noted the father built the shed. This was not a "casual delivery," but one which involved considerable preparatory work by a family member.

Often the birth took place in the home of the mother's or the father's mother. Thus, the care of the heavily pregnant and newly delivered woman fell on the grandmother and her younger daughters. Frequently even when later births took place away from the original home, special efforts were made to return the primipara to her own mother for her first confinement. The Punjab girl left her husband and mother-in-law, with whom she still felt shy, and traveled to the home of her birth to be with her own mother and the village midwife, whom she had known for years.[30] Thousands of miles away, in Africa,[50] North America,[103] South America,[36] the Middle East,[33] and in the Pacific Islands,[9] the same return to [the] mother's home for the first baby took place.

In primitive cultures all over the world, the elderly woman, rather than the skilled man, is the predominant attendant at normal labor. Ford[27] found elderly women assisting at birth in 58 cultures and not assisting in only two. In only four of his cultures was information lacking.

When social role differentiation has developed to such an extent that there is a person designated as a regular midwife, her personality and character are usually taken into account. Thus the Ojibwa felt that the midwife "should be a woman of mature years, preferably not under thirty-five. She should have had a few children of her own and be known to have had easy deliveries. She should be of calm temperament."[48] Among the Yahgan some women had the reputation of being good at delivery. "They get this reputation because of their frequent assistance and personal skill. . . . In general a woman will always be attended by the same midwife, because the latter has learned her physical characteristics from experience."[35]

Knowledge does not always come from personal experience, however; Graybull's wife, a North American Crow Indian, gave a horse as payment to obtain her obstetrical knowledge from a visionary.[52] At Tau in Samoa, barren women past childbearing age compensated for their barrenness by acting as midwives and were reputed to be very wise.[61]

In modern American culture there may be a tendency to mute the help available from older experienced women. Young couples often living many miles from their parents find the help of relatives at the time of child-bearing difficult to obtain. Among some families there is even a feeling that it is somehow better to try to manage alone without feeling "dependent" on the help and experience of the older generation. During labor in America, female relatives of the parturient are often excluded. Other women—practical nurses or registered nurses—do look after women in the hospital in the first stage of labor and postpartum, but these women are strangers, not friends or relatives. There is no requirement that a nurse have experienced childbearing herself. A registered nurse who has never had a baby is usually considered more desirable as a labor attendant in normal labor than the practical nurse who has experienced several labors and deliveries.

Although females all over the world attend women in labor, giving them emotional support by their presence as well as ministering to their simple needs, the role of males in labor is extremely variable.

The tendency to feel that birth is woman's business is so strong that men, other than husbands, are usually excluded from entering the same abode as the laboring woman. Even the male healer is frequently excluded. For example, in Africa, the Tuareg midwife, in case of abnormality, may ask for the help of a marabout (a Mohammedan hermit or saint), but he must stand outside the tent, for he may not go near the parturient woman.[50] The Cuna, who consider all labor a fearful ordeal, do call on the shaman for supervision regularly, but he must stay away from the laboring woman and depend on the female attendant's description.[58]

However, the feeling against males attending labor is by no means universal or absolute. In some industrial countries males command a much higher price for officiating at a delivery than does the midwife, and affluent women prefer to have such prestigious persons assist them even in normal deliveries, although the emotional support during labor is still usually left to women.

In preliterate cultures males may be called in under certain circumstances. Quite frequently, when labor is abnormal, male healers participate actively. When the Aranda woman had delayed labor, the male Mura took a hair girdle, and, violating the usual prohibition against men, went to her and tied the belt around her body.[90] The Sakai of Malaya have made the midwife role a hereditary one which both men and women inherit.[104] The Lepcha of the Himalayan mountain region appeared to have no sex preferences—the parents-in-law or anybody who knew how would help the woman in labor.[31] The pattern of the Araucanians of South America was changing at the time they were studied. In one area they had not yet developed a word for male obstetrician, but several middle-aged men were actually assisting at deliveries.[41] The Araucanian husbands also assisted their wives in dire necessity, such as when everyone else had gone to a fiesta or when they were too poor to hire a midwife.

The father very frequently had a patterned role to play, but not necessarily as an emotional supporter and companion to his wife. The Pacific Ocean Easter Islander father got a real sense of participation in birth by having his wife recline against him during labor and delivery.[71] The Kurtatchi father of the Pacific Islands was excluded from the labor, which took place in another hut, but the importance of his impending fatherhood was emphasized by the fact that he must stop work and remain in seclusion. On no account might he lift anything heavy or touch a sharp instrument.[8]

The custom of couvade occurred in many parts of the world. Essentially it involved a period of activity restriction and "regulation" for the father as well as the mother for a time after birth. Ford's sample[27] of 64 cultures contains records of the customs of 18 tribes in this regard. Seventeen tribes from Asia, North America, Oceania, and South America involved the father in couvade after delivery. In only one group was it definitely recorded that there was no couvade. There may be real survival value in this custom, as it may particularly emphasize the father's role and responsibilities at the crucial time as each child is born. It may help him to identify with mother and baby.

Delivery Position

The most essential aspect of birth is the movement of the baby from the uterus to the outside. Thus the body mechanics of second-stage labor are fundamental to the whole problem of normal, spontaneous birth. One would perhaps expect that biological factors would determine the position and movements of the woman at this time but even here ideas and cultural patterning or customs may overrule physiological and anatomical cues.

Delivery is possible in a great variety of positions.[26] A recent cross-cultural survey of 76 non-European societies in the Human Relations Area Files found that 62 used upright positions.[26] Of these upright positions, the most common was kneeling, with

21 cultures represented. The next most common position was sitting, with 19 cultures using this method. Fifteen cultures used squatting, and 5 used standing positions.

Sometimes the culture patterns delivery in more than one way.[82] The Siriono woman lies in her hammock for the delivery of the baby but kneels for the delivery of the placenta.[43] The Sierra Tarascans[7] use both kneeling and flat deliveries depending on "circumstances," according to a midwife. It is reported that the mother makes the choice for herself. A 1948 report indicated that the Goajiro woman had four different positions to choose from, for the sitting, kneeling, and squatting positions are all included in the traditional cultural pattern, and the supine position was also used occasionally.[36]

Among primitive peoples, the curved back is typical of most birth positions. In the sitting, squatting, and kneeling positions, the back automatically curves forward unless unusual effort is made. Bearing down in the standing position almost automatically forces some curving of the back. It is probable that many supine deliveries also involve a curve in the back. Thus the hammock-deliveries[43,57] may take place with backs curved forward. However, two peoples clearly have an opposite pattern. The Bambara woman[78] kneels with her hands thrown behind her while the midwives support the small of her back. The Jordan city woman sits on the side of her bed leaning backwards.[33]

Unfortunately, since most material dealing with primitive peoples does not indicate how far apart the legs were at the time of delivery, there is no way of knowing how much tension is usually put on the perineum at this time. The Laotians were reported to sit with legs folded and spread wide apart.[83] Blackwood[9] reports a Kurtatchi delivery with knees drawn up and wide apart. However, the birth description of the Hottentots, although not specific, suggests that the legs may be together, since a hand is kept constantly between the legs of the woman to ascertain the progress of the child's head.[86]

Many primitive peoples used pushing, pulling, and bracing devices to help the parturient in her expulsive efforts. Ropes, which furnish firm resistance to pulling but are easily adjustable in regard to angle and height, are used by groups in Asia,[31] North Africa,[10] North America,[7] and South America.[41,43] Poles and stakes are also used for grasping during delivery.[96,102] In Manus houses, where labor takes place, an extra post or board will be fastened firmly to the leaf wall so that the laboring woman will have something to push her feet against.[64] The Yahgan woman squats, spreading her legs wide apart, and braces herself with hands and feet flat on the ground.[35]

Today in the United States the position for delivery is similar to that used for surgical operations. The body is flat and neck is straight without a pillow to support it, as is the custom on operating tables. Arms are tied so that they will not stray into the sterile field. The legs are mechanically spread wide apart with leg braces to allow the physician to have an unobstructed view of the operative area.

This rigid surgical structuring of position for normal delivery is quite new in American obstetrics. The 1913 edition of the DeLee textbook illustrates delivery with the woman lying on her side in the lateral Sims position, her back curved and her legs only a few inches apart.[18] Lusk[54] in 1894 expressed a permissive attitude toward the position of the woman for delivery: "During the second stage, the patient's posture should be left in general to her own volition. The physician should accustom himself to conduct labor with equal facility, no matter where the woman lies, upon her side or upon her back."

The problem of the body mechanics of labor is mentioned by earlier American obstetrical textbook writers. Adequate foot support to use for bracing during contractions is considered a matter of concern.[12,54] As late as 1947, some thought was being given to labor as a muscular event. In that year, Beck's[8] obstetrical textbook advocated "pullers" and snug abdominal binders to facilitate the body mechanics of delivery and to "retain the advantages of the squat position."

Recent American texts, however, do not appear to give much consideration or discussion to problems of efficient body position and bracing for effective expulsive effort. In a few hospitals a triangular pillow or backrest is occasionally used to help the women achieve a curved back position, but the need for the parturient to push or pull by bracing and holding is almost entirely muted in American hospital practice today.

Concluding Comments

In seeing the possibility of other ways of feeling and acting, one's own way is more clearly delineated. Basically, the questions raised can only be answered by each individual for himself. Questions similar to the following are pertinent. What are my personal attitudes toward birth? What are the attitudes of the majority of persons working with me? Are the attitudes of childbearing women different in my group from those of males and non-reproducing women?

To be sure obstetrical *behavior* is also noteworthy. In so far as it mutes or develops emotional support, sensory stimulation, body mechanics, and biochemical manipulation, it can have a profound influence on the emotions of the parturient and those around her. However, emphasis on the varying patterns possible for birth behavior should not obscure the fact that behavior tends to reflect culturally determined attitudes.

An example of the force of attitudes in determining birth behavior is the fate of research studies which conflict with current obstetrical attitudes. For instance, considerable research on the problem of position in labor in relation to ease of delivery suggests that the flat supine position for delivery may make spontaneous delivery more difficult. Mengert and Murphy,[68] in an extensive experimental study, recorded actual intra-abdominal pressure at the height of maximum straining effort in more than 1,000 observations with women placed in 7 postures. The researchers used sophisticated statistical techniques to analyze their data. They found that the greatest intra-abdominal pressure was exerted in the sitting position. This was due not only to major visceral weight but also to increased muscular efficiency. Vaughan presented X-rays and measurements that indicate that squatting alters the pelvic shape in a way that makes it advantageous for delivery. Had Mengert and Murphy[68] and Vaughan[100] advocated a new drug to speed labor, it is likely that culturally accepting attitudes would have resulted in adoption of their findings—even with far less scientifically controlled data.

However, instead, the proposition of improving labor efficiency through sitting and squatting conflicted with the strongly held cultural attitude that birth is an event experienced lying down. This extensive research, instead of becoming part of the fundamental knowledge required of obstetricians, was ignored.

The importance of cultural attitudes in determining birth patterning can also be seen in the history of the "natural childbirth" program set up at Yale University under the leadership of Dr. Herbert Thoms. While Dr. Thoms continued work at Yale, published statistics indicated that 88% of the mothers had spontaneous deliveries and 29% had no anesthesia at birth.[97] Dr. Thoms retired, and some others working closely with him left. The formal patterns of education for childbirth and support during labor continued, but they no longer appeared to influence patterning of birth. A follow-up study,[16] published just eight years after the previous study, indicated that the once deviant Yale practice had quickly changed in the direction of the norm of the surrounding culture. Now only 47% of the women had normal spontaneous deliveries, and less than 1% of the women received no anesthesia at birth, although all of these still received pre-natal training and support in labor.

Socially determined attitudes may also determine how the mother behaves in labor, even to the point of possibly regulating her uterine contractions. Heyns[39] presents statistics showing that Bantu women of South Africa, although their pelves are so small that Western women would require cesarean sections, deliver babies spontaneously. This seems to be accomplished by a moulding of the fetal head by extraordinarily forceful contractions. In extreme cases the baby may be born dead, but the mother's life may be saved through her ability to get rid of the products of conception.

Heyns[39] believes that psychological differences may account for the differences in uterine contractions. "It is submitted that in the European there is an unfavorable emotional background, which has an inhibitory effect on efficient uterine action. . . . Where in any individual parturient there is emotional stability supported by an unwavering resolution to push through with the task of spontaneous delivery, and where the realization that obstetric aid is readily available is not over-emphasized, the achievement of the Bantu woman may always be equaled. . . . Simple dystocia, due to contracted bony passages, can almost be eliminated by fostering the will in the parturient to deliver herself."

This illustration particularly shows the interaction of birth behavior and birth attitudes. The availability of forceps and cesarean sections depends on cultural attitudes that accept the idea of non-spontaneous birth. In turn, the widespread use of operative procedures may decrease the desire to push the baby out spontaneously. The close interrelation of attitudes and behavior emphasizes that attempts to change obstetrical patterning may meet with unanticipated ramifications.

A broad view is required, which takes both attitudes and procedures into account. Perhaps the chief value of reviewing patterns of behavior surrounding birth is that it widens the perspective in the same way as historical knowledge increases understanding. In learning how others have done it, it is possible to get new insight into current patterns, their possible origin and interactions.

References

1. Adaua, K. V. 1940. Ayurvedic midwifery. *E. Afr. med. J*, 17, 142.

2. Atlee, H. B. 1963. Fall of the Queen of Heaven. *Obstet. Gynec.*, 21, 514.

3. Bailey, F. L. 1950. Some sex beliefs and practices in a Navaho community. *Papers of the Peabody Museum of American Archaeology und Ethnology*, 40, 2. Cambridge: Harvard University Press.

4. Bartos, F. 1897. Volksleben der Slaven. In *Die Osterreichisb-Ungarische Monarchie in Wort und Bild: Mähren und Schlesien*. Vienna: Kaiserlich-Koniglichen Staatsdruckerei.

5. Beaglehole, E., and Beaglehole, P. 1938. Ethnology of Pukapuka. *Bernice P. Bishop Museum Bulletin*, ISO, Honolulu.

6. Beaglehole, E., and Beaglehole, P. 1939. Brief Pukapukan case history. *J. Polynesian Soc.*, 48, 135.

7. Beals, R. L. 1946. *Cherán: A Sierra Tarascan village.* Pub. No. 2, Smithsonian Institute of Social Anthropology, Washington.

8. Beck, A. C. 1947 *Obstetrical practice*, 4th ed. Baltimore: Williams & Wilkins.

9. Blackwood, B. 1935. *Both sides of Buka Piissage.* Oxford: Clarendon Press.

10. Blangueron, C. 1955. *Le Hoggar.* Paris: Arthaud.

11. Bounder, G. 1957. *Indians on horseback.* London: Dennis Dobson.

12. Burns, J. (with improvements and notes by James, T. C.) 1831. *The Principles of midwifery: including the diseases of women and children.* New York: Clafton and Van Norden.

13. Cane, L. B. 1945. African birth customs. *St. Bartholomew's Hosp. J*, 49, 94.

14. Chertok, L. 1959. *Psychosomatic methods in painless childbirth.* New York: Pergamon Press.

15. Chertok, L. 1961. Relaxation and psychosomatic methods of preparation for childbirth. *Amer. J. Obstet. Gynec.*, 82, 262.

16. Davis, C. D., and Morrone, F. A. 1962. An objective evaluation of a prepared childbirth program. *Amer. J. Obstet. Gynec.*, 84, 1196.

17. De, T. D. 1951. Notes on birth and reproduction in Vietnam. Unpublished manuscript by Margaret Coughlin.

18. DeLee, J. B., 1913. *The Principles and practices of obstetrics.* Philadelphia: Saunders.

19. De Lery, J. 1906. Extracts out of the Historie of John Lerius, a Frenchman, who lived in Brasil with Mons., Villagagnon, Ann. 1557 and 1558. In *Hakluvtus Posthumus of Purchas His Pilgrimes*, 16, 518. Glasgow: MacLehose.

20. De Vidas, J. 1947. Childbirth among the Aranda, Central Australia. *Oceania*, II, 117.

21. Deydier, H. 1952. *Introduction à la connaisance du Laos.* Saigon: Imprimerie française d'Outre-Mer.

22. Dorsey, G. A., and Murie, J. R. 1940. Notes on Skidi Pawnee society. *Field Museum of Natural History, Anthropology Series*, 27, 2, 65. Chicago: Field Museum Press.

23. Du Bois, C. 1944. *The people of Alor.* Minneapolis: University of Minnesota Press.

24. Eastman, N. J., and Hellman, L. M. 1961. *Williams' Obstetrics*, 12th edn. New York: Appleton-Century-Crofts.

25. Engel, E. L. 1963. Family-centred hospital maternity care. *Amer. J. Obstet. Gynec.*, 85, 260.

26. Englemann, G. J. 1883. *Labor among primitive peoples*, 2nd edn. St. Louis: Chambers.

27. Ford, C. S. 1945. *A Comparative study of human reproduction.* Yale University Publications in Anthropology, No. 32: New Haven.

28. Gabb, W. M. 1876. On the Indian tribes and languages of Costa Rica. *Proc. Amer. Philosoph. Soc.,* 14, 483.

29. Gamble, D. P. 1957. *The Wolof of Senegambia.* London: International African Institute.

30. Gideon, H. 1962. A baby is born in the Punjab. *Amer. Anthropol.,* 64, 1220.

31. Gorer, G. 1938. *Himalayan village: an account of the Lepchas of Sikkim.* London: Michael Joseph.

32. Granqvist, H. 1935. Marriage conditions in a Palestinian village. *Commentationes humanarum litterarum,* 6, No.8.

33. Granqvist, H. 1947. *Birth and childhood among the Arabs: Studies in a Muhammadan village in Palestine.* Helsingfors: Söderström.

34. Grodekov, N. I. 1889. *Kirgizy i Karakirgizy Syr-Dar'inskoi Oblasti,* Vol. I. Tashkent: The Typolithography of S. I. Lakhtin.

35. Gusinde, M. 1937. *Die Yamana: vom Leben und Denken der Wassernomaden am Kap Hoorns,* Vol. II. Mudling, near Vienna: Anthropos-Bibliothek.

36. Gutierrez De Pineda, V. 1948. Organizacion social en la Guajira. *Rev. Inst. Etnolog. Nac. (Bogota),* 3.

37. Gutmann, B. 1926. *Das Recht der Dschagga.* Munich: C. H. Beck.

38. Henry, J. 1910. L'aime d'un peuple Africain. *Bibliotheque-Anthropos,* I, No.2.

39. Heyns, O. S. 1946. The superiority of the South African negro or Bantu as a parturient. *J. Obstet. Gynaec. Brit. Emp.* 53, 405.

40. Hilger, M. I. 1951. *Chippewa child life and its cultural background.* Washington: Bulletin 146, Bureau of American Ethnology, Smithsonian Institution.

41. Hilger, M. I. 1957. *Araucanian child life and its cultural background.* Washington: Smithsonian Miscellaneous Collection, Vol. 133, Smithsonian Institution.

42. Hoernle, A. W. 1923. The expression of the social value of water among the Naman of South-West Africa. *S. Afr. J. Sci.,* 20, 514.

43. Holmberg, A. R. 1950. *Nomads of the Long Bow: the Siriono of Eastern Bolivia.* Washington: Publication No. 10, Smithsonian Institute. Institute of Social Anthropology.

44. Jelliffe, D. B., Jelliffe, E. F. P., Garcia, L., and De Barrios, G. 1961. The children of the San Blas Indians of Panama. *J. Pediat.,* 59, 271.

45. Kinietz, W. V., 1947. *Chippewa village: The story of Katikitegon.* Bloomfield Hills: Cranbrook Press.

46. Kinsey, A. C., Pomeroy, W. B., Martin, C. E., and Gebhard, P. H. 1953. *Sexual behavior in the human female.* Philadelphia: Saunders.

47. Koenig, S. 1939. Beliefs and practices relating to birth and childhood among the Galician Ukrainians. *Folklore,* SO, 272.

48. Landes, R. 1937. *Ojibwa Society.* New York: Columbia University Press.

49. Levin, S. 1960. Obstetrics in the Bible, *J. Obstet. Gynaec. Brit. Emp.,* 67, 490.

50. Lhote, H. 1944. *Les Touaregs du Hoggar.* Paris: Payot.

51. Lockett, C. 1939. Midwives and childbirth among the Navajo. *Plateau,* 12, 15.

52. Lowie, R. H. 1922. The religion of the Crow Indians. *Anthropological Papers of the American Museum of Natural History,* 25, 309.

53. Lowie, R. H. 1935. *The Crow Indians.* New York: Farrar and Rinehart.

54. Lusk: W. T. 1894. *The science and art of midwifery.* New York: Appleton.

55. Luzbetak, L. I. 1951. *Marriage and the family in Caucasia: a contribution to the study of North Caucasian ethnology and customary law.* Vienna-Modlin: St. Gabriel's Mission Press.

56. Marchand, L. 1932. Obstetrics among South African natives, *S. Afr. Med., J.,* 6, 329.

57. Marshall, D. S. 1950. Cuna Folk. A Conceptual Scheme Involving the Dynamic Factors of Culture, as Applied to the Cuna Indians of Darien. Unpublished manuscript, Department of Anthropology, Harvard University.

58. Marshall, H. I. 1922. The Karen people of Burma: a study in anthropology and ethnology. *Ohio State University Bulletin,* 26, No. 13.

59. Maxwell, P. 1927. Obstetrics in China in the 13th century. *J. Obstet. Gynaec. Brit. Emp.,* 34, 481.

60. McCammon, C. S. 1937. Study of four hundred seventy-five pregnancies in American Indian women. *Amer. J. Obstet. Gynec.,* 61, 1159.

61. Mead, M. 1928. *Coming of age in Samoa.* New York: William Morrow.

62. Mead, M. 1935. *Sex and temperament in three primitive societies.* New York: William Morrow.

63. Mead, M. 1939. *From the South Seas.* New York: Morrow.

64. Mead, M. 1956. *New Lives for Old.* New York: Morrow.

65. Mead, M., and Newton, N. 1965. Conception, pregnancy, labor and the Puerperium in cultural perspective. In *First International Congress of Psychosomatic Medicine and Childbirth,* p. 51. Paris: Gauthier-Villars.

66. Mead, M., and Newton, N. 1967. Cultural patterning of perinatal behavior. In *Childbearing —its social and psychological aspects,* edited by S. A. Richardson and A. F. Guttmacher. Baltimore: Williams and Wilkins.

67. Medical Exchange Mission to the U.S.S.R. 1960. Maternal and Child Care. *Public Health Service Publication,* 954. U.S. Government Printing Office.

68. Mengert, W. F., and Murphy, D. P. 1933. Intra-abdominal pressures created by voluntary muscular effort. *Surg. Gynec. Obstet.,* 57, 745.

69. Merriman, S. (with notes and additions by James, T. C.). 1816. *A synopsis of the various kinds of difficult parturition, with practical remarks on the management of labours.* Philadelphia: Stone House.

70. Messing, S. D. 1957. The Highland-plateau Amhara of Ethiopia. Philadelphia: Doctoral (anthropology) dissertation, University of Pennsylvania.

71. Metraux, A. 1940. Ethnology of Easter Island. Honolulu: *Bernice P. Bishop Museum Bulletin,* 160.

72. Miller, J. S. 1970. The role of the physician. Unpublished paper given April 30 at Jefferson Medical College: Continuing Medical Education Symposium on Safety and Satisfaction in Childbearing.

73. Moller, M. S. G. 1958. Bahaya customs and beliefs in connection with pregnancy and childbirth. *Tanganyika Notes, Records,* 50, 112.

74. Moller, M. S. G. 1961. Custom, pregnancy and child rearing in Tanganyika. *J. Trop. Pediat.,* 7, 66.

75. Morris, J. 1938. *Living with Lepchas: A book about the Sikkim Himalayas.* London: Heinemann.

76. Naroll, F., Naroll, R., and Howard, F. H. 1961. Position of women in child-birth. *Amer. J. Obstet. Gynec.,* 82, 943.

77. Newton. N. 1955. *Maternal emotions.* New York: Hoeber.

78. Paques, V. 1954. *Les Bambara.* Paris: Presses Universitaires de France.

79. Philipp, E. E. 1962. *Obstetrics and gynaecology combined for students.* London: Lewis.

80. Rao, K. 1952. Obstetrics in ancient India. *J. Indian Med. Ass.,* 21, 210.

81. Raum, O. F. 1940. *Chaga childhood.* London: Oxford University Press.

82. Raynalde, T. 1626. *The Byrthe of mankyndt.* London: Boler.

83. Reinach, L. De. 1901. *Le Laos.* Paris: Charles.

84. Robbins, W. W., Harrington, J. P. and Freire-Marreco, B. 1916. *Ethnobotany of the Tewa Indians.* Washington: Smithsonian Institution.

85. Sanders, I. T. 1949. *Balkan village,* Lexington: University of Kentucky Press.

86. Schultze, J. 1907. *Aus Nanaland und Kalahari.* Jena: Fischer.

87. Sewall, S. 1878. *The diary of Samuel Sewall, 1674–1729.* Boston: Massachusetts Historical Society.

88. Smith, E. W. and Dale, A. M. 1920. *The Ila-speaking peoples of Northern Rhodesia.* London: Macmillan.

89. Soranus. 1956. *Gynecology,* translated by O. Temkin. Baltimore: Johns Hopkins Press.

90. Spencer, W. B., and Gillen, F. J. 1927. *The Arunta: a study of a Stone Age people.* London: Macmillan.

91. Spier, L. 1933. *Yuman tribes of the Gila River.* Chicago: University of Chicago Press.

92. Srinivas, M. N. 1942. *Marriage and family in Mysore.* Bombay: New Book.

93. Stone, A. 1953. Fertility problems in India. *Fertil. Steril.,* 4, 210.

94. Stout, D. B. 1947. *San Blas Cuna acculturation: an introduction.* New York: Viking Fund Publications.

95. Stout, D. B. 1948. The Cuna. *Handbook of South American Indians,* 4, 257. Bureau of American Ethnology Bulletin 143, edited by Julian H. Steward. Washington: Smithsonian Institution.

96. Teit, J. A. 1956. *Field notes on the Tahltan and Kaska Indians,* 1912–15. Ottawa: The Research Center for American Anthropology.

97. Thoms, H. and Karlovsky, E. D. 1954. Two thousand deliveries under training for childbirth program: a statistical survey and commentary. *Amer. J. Obstet. Gynec.,* 68, 279.

98. Tomasic, D. 1948. *Personality and culture in eastern European politics.* New York: Stewart.

99. Van Patten, N. 1932. Obstetrics in Mexico prior to 1600. *Ann. med. History, 2d series,* 4, 203–12.

100. Vaughan, K. O. 1937. *Safe childbirth: the three essentials.* London: Bailliere, Tindall and Cassell.

101. Voegelin, E. W. 1938. *Tübatulabal ethnography.* University of California Anthropological Records, 2, 1–90. Berkeley: University of California.

102. Wallace and Hoebel, E. A. 1952. *The Comanches: lords of the South Plains.* Norman: University of Oklahoma Press.

103. Whitman, W. 1947. *The Pueblo Indians of San Ildefonso.* New York: Columbia University Press.

104. Williams-Hunt. P. D. R. 1952. *An introduction to the Malayan aborigines.* Kuala Lumpur: Government Press.

105. Wright, J. 1921. Collective review—the view of primitive peoples concerning the process of labor. *Amer. J. Obstet. Gynec.,* 2, 206.

Editor's Introduction 2
Evolutionary Environments of Human Birth and Infancy: Insights to Apply to Contemporary Life

WENDA R. TREVATHAN AND JAMES J. MCKENNA

FOR MANY ASPECTS SURROUNDING BIRTHING and care of neonates, there is no right or wrong. Rather it is a matter of custom. Nonetheless, practices from other cultures that are unfamiliar may seem to be not only strange, but also dangerous. The next two chapters in this book, however, provide illustrations of this phenomenon, but from the perspective of residents of *non-Western* countries who might examine Western birthing practices. Thus these articles provide a counter-argument to Americans' sense of cultural superiority by demonstrating that certain common Western practices may have disadvantages when compared to practices in those countries deemed "less advanced."

Chapter 2 (taken from *Children's Environment* 11 [1994]: 88–104), by Trevathan, a biological anthropologist who is a regents professor at New Mexico State University, and McKenna, a professor at the University of Notre Dame, explains how the evolution of human birth (versus the delivery of smaller-brained primates) affects the need for birth attendants who meet both practical and social needs. This purported need raises questions about the usual relatively sterile and isolated solitary environment in which women in the United States give birth. The authors also examine the evolutionary course of infancy as it pertains to maternal-infant physical proximity. When American parents insist upon having their infants sleep some distance away from them in a separate crib or bed rather than co-sleep or bed-share (presumably to encourage independence, even as early as in infancy), the infant's sleep patterns and social and emotional development are compromised, according to the authors.

For the implications of co-sleeping on Sudden Infant Death Syndrome (SIDS), see chapter 9 by McKenna in this book. For a full discussion of the importance of touch, see D. Morris, *Intimate Behaviour* (New York: Random House, 1971). See also K. R. Rosenberg, "The Evolution of Modern Human Childbirth," *Yearbook of Physical Anthropology* 35 (1992): 89–124 for a comparison of human birth to other primates' birth including a detailed delineation of the physical aspects of parturition and how they impact the emotional experience of this event.

For additional essays by Trevathan, see "The Evolutionary History of Childbirth: Biology and Cultural Practices," *Human Nature* 4 (1993): 337–350; "The shoulders follow the head: postcranial constraints on human childbirth," *Journal of Human Evolution*, 39 (2000): 583-586 (by Wenda Trevathan and Karen Rosenberg); as well as such earlier articles as "Maternal Touch at First Contact with the Newborn Infant," *Developmental Psychobiology* 14 (1981): 549–558; "Maternal Lateral Preference at First Contact with Her Newborn Infant," *Birth* 9 (1982): 85–90; "Maternal *en face* Orientation during the First Hour after Birth," *American Journal of Orthopsychiatry* 53 (1983): 92–99; and "Factors Influencing the Timing of Initial Breastfeeding in 954 Out-of-Hospital Births," *Medical Anthropology* 8 (1984): 302–307; as well as the following books: *Human Birth: An Evolutionary Perspective* (New York: Aldine de Gruyter, 1987); *Evolutionary Medicine* (Oxford University Press, 1999), edited by Wenda Trevathan, James J. McKenna, and Euclid O. Smith; and *Introduction to Physical Anthropology* (West/Wadsworth, 2000), by Robert Jurmain, Harry Nelson, Lynn Kilgore, and Wenda Trevathan.

Evolutionary Environments of Human Birth and Infancy
Insights to Apply to Contemporary Life

2

WENDA R. TREVATHAN AND JAMES J. MCKENNA

Introduction

IN THIS PAPER WE REVIEW THE EVOLUTIONARY HISTORY of human birth and infancy and situate it within the context of modern life. We describe how these two life cycle stages were experienced during the approximately 5 million years of existence of the human (hominid) family, and suggest how this knowledge can be applied to improve the lives of infants and parents.

Most discussions of childbirth and infancy relate to the ways these two events play out in contemporary industrialized societies such as the United States, Canada, Great Britain, and Australia. Only occasionally will a review make serious reference to childbirth or infancy in traditional cultural settings, or among other primate species, and usually these examples serve only to illustrate novel, if not bizarre, variations.

The concepts and data we present below, however, demonstrate just how enriching and, indeed, necessary human evolutionary (including cross-cultural and cross-species) studies are to fully understanding social, psychological, and physiological processes underlying birth and infant development. We hope to surprise the reader just a bit, too, by demonstrating how evolutionary studies often reveal mistaken cultural assumptions that underlie even the "best" of contemporary scientific research, thereby constraining it. Finally, we use evolutionary reconstructions to show how extraordinarily different past environments for mothers and infants are from environments they experience today in urban, industrialized areas. This is important because maternal and infant biology has not changed as quickly or as much as the environments within which that biology unfolds. Our point is that by recognizing these differences, and by acting, where appropriate, to ameliorate some of the differences between ancient and recent environments, we can improve maternal and infant well being.

Others have argued, for example, that an evolutionary perspective is important for understanding many of the physical ills of modern civilization, including diabetes, atherosclerosis, coronary heart disease, and many lifestyle-linked cancers. To a great extent, many aspects of our twentieth century lifestyles are incompatible with our Paleolithic bodies. For example, our nutritional needs co-evolved with diets that were characteristically low in fats (especially saturated fats), moderately high in protein, and high in complex carbohydrates. Contemporary Western diets are high in fat and in simple carbohydrates such as refined white sugar. Our bodies were also "designed" for higher levels of physical activity than most of us practice today. Those who study the evolutionary history of human diet, physical fitness, and diseases argue that comparison of modern lifestyles with those of our hypothesized ancestors may lead to solutions to many of the modern "diseases of civilization" which result from the mismatch between our current lifestyles and the lifestyles our bodies were designed by natural selection to experience (Eaton, Shostak, and Konner, 1988).

For the same reasons, we argue that an understanding of the evolutionary history of birth and infancy may lead to solutions to several of the dissatisfactions women have with the way birth is treated in medical environments and some of the problems that appear in infancy and early childhood. Just as the human species as a whole has an evolutionary history, birthing women and infants have evolutionary histories too, and it is time for both social and natural scientists to accord both mothers and infants their unique evolutionary pasts.

The goal of the first part of this paper is to construct a scenario for the way in which labor, delivery, and the early postpartum period may have been experienced by our ancestors for the long period of time (perhaps as long as 95%) of our history (and prehistory) during which we were mobile gatherers of game and other wild foods, living in small bands of close relatives. The second part of the paper will do the same for infancy, especially through an examination of forms of contact and care which includes sleeping arrangements. Although such evolutionary reconstructions are to a degree speculative, anthropological data collected during the last fifteen years especially makes comparisons between modern and ancient environments meaningful and scientifically more accurate.

To examine contemporary human behavior, either to reconstruct its evolutionary origins or to understand it more fully, anthropologists rely on several independent lines of evidence. Observations of birth, breastfeeding, and infant care practiced among our closest animal relatives, the nonhuman primates, constitute one important data set. The fossil record provides another source of information. For example, ancient human and prehuman fossils provide evidence of birth canal morphology and infant childhood developmental stages. Finally, cross-cultural studies of contemporary humans in diverse ecological and economic settings provide comparative information about birth and the postpartum period for contemporary humans, ranging from those who live in environments somewhat similar to those of our ancestors to those giving birth in modern urban hospitals with the most advanced medical technology available. Together these lines of evidence present a broad species-wide perspective on the likely patterns of birth, infancy, and infant care practices favored by natural selection throughout most of our existence as a species.

Childbirth in Evolutionary Perspective

Birth in Nonhuman Primates

A common misconception about birth in mammals other than humans is that it is relatively pain- and stress-free; however, head size in other primates, most especially monkeys, is also large relative to body size, making the fit between neonatal heads and maternal birth canals a tight one, indeed. In fact, neonatal death due to fetal head size and maternal pelvic size disproportion is not particularly uncommon. Chimpanzees, orangutans, and gorillas are exceptions to this generality about primate births; their birth canals are much larger than the neonatal heads, making birth easier and safer.

Contractions of labor are similar in human, monkeys, and apes, although the total length of labor appears to be longer for humans. When labor begins for monkeys and apes, the female tends to seek isolation if circumstances permit. Behaviors interpreted as indicating pain have been described for many observed deliveries. These include grimaces, contorted postures, grasping "blindly" at objects, and moaning (Tinklepaugh & Hartman, 1930). Observers know that delivery is imminent when the female increases movement and position changes. She also spends more time exploring her perineum, the area between her vulva and anus. The monkey mother delivers in a squatting position and helps to guide the infant from the birth canal as it emerges. Often the mother wipes mucus from the baby's mouth and nose to assist its breathing.

In almost all monkey deliveries observed, the infant presents facing the mother (occiput posterior). In most monkey species, the newborn's motor skills are such that, once the hands are free, it can assist in its own delivery. After delivery the monkey mother licks the infant until the placenta delivers, at which time she devotes almost all of her attention to its consumption. The infant is often ignored during this time, but once the placenta and related birth fluids have been consumed, the mother returns her attention to the infant, further cleaning it and allowing it to begin nursing. Throughout this time, the infant never breaks contact with the mother, or vice-versa. Delivery and initial care of the newborn infant almost always occur in isolation that the mother seems actively to maintain. Once the infant has been cleaned up, however, the mother and newborn often become the centers of attention from the rest of the social group. Infants act as social magnets drawing together many individuals in the group.

In short, birth among monkeys and apes most often takes place in the trees away from predators and the mother is almost always alone during delivery, although other group members may exhibit intense interest in mother and newborn soon after delivery is completed. In most monkey species, the females in the group are often closely related, so that monkey mothers usually have their matrilineal relatives nearby. Most monkeys mate promiscuously, so the father of the infant is likely unknown by the mother or himself. Adult males virtually never play a role in either birth or early infant care and typically they exhibit only mild interest in this event. The few births which have been observed in the wild have usually been described as quiet. Although signs of painful contractions are evident, most births in the wild appear to be relatively stress-free. Births in captive species appear to be more stressful, likely due to the circumstances of captivity (lack of privacy and obscurity) and the presence of human observers.

The Fossil Record of Childbirth

Fortunately, several examples of fossilized birth canals exist, making it possible to reconstruct the likely birth process of our earliest hominid ancestors, those known as australopithecines. "Hominids" represent the taxon Hominidae, a "family" designation defined by the unique characteristic of upright locomotion (bipedalism) and its associated anatomy. Only members of this family habitually walk upright on two legs. Both the vertebral column and the pelvis are structured to permit this specialized form of locomotion. While most other primates have the ability to walk upright, they can do so for only short periods of time. Their pelvic morphology is designed for quadrupedalism (four-legged walking) or swinging through the trees, and not for efficient bipedal walking.

The earliest evidence we have of bipedalism is the fossil known as "Lucy" from Ethiopia, found by Donald Johanson in 1974. She is a member of a taxon called *Australopithecus afarensis,* and is thought by most anthropologists to be the probable ancestor of all other hominids. Dated to 3.6 million years of age, her pelvis indicates that she definitely walked on two legs. Relative to the ape or monkey pelvis which is long and narrow, the bipedal pelvis is rather broad, and the hip bones are rotated forward. This means that by at least 3–5 million years ago, fundamental changes had occurred in the way our human ancestors experienced birth.

The birth canal can be considered a passageway with an entrance (inlet) and an exit (outlet). In quadrupedal species like monkeys, the entrance and exit have their greatest length in the front-to-back or sagittal dimension. The infant, whose head is also longest in the front-to-back dimension, passes straight through the birth canal without rotating. (Monkey shoulders are not as broad as those of apes and humans, so they do not hinder the birth process.) As noted above, the baby emerges facing toward the front of the mother's body. In a bipedal pelvis, the birth canal is twisted in the middle so that the inlet to it is longest in the transverse or side-to-side dimension and the outlet is longest in the sagittal dimension. Thus, the greatest dimensions of the entrance and exit are perpendicular to each other. The greatest fetal dimensions are also perpendicular to each other: the head is longest in the sagittal dimension, the broad, rigid shoulders in the transverse dimension. This means that the human infant must undergo a series of rotations in order to pass through the birth canal without hindrance.

The anatomical change that has even greater significance for behavior at birth is that the human infant must emerge from the birth canal facing away from the mother. This is because the back of the fetal head must fit against the front of the mother's pelvis in order to pass through. Since the baby emerges facing away from her, this hinders the mother's ability to reach down and clear a breathing passageway for the infant and to remove the cord from around the neck if it interferes with breathing or continued emergence. If she attempts to guide the infant from the birth canal, thereby assisting in the delivery of her own infant, she risks pulling it against the body's angle of flexion, perhaps damaging the emerging infant's nerves and muscles in the process (Trevathan, 1988). This is why it has been suggested that having another person in the vicinity of the birth who could assist in this final stage of delivery could reduce mortality. That is, it is suggested that birth in humans is an inherently social event rather than a solitary event as in monkeys, apes, and most other mammals.

With increased brain size in the genus *Homo*, approximately 2 million years ago, the already-tight fit between infant head and maternal pelvis became even tighter, although one of the compromises to the conflict between selection for large brains and narrow birth canals was to delay most of brain growth until the infant is born, i.e., the postnatal period. The result of this adaptation is that human infants today are more helpless at birth than those of monkeys and apes. They are born with only 25% of their adult brain size, compared with 45% attained by infant chimpanzees at birth. Giving birth to more helpless infants, unable to assist themselves during delivery, poses more challenges to ancestral hominid females, adding to the advantages of having another person present at delivery. This also means that the early months of infancy are very different for humans than for nonhuman infants and this has an array of implications for developmental needs in relation to caregiving practices as discussed below.

Cross-cultural Environments of Childbirth

The cultural significance of childbirth is highly variable, but one of the commonalities worldwide is that it almost always takes place in the presence of another person. Most often the other people present are relatives of the birthing woman or of her husband. In other words, rarely do women give birth alone or in the presence of strangers. It is also rare for a woman to give birth in unfamiliar surroundings. Although the prescribed location of delivery varies from culture to culture, it is most commonly the woman's own home or that of a close relative or in-law. Less common birth locations include menstrual huts, specially built structures, or in the open.

Beliefs about appropriate temperature, nutritional supplementation, and physical support also vary, but, in general, the goal of those attending a woman at delivery is to reassure her and to ease the process as much as possible. Support of the birthing woman may include massages, herbal teas, chanting, ritual activities, and music. Restraint of the woman in labor is far less common than allowing her to move about at will. For the delivery itself, she may be required to kneel, squat, or sit in a special bed or chair, but she is usually supported in her efforts by another person who most commonly sits or stands behind her.

In most cultural settings there is a woman who is recognized for her skills as a midwife. These skills are most often gained through experience, although formal training in Western-style midwifery techniques is increasingly available. The presence of males at birth is unusual across human cultures, just as it is in nonhuman primates. Birth is most commonly viewed as an activity restricted to women. Often only women who themselves have given birth are allowed to attend deliveries, but in some places, births are open to anyone who cares to attend.

The Evolutionary Environment of Birth

As noted above, the fossil remains of early hominids suggest that their infants emerged from the birth canal facing away from the mother. This phenomenon alone made it advantageous to have another person present at birth and the reassuring emotional bases for the behavior would have been favored by natural selection. Thus, we conclude that birth was transformed from a solitary to a social event during the earliest phases of human evolution (Trevathan, 1992). Perhaps having an attendant at birth was somewhat opportunistic at first, but it gradually became more common as those who sought assistance had lower mortality associated with birth than those who continued the ancient pattern of delivering alone. It is not likely, however, that early hominid females consciously sought assistance during labor because of desire to reduce mortality. Rather, assistance was most likely sought because of the uncertainty and anxiety that resulted from increased awareness of vulnerability during labor and delivery. This awareness may have been one of the consequences of increased brain size and intelligence that evolved with the genus *Homo.* The pains of labor contractions were the likely signals that led early hominid females to seek out companionship during labor. Because the risks of mortality from unattended deliveries are generally far higher than those for attended deliveries, we would argue that humans have inherited the characteristic of "obligate midwifery" from their earliest bipedal ancestors (Trevathan, 1987).

How Well Do the Environments of Modern Birth Meet the Evolved Needs of Mothers and Infants?

Today in many Western nations women complain that their emotional and social needs during labor and delivery are not met. One of the consequences of this dissatisfaction is that during the last twenty years hospitals have relaxed restrictions against having husbands and other support persons present at birth. In other instances, women have chosen home delivery to ensure a birth experience in environments with elected companions. But the vast majority of women giving birth in the United States and Canada still do so in environments that are not familiar to them and in the presence of people who are not close relatives or friends. In other words, many contemporary women give birth under very different circumstances from those which characterized most of human evolutionary history. In general, their fears and uncertainties at the time of birth are not being met by the busy professionals who attend them; among the consequences of these unmet emotional needs are impeded delivery, greater medical intervention, and other less desirable outcomes (Klaus et al., 1992). It is also possible that negative emotional experiences during delivery have an effect on subsequent mother-child interaction and family relations for many women (Klaus et al., 1992).

In summary, we would argue that the evolutionary process has resulted in heightened emotional needs during labor which lead women to seek companionship at this time. Having someone else present at delivery leads (as studies show) in turn to lowered mortality and greater reproductive success for the women who respond to the stress of birth in this manner. The desire for supportive, familiar people at birth is deeply rooted in human history and it is a need that is often not met today.

Infancy in Evolutionary Perspective

"There is no such thing as a baby; there is a baby and someone."

—D. WINNICOTT

The Question of Infant Autonomy in Western Society

Infancy for mammals is defined as the time from birth to weaning. For monkeys this phase of the life span averages 10 months (range from 3 to 16 months); for the great apes it averages 46 months (range 36–53 months); and for most humans the average duration of nursing is two years (figures from Harvey & Clutton-Brock, 1985), although it is much less than this in urban, Western societies and the latest figures suggest that its duration is becoming even shorter. Humans in hunting and gathering societies and for most of evolutionary history nursed their infants approximately four years, a figure similar to that cited for apes (Short, 1984).

Unlike human infants, most primates are born with relatively developed motor skills and are able to cling to their mothers within minutes after birth. Hence, maintaining contact between mother and infant is a joint undertaking. The infant spends its first several months of life on its mother's body or in the arms of other group members in species for which "infant sharing" is tolerated. Because infants are never left alone and are able to nurse whenever they are hungry, crying is rare in nonhuman primates, except in association with illness or injury. It is a sensory rich social universe into which nonhuman primate infants are born and within which they are nurtured during the first few years of life.

The Evolutionary Environment of Infancy

Like nonhuman primate mothers, human mothers engage in a number of actions immediately following birth which likely served to increase survival of mother and infant in the past as they do in many environments today. These actions include rubbing and massaging the infant which serves to dry and warm it. Rubbing and tactile stimulation in general also activate respiration, digestion, and elimination, just as licking the infant does for most other mammals. The neonatal thermoregulatory system is poorly developed at birth so continual warming through close contact with the mother's body reduces the chances of hypothermia. Other behaviors probably serve to calm and reassure the infant, thus reducing energy expenditure and, in the evolutionary past, reducing the chances of detection by predators. Calming behaviors include holding the infant on the left side of the body so it is exposed to the soothing heartbeat (Salk, 1960; Weiland & Serber, 1970), talking to the infant in a high pitched voice (Eisenberg et al., 1964), maintaining eye contact (Robson, 1960), and nursing. All of these have been described as species characteristic or universal behaviors exhibited by human mothers immediately after birth (Klaus & Kennell, 1982; Trevathan, 1987).

Using cross-cultural and nonhuman primate examples, it is clear that human mothers and infants in the evolutionary past spent the first several hours, days, and weeks after birth in continual contact. Infants likely nursed whenever they wanted to, and crying was probably rare except for illness or injury as it is for nonhuman primate infants today.

Frequent and regular breast milk was necessary for adequate nutrition during infancy when the human brain was growing at its most rapid rate, doubling in size in the first year of life. Besides providing nutritional support, breast milk was the best source of antibodies to protect the infant from pathogens in its environment. Relative to the milk of most other mammalian species, primate (including human) milk is low in fat and protein, thereby assuring that infants and mothers must remain in constant physical proximity.

Considering that approximately four years is the duration of nursing for our closest living relatives, most anthropologists conclude that about four years between births represents the normal birth interval for most humans for most of evolution (Eaton, Shostak, and Konner, 1988). Moreover, until the domestication of plants and animals approximately 10,000 years ago, few foods were safely digestible by infants and children, further supporting the proposals of long periods of breastfeeding and four years between infants. In fact, if the mother died in the evolutionary past, it is likely that the infant also died unless there was another woman available to serve as a wet nurse.

Since frequent mouthing of the mother's nipples by the infant can suppress ovulation, women in the evolutionary past who nursed their infants in the way great apes do today may have had healthier children. A four-year period between children meant less direct nutritional and/or emotional competition between siblings.

Infancy Western Style: Culture and Biology in Conflict

In Western society it is clear that psychological, developmental, clinical and pediatric research begins with the false assumption that human infants are, at birth, prepared to be independent (socially, psychologically, and physiologically) and that, in fact, it is in the infant's best interest for parents to practice forms of care which minimize various forms of physical contact—especially sleep contact (see McKenna et al., 1993; Spock & Rothenberg, 1985).

Given our society's emphasis on the importance of autonomy and independence as compared with familial interdependence, this bias in infant care recommendations is not surprising. However, when the infant's evolution (i.e., its biology) is considered, just how much our cultural values have led us away from conceptualizing the true needs of infants is made more clear. An evolutionary perspective forces us to ask: To what extent do we push some fragile infants to their adaptive limits and beyond? To what extent have our non-conscious cultural ideologies limited developmental research to questions aimed at confirming who we "want" infants to be, rather than to questions aimed at discovering who infants really are?

Consider, for example, that the human infant is one of the least neurologically mature mammals at birth. It experiences the longest delays in both social and biological maturation, a fact not likely to be appreciated without a comparative analysis of mammalian evolution and development and known physiological effects of short-term separation from a caregiver. As noted above, an astonishing 75% of human brain growth occurs postnatally. As a consequence of its immaturity, the human infant is forced to rely on a significant amount of external regulation and support, especially at the beginning of life. The extent to which, on a minute-to-minute basis, the infant's most fundamental physiology, such as heart rate, body temperature, breathing, sleep, and arousal, is influenced by a caregiver constitutes one of the most important discoveries made during the last twenty years, an insight that Western researchers need to incorporate into their research strategies (see Trevathan, 1987; McKenna, 1986). In our enthusiasm to view the infant as the clearly competent organism it is, McKenna (1986) argues that we have pushed too far the notion of the infant's physiological independence from the caregiver, thereby confusing its preparedness to adapt with actual adaptation, taken here to mean the assumption of the infant's physiological autonomy at much too early an age in development.

As with birth, evidence comes from both human and nonhuman primates. For example, short-term separation of monkey infants from their mothers causes changes in the fundamental efficiency of systems not previously thought to be regulated by the presence or absence of a caregiver. When experimentally separated from their caregivers for periods as short as three hours, monkey infants can experience significant detrimental effects, such as a decrease in body temperature, a release of stress hormones (ACTH), cardiac arrhythmias (Coe et al., 1985), sleep disturbances, and compromises to the immune system. Among human infants, Keefe (1987) found that "rooming-in" newborns spent more time in quiet sleep than infants sleeping away from their mothers in the hospital nursery. Another study by Fardig (1980) showed that the human newborns placed in incubators lost up to 1.5 degrees of body temperature compared with newborns placed directly (skin-to-skin) on their mothers' stomachs immediately following birth. And Ludington-Hoe et al. (1991a; 1991b) and Anderson's (1991) innovative studies of the beneficial effects of skin-to-skin contact (kangaroo care) for preterm infants reminds us of just how important touch is as a mediator of physiological systems during both pre- and post-natal life (McKenna, 1986).

Walkie-Talkie Babies and the Need to Switch the Amplifiers Around

Fisher-Price walkie-talkies are a hot item on the baby care technology market. As caregivers dash around the house, or while they sleep in distant bedrooms at night, one-way monitors placed in the babies' bedrooms near their cribs broadcast the infants' stirrings to parents, thereby compensating for the loss of sensory access. Guided by the evolutionary, cross-species, and cross-cultural perspectives, we are amused by this baby monitor phenomenon, primarily because it seems that modern technology has it all backwards.

A great number of developmental studies of infants suggests that rather than the parents having auditory access to the infant, it should be the other way around, with the infant having access to parental stirrings (especially breathing sounds and vocalizations). Infant sleep, heart rate, breathing, and arousal levels are all affected by such stimuli, probably in adaptive ways to facilitate development and to maximize adjustment to environmental perturbations (cf. Stewart & Stewart, 1991; Chisholm, 1983). At the very least, monitors should be broadcasting sound in both directions (McKenna, 1993).

The Chronic, Simultaneous, Over- and Understimulation of Western Infants

Pediatricians and developmental psychologists in Western societies constantly warn parents against overstimulating infants. Yet, contact and caregiving, which assures a steady stream of gentle stimulation, characterized the infant's microenvironment throughout all of human evolution up until about a few hundred years ago. Recent changes in the infant's sensory world represent too short a period of time for infants to become genetically "adjusted" or fine-tuned biologically to the long periods of separation and sensory isolation they often experience in urban Western societies. In fact, a strong case can be made for the fact that, in the short term, Western infants are often overstimulated, and in the long term, chronically neglected—and understimulated. That is, American parents spend a great deal of money buying gadgets to stimulate their infants visually and auditorially (e.g., with mobiles, toys, music boxes, and colored wall paper); and stimulation is thought to be an activity induced by the parents, restricted to concentrated and intense play periods. After "playtime" the infant is thought to need a rest—to be allowed to turn off—and to be calmed and "put down for sleep" usually in a room separate from normal family noise and activity.

This pattern of "on and off" stimulation, followed by complete isolation, is very different from the more gentle but consistent stimulation which emerges naturally from constant sensory proximity and care. From our perspective, infant developmental health and physiology are threatened more by long periods of social isolation (sleeping in a quiet room) than by overstimulation derived from constant, even-paced contact and proximity—stimulation to which the human infant is well adapted and "expects" to experience (see Konner & Worthman, 1980; Elias et al., 1986).

Infant Sleep Environments: A Quintessential Conflict between Biology and Present Cultural Context

In no other area of birth and infancy research are the values and ideologies of researchers so well-entrenched, and so fundamentally flawed, as they are in the field of infant sleep research. In fact, infants sleeping for long periods in social isolation from parents constitutes an extremely recent cultural experiment, the biological and psychological consequences of which have never been evaluated. Most Americans and health professionals assume that solitary sleep is "normal," the healthiest and safest form of infant sleep. Psychologists as well as parents assume that this practice promotes infantile physiological and social autonomy. Recent studies challenge the validity of these assumptions, however, and provide many reasons for postulating potential benefits to infants sleeping in close proximity to their parents—both physiological and psychological benefits that are not possible with solitary sleeping (see McKenna et al., 1993; Medoff & Schaefer, 1993; Abbott, 1992; Morelli et al., 1992; Forbes et al., 1992).

Current clinical models of the development of "normal" infant sleep are based exclusively on studies of solitary sleeping infants. Since infant-parent co-sleeping represents the species-wide pattern, and is practiced by the vast majority of contemporary peoples, the accepted Western clinical model of the "ontogeny" of infant sleep is not accurate, but rather reflects only how infants sleep under solitary conditions. New studies are needed to determine just how different social and solitary sleep environments are in changing the developmental trajectory of infant sleep and concomitant behaviors in the first year of life. Without such studies of infants sleeping with a caregiver, we cannot claim to understand the true normal development of infant sleep, but rather only infant sleep as it unfolds in a sensory-deprived solitary condition—a novel, if not aberrant, infant sleep environment for the human primate.

Most Infant-Parent Sleep Struggles Are Culturally Induced

Parents struggling with infants and children to get them to sleep alone and through the night, as early in life as possible, is the leading complaint heard by pediatricians in the United States (Lozoff et al., 1984). But given the human infant's evolutionary past, where even brief separations from the parent could mean certain death, we need to reconsider why infants protest sleep isolation and reinterpret its meaning. Surely infants are acting adaptively, rather than pathologically. Perhaps infant "signalers," as Tom Anders (Thomas F. Anders, M.D., a child psychiatrist who is the associate dean for Academic Affairs at UC Davis School of Medicine, studies the disorders of regulation that affect infants and their families, especially sleep disorders. See, for example, T. F. Anders, Infant sleep, nighttime relationships, and attachment, *Psychiatry* 57 [1994]: 11–21; B. L. Goodlin-Jones, M. M. Burnham, E. E. Gaylor, and T. F. Anders, Night waking, sleep-wake and organization, and self-soothing in the first year of life, *J Dev Behav Pediatr* 22 [2001]: 226–233) calls them, have unique needs and require parental contact more than do some other infants, who fail to protest. Perhaps those who protest sleep isolation from their parents are among the most adapted infants and children of all.

McKenna's work (1986) suggests that we reexamine the cultural meanings that parents and researchers place on nighttime awakening and reconsider the role that values and misguided cultural expectations play in creating the problems themselves. He does not question the fact that biologically based sleep problems can exist in infants, but that they are rare, indeed. He suggests that, depending on the infant or child's age, both parents and professionals may be interpreting awakenings in an unnecessarily negative way and promoting unrealistic expectations that not all infants can, or necessarily should, meet (see also Mosko et al., 1993).

Accordingly, infants are encouraged by solitary sleep environments, and culturally based models of normal infant sleep, to sleep too long per sleep bout, and too deeply, possibly before their arousal mechanisms may be best able to handle it physiologically. In short, too much infant sleep, isolated from sensory stimuli from caregivers that helps to keep infants in deeper stages of sleep, may be dangerous to some particularly vulnerable infants (see McKenna et al., 1990; 1993). He and his colleagues are studying physiological differences between solitary and social (same-bed) sleeping human mother-infant pairs, in a sleep laboratory, to determine if significant differences exist, and if the differences that are found may shed light on co-factors involved in some cases of the sudden infant death syndrome (SIDS) (see McKenna & Mosko, 1993).

Infants and Parents Sleeping in Proximity and Contact: Why "Co-Sleeping" Is Misunderstood and Condemned

One reason why Western parents and health professionals react so negatively when the issue of co-sleeping is raised is because it is mostly discussed as if it were a discrete, unitary, all-or-nothing phenomenon. It isn't. The question should not be, should I sleep or not sleep with the baby? A better question is, how can parents and infants safely and comfortably benefit from sleep proximity with one another? Since social sleep is evolutionarily and biologically normal infant sleep, how can urban, modern parents act to fit better the evolutionary (here, biological) expectation of the infant?

McKenna (1993) conceptualizes infant sleep arrangements in terms of a continuum ranging from same-bed contact to the point where infant-parent sensory exchanges are eliminated altogether, as, for example, infants sleeping alone in a distant room with the door closed. An infant sleeping in proximity alongside the parental bed, or with a caregiver in a rocking chair, or next to a parent on a couch, in a different room other than a bedroom, or in a caregiver's arms, all constitute forms of infant co-sleeping. From the standpoint of the infant, any form of sensory contact, however limited, is better than none. McKenna's research suggests that infants should sleep in the context of family activities and not in an isolated room (McKenna et al., 1993).

Does Co-Sleeping Create Increased Infant or Child-Parent Sleep Struggles?

Only a few studies exist that provide data on this subject; but unfortunately the findings are misleading and cannot be interpreted in a simple way (see Medoff & Schaeffer, 1993). This is because randomized studies include parents who often accept infants into their beds in response to existing sleep problems, rather than as a favored, preferred, or elected infant sleep management strategy. The result is that many parents who permit children into their bed do not accept the values that define the behavior positively. Rather, these parents see this behavior as a last-resort strategy, and as an indication of their own parenting deficits, or as deficits in their children. Indeed, these parents assume that co-sleeping is in the long run detrimental so they practice an erratic pattern of co-sleeping. Rather than solving the preexisting struggles they often reinforce or worsen them (see Mandansky & Edelbrock, 1990).

When co-sleeping is accepted as a favored and preferred sleep pattern, however, and infant awakenings are not *culturally* defined as a "problem," even when infants or children awaken frequently it is not perceived as a "sleep problem" (Lozoff et al., 1984; Elias et al., 1986; Morelli et al., 1992; Abbott, 1992). From our perspective it is unfortunate that we have constructed culturally based models of infant sleep expectations which are quite at odds with the infant's biology and emotional needs. When they cannot conform to this unrealistic model, both infants and children are considered in a crisis, as are their parents who often seek professional advice (see Ferber, 1986).

Infant Sleep Environments and Cultural Values: How It Works

Recommendations as to where babies should sleep depend on the developmental outcomes that society favors, and the perceived value of particular care-giving practices thought to help achieve those outcomes. They do not take into consideration infant biology and, unfortunately, neither health professionals nor parents are aware of this fact. The relationship between cultural values, developmental outcomes, and recommended sleeping arrangements for infants and children is made abundantly clear by considering differences between Japan and the United States. For example, interdependence and group harmony are two values positively sanctioned in Japan where co-sleeping occurs in large measure to create a social environment which fosters the very kind of socioeconomic interdependencies which Americans attempt to inhibit or suppress. According to Christopher (1983: 70): "One monkey that does perch on the back of nearly all Japanese is a deeply ingrained feeling that individual gratification is possible only in the group context—a feeling which, like the taste for dependence, clearly stems from childhood experiences."

The fact that American children are taught to be self-reliant and display their individuality (and, thus, learn to sleep alone) and Japanese children are taught to "harmonize with the group" (and, hence, sleep with their parents) is best understood by the very different attitudes and values Japanese and American parents have concerning the "nature" of the infant at birth. Caudill and Weinstein, cited in Shand (1985) explain:

> In Japan the infant is seen more as a separate biological organism who from the beginning, in order to develop, needs to be drawn into increasingly interdependent relations with others. In America, the infant is seen more as a dependent biological organism who, in order to develop, needs to be made increasingly independent of others.

It is important, of course, that infant sleep patterns fit into other cultural patterns as, for example, parental work schedules and attitudes about their infant's sleep and their own needs for privacy. We realize that infants must fit into a complex of social and psychological constellations of each unique family. But responsible scientists must begin to acknowledge that the infant's biological needs are not necessarily the same as the parents' best social interests in any given cultural setting. Infant biology changes much more slowly than do parental lifestyles, including infant care-giving patterns and the attitudes that underlie them.

At very least it is important for parents to be informed that they have a range of options as to where their infants or children can sleep, including sleeping in proximity in a responsible way. It is important for parents to know that when pediatricians give advice as to where their infants and children should sleep, they are dispensing cultural judgments and not advice based in scientific findings. It is important for researchers to know that the infant's body was designed by natural selection to sleep next to its mother and that nursing and co-sleeping are part of the same adaptive complex. It has only been since the introduction of substitutes for mothers' milk some fifty years ago, and/or dwellings with multiple bedrooms, that we came to consider the possibility that infants and parents could or should sleep in separate locations. Just as we have rediscovered the benefits of nursing, so too, we predict, in the next ten years we will discover the benefits of the other half of it, infant-parent sleep contact and proximity.

Where Did the Ideology of Solitary Infant Sleep As Natural, Safe, and Healthy Come From?

Where Western attitudes about co-sleeping actually come from is a question that cannot be answered in any simple way. Our beliefs about the practice stem from a diffuse confluence of historical, socioeconomic, ideological, and religious factors, including a concern for children's safety (protection from infanticide), that carries over in a distorted way, mostly from historical events in Europe centuries ago (see table 2.1). For example, moralist philosophers writing in seventeenth-century France were concerned with the sexual "purity" of children. Incest between teenagers (not infants) and par-

Table 2.1.   The Ideology of Solitary Infant Sleep As Normal/Safe/Good Sleep: Where did it come from?

1. Laws and proclamations passed from the sixteenth through the eighteenth century protecting infants from *infanticide*—purposeful overlying in conditions of poverty
2. Seventeenth-century "Moralists" and concerns of the Catholic Church in getting teenage daughters out of parents' bed to protect from *father's sexual abuse*
3. The emergence of the importance of the *"conjugal bond"* at the expense of the child-parent bond, early seventeenth- into eighteenth-century Europe and France
4. The emergence in the eighteenth century of *"romantic love"*
5. Seventeenth- and eighteenth-century European socio-political changes re-defining patriarchy and the *socio-sexual privacy* of the family/husband-wife from the public
6. American values of *individualism, separateness, autonomy*—the "All American Infant" idea—our own socialization and experience

References: Aries, 1962; Flandrin, 1979; Kellum, 1974; Stone, 1977; Vinovskis, 1987.

ents who slept together became a concern, particularly during the seventeenth and eighteenth centuries. The Catholic Church advocated separate sleeping places for older children when tales of incestuous relationships between pubescent daughters and their fathers were making their way into the confessionals (Flandrin, 1979). Moreover, the rise of the notion of romantic love and the preeminence of the conjugal (husband-wife) bond over the parent-child relationship which also occurred in Western cultures at around the same time (see Stone, 1977) also influenced attitudes concerning parent-infant co-sleeping. The infant-child came to be seen as a competitor of the patriarch who threatened the sanctity of affection and love between the husband and wife—a view not too unlike what later became formalized in Freudian psychology as the Oedipus complex.

A common reason given by contemporary pediatricians and health officials as to why co-sleeping should not be practiced concerns fears of "overlying" or suffocating the infant—a reason that may have some historical connection to the fact that in England, Germany, and France during the seventeenth century, proclamations were written and laws were passed threatening parents with jail should they be caught in the same bed with their infants. These laws were aimed at preventing infanticide—a serious problem among the extreme poor of England and France during this period. Not able to provide food for more than one child at a time, many parents claimed to have accidentally rolled over, killing their infants while sleeping with them. (In many human cultures, when conditions of resource deprivation exist, infanticide has been a form of birth control when an infant is born before the previous one is weaned.) Infanticide by suffocation was a serious problem in urban centers of Paris, London, and Germany during the sixteenth, seventeenth, and eighteenth centuries (see Aries, 1962; Flandrin, 1979), leading to legislation outlawing infants less than two years of age from their parents' bed (see Kellum, 1974). The important point is that it was not accidental suffocation that induced such laws, but purposeful suffocation.

While it is, of course, possible to suffocate an infant by rolling over on it, especially by irresponsible parents desensitized by drugs or alcohol, under normal circumstances it is very difficult to do so and probably no more likely than an infant strangling itself in a crib (see McKenna, 1986, for discussion). Infants are very strong and vocal when their oxygen is threatened. If infant suffocation had ever been a serious problem for our species, none of us would be here today because our ancestors would have died as the result of co-sleeping. Certainly the fear of overlying or suffocating the infant during co-sleeping is exceedingly prevalent in the United States but it is a fear that is disproportionate to the likelihood of it ever occurring. It is a fear exacerbated by myth, socialization, and ideology, not facts.

Finally, in the United States, baby care books are mostly written by men who have long advocated separate sleep for parents and infants (see Spock & Rothenberg, 1985). Too much dependence by infants and toddlers on parents during the night is seen as limiting the infant's growth toward autonomy, as in the form of self-soothing and self-regulation of sleep. So too does the misplaced fear that infants will be traumatized by hearing the sounds and possibly seeing their parents' lovemaking (see Robertiello, 1975). Not one of these speculations has been verified through systematic study. In fact, several recent studies find no support for negative effects of co-sleeping; while several suggest possible benefits (see Lewis & Janda, 1988; Abbott, 1992; Morelli et al., 1992).

In sum, contemporary infant sleep researchers and other scientists live in a culture where co-sleeping is assumed to be physically dangerous for the infant, potentially deleterious for the infant's psychological and socio-emotional development, and simply not "natural." Furthermore, it is highly unlikely that Western researchers slept with their own parents or children. Within this cultural context it is not surprising then that questions such as the following have not often been asked: Does co-sleeping have any significant beneficial effects on infants? Might some infants *need* nocturnal contact with parents more than others? Could co-sleeping make it more difficult for the SIDS deficit to find expression?

Summary and Conclusions

Although we enjoy tremendous medical advantages over non–industrial Western people, the link between the infant's biological status and coevolved patterns of birth and parental care cannot be clearly understood by examining mothers and infants in their contemporary biocultural context. Hunting, collecting, and foraging, birth with women assistants, and, indeed, parent-infant co-sleeping represent the evolutionary context within which modern humans were sculpted and designed biologically and psychosocially for well over 95% of our existence as a species (see figure 2.1). Mismatches between recent cultural changes and the more slowly changing biological needs of mothers and infants may be more significant than we realize. These mismatches may emerge as the source of many physiological and psychological disorders.

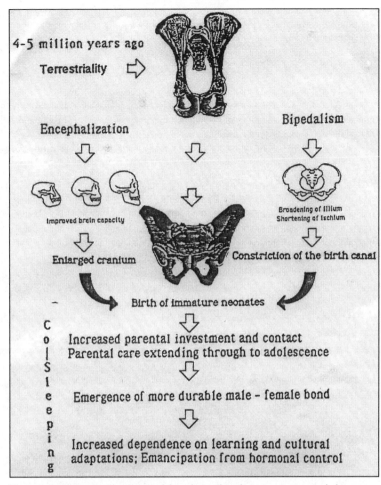

Figure 2.1. *Schematic illustration of the relationships between anatomical changes required for upright walking, the birth of neurologically immature infants, and the need for prolonged and intense parental contact and care, including co-sleeping.*

Evolution never promised us a rose garden and we need not, indeed cannot, stop cultural changes; but our evolutionary past has much to teach us, too. It can't be all wrong. Future research on infants, children, and adult environments using evolutionary data promises to reveal some unexpected new relationships tying social behavior, birth, and infant physiology together in unanticipated ways.

References

Abbott, S. (1992). How can you expect to hold onto them later in life if you begin their lives by pushing them away? *Ethos*, 20(I), 33-65.

Anderson, G. C. (1991). Current knowledge about skin-to-skin (kangaroo) care for preterm infants. *Journal of Perinatology*, 11, 216-226.

Aries, P. (1962). *Centuries of Childhood*. New York: Vintage.

Chisholm, J. S. (1983). *Navajo Infancy*. Hawthorne, NY: Aldine.

Christopher, R. C. (1983). *The Japanese Mind: The Goliath Explained*. New York: Linden Press/ Simon & Schuster.

Coe, C. L., Wiener, S. G., Rosenburg, L T., and Levine, S. (1985). Endocrine and immune responses to separation and maternal loss in non-human primates. In M. Reite and T. Field (Eds.), *The Psychobiology of Attachment and Separation*, 163-196. Orlando: Academic Press.

Eaton, S. B., Shostak, M., and Konner, M. (1988). *Paleolithic Prescription*. New York: Harper and Row.

Eisenberg, R. B., Griffin, E. J., Coursin, D. B., and Hunter, M. A. (1964). Auditory behavior in the human neonate: a preliminary report. *Journal of Speech and Hearing Research*, 7, 245-269.

Elias, M. F., Nicholson, N., Bora, C., and Johnston, J. (1986). Sleep-wake patterns of breast-fed infants in the first two years of life. *Pediatrics*, 77(3), 322-329.

Fardig, J. A. (1980). A comparison of skin-to-skin contact and radiant heaters in promoting neonatal thermoregulation. *Journal of Nurse-Midwifery*, 25, 19–28.

Ferber, R. (1986). *Solve Your Child's Sleep Problems*. New York: Simon & Schuster.

Flandrin, J. L. (1979). *Families in Former Times: Kinship, Household and Sexuality*. New York: Cambridge University Press.

Forbes, J. F, Weiss, D. S., and Folen, R. A. (1992). The co-sleeping habits of military children. *Military Medicine*, 157, 196-200.

Harvey, P. H., and Clutton-Brock, T. H. (1985). Life history variation in primates. *Evolution*, 39, 559-581.

Keefe, M. R. (1987). Comparison of neonatal night-time sleep-wake patterns in nursery versus rooming-in environments. *Nursing Research*, 36, 140-144.

Kellum, B. A. (1974). Infanticide in England in the Later Middle Ages. History of Childhood Quarterly. *The Journal of Psychohistory*, 1, 367–388.

Klaus, M. H., and Kennell, J. H. (1982). *Parent-Infant Bonding*. St. Louis: Mosby.

Klaus, M., Kennell, J., Berkowitz, G. & Klaus, P. (1992). Maternal assistance and support in labor: father, nurse, midwife, or doula? *Clinical Consultations in Obstetrics and Gynecology*, 4, December, 211-217.

Konner, M., and Worthman, C. (1980). Nursing frequency, gonadal function, and birth spacing among !Kung hunter-gatherers. *Science*, 207, 788-791.

Lewis, R. J., and Janda, L. H. (1988). The relationship between adult sexual adjustment and childhood experience regarding exposure to nudity, sleeping in the parental bed, and parental attitudes toward sexuality. *Archives of Sexual Behavior*, 17, 349–363.

Lozoff, B., Wolf, A., and Davis, N. (1984). Co-sleeping in urban families with young children in the United States. *Pediatrics*, 74, 171–182.

Ludington-Hoe, S. M., Hadeed, A., & Anderson, G. C. (1991a). Physiologic responses to skin-to-skin contact in hospitalized premature infants. *Journal of Perinatology*, 11, 19–24.

Ludington-Hoe, S. M., Hadeed, A., and Anderson, G. C. (1991b). Randomized trials of cardiorespiratory, thermal and state effects of kangaroo care for preterm infants. Paper presented at the biennial meetings of the Society for Research in Child Development, Seattle, April 19.

Mandansky, D. & Edelbrock, C. (1990). Co-sleeping in a community of 2- and 3-year-old children. *Pediatrics*, 86, 1987-2003.

McKenna, J. J. (1986). An anthropological perspective on the sudden infant death syndrome (SIDS): The role of parental breathing cues and speech breathing adaptations. *Medical Anthropology*, 10, 8–92.

McKenna, J. J. (1993). Rethinking healthy infant sleep. *Breastfeeding Abstracts*, 12, 27.

McKenna, J. J. & Mosko, S. (1993). Evolution and infant sleep: An experimental study of infant-parent co-sleeping and its implications for SIDS. *Acta Paediatrica Supplement*, 389, 31–36.

McKenna, J. J., Mosko, S., Dungy, C. & McAninch, P. (1990). Sleep and arousal patterns of co-sleeping human mothers/infant pairs: A preliminary physiological study with implications for the study of Sudden Infant Death Syndrome (SIDS). *American Journal of Physical Anthropology*, 83, 331–347.

McKenna, J. J., Thoman, E., Anders, T., Sadeh, A., Schechtman, V. & Glotzbach, S. (1993). Infant-parent co-sleeping in evolutionary perspective: Implications for understanding infant sleep development and the Sudden Infant Death Syndrome (SIDS). *Sleep*, 16, 263–282.

Medoff, D. & Schaefer, C. E. (1993). Children sharing the parental bed: A review of the advantages and disadvantages of co-sleeping. *Psychology: A Journal of Human Behavior*, 30, 1–9.

Morelli, G. A., Rogoff, B., Oppenheim, D. & Goldsmith, D. (1992). Cultural variation in infant's sleeping arrangements: Questions of independence. *Developmental Psychology*, 28, 604–613.

Mosko, S., McKenna, J., Dickel, M. & Hunt, L. (1993). Parent-infant co-sleeping: The appropriate context for the study of infant sleep and implications for SIDS research. *Journal of Behavioral Medicine*, 16(6): 589–610.

Reite, M. & Field T. (eds.). (1985). *The Psychobiology of Attachment and Separation*. Orlando, Fla.: Academic Press.

Robertiello, R. C. (1975). *Hold Them Very Close, Then Let Them Go*. New York: The Dial Press.

Robson, K. S. (1967). The role of eye-to-eye contact in maternal-infant attachment. *Comments on Contemporary Psychology and Psychiatry*, 8, 13–25.

Salk, L. (1969). The effects of the normal heartbeat sound on the behavior of the newborn infant: Implications for mental health. *World Mental Health*, 12, 168–175.

Shand, N. (1985). Culture's influence in Japanese and American maternal role perception and confidence. *Psychiatry*, 48, 52-67.

Short, R. V. (1984). Breastfeeding. *Scientific American*, 250, 35-41.

Spock B. & Rothenberg, M. (1985). *Dr Spock's Baby and Child Care*. New York: Pocket Books.

Stewart, M. & Stewart, L. (1991). Modification of sleep respiratory patterns by auditory stimulation: Indications of a technique for preventing Sudden Infant Death Syndrome? *Sleep*, 14, 241–248.

Stone, L. (1977). *The Family, Sex and Marriage in England, 1500–1800*. New York: Harper & Row.

Tinklepaugh, O. L. & Hartman, C. G. (1930). Behavioral aspects of parturition in the monkey *(Macaca rhesus)*. *Comparative Psychology*, 11, 63–98.

Trevathan, W. R. (1987). *Human Birth: An Evolutionary* Perspective. Hawthorne, NY: Aldine de Gruyter.

Trevathan, W. R. (1988). Fetal emergence patterns in evolutionary perspective. *American Anthropologist*, 90, 19-26.

Trevathan, W. R. (1992). Before birth was social. Paper presented at the Annual Meeting of the American Anthropological Association, San Francisco.

Vinovskis, M. A. (1987). Historical perspectives on the development of the family and parent-child interactions. In *Parenting Across the Life Span: Biosocial Dimensions*, Jane B. Lancaster, Jeanne Altmann, Alice S. Rossi, Lonnie Sherrod (eds.) Hawthorne, NY: Aldine de Gruyter, pp. 295–314.

Weiland, I. & Serber, Z. (1970). Patterns of mother-infant contact: The significance of lateral preference. *Journal of Genetic Psychology*, 117, 157–165.

Editor's Introduction

3

The Evolution of Maternal Birthing Position

LAUREN DUNDES

LIKE THE PREVIOUS CHAPTER IN THIS BOOK, this selection raises questions about the underlying validity of a modern Western approach to birthing that many assume to be the optimal standard of practice. By adopting a supine maternal birthing position, Westerners have abandoned a logical technique (upright birthing posture) in favor of one that has disadvantages that few recognize. The following chapter (taken from the *American Journal of Health* 77 [1987]: 636–641) explores how and possibly why Western maternal birthing posture changed from upright positions such as kneeling, squatting, standing, sitting, and so forth to a reclining posture, further exacerbated when the woman is required to have her legs up in stirrups (the lithotomy position).

The supine position inhibits the otherwise helpful force of gravity and impedes blood circulation. To better understand the seriousness of this issue, one need only ask the reader to imagine the act of defecating while lying down in order to demonstrate that such a position is unquestionably inferior with respect to expelling any substance from the body (i.e., pushing power is markedly reduced). The physiological disadvantages of lying down during birth are succinctly discussed in L. Fenwick in "Birthing," *Perinatology/Neonatology* 8 (1984): 51–62. It is important to note, however, that the use of various monitors or anesthesia may preclude the use of an upright posture; yet even sitting rather than lying flat can alleviate some of the adverse symptoms that arise from an unnatural supine birthing position.

In addition, the disadvantages of a horizontal maternal birthing position may result in the necessity of using other invasive procedures. For example, when a woman has her legs in the lithotomy position, the narrowing of the vaginal outlet makes the emerging infant's head more likely to tear the mother's perineum, thereby increasing the likelihood of unnecessary surgical widening of the perineum (an episiotomy).

The supine maternal birthing position continues as the norm in the United States partly because the medical establishment is resistant to change. Analogous examples of this intransigence in the 1990s include physicians' initial unwillingness to accept new evidence that ulcers were bacterial in origin (not stress related) and that mad cow disease was caused by a mutated protein—a prion—rather than viruses, bacteria, or parasites.

A number of scholars have pointed out that the Western maternal birthing position is both distinct from the positions traditionally assumed for birth in most other cultures as well as possibly disadvantageous physiologically and psychologically. Few authors, however, discuss factors that may have led to the American use of the supine position, particularly the lithotomy position.

This chapter speculates how the current maternal birthing position evolved, an interesting question since the change from an upright to a horizontal birthing position may be an instance where the "advances" of modern medicine could benefit from a reconsideration of "primitive" or early ways. Nevertheless, Western influence is clear: Beverly Chalmers in her "Changing Childbirth Customs" (*Pre- and Peri-Natal Psychology* 5 [1991]: 221–232) found that over 90 percent of Pedi women in South Africa preferred the supine maternal birthing position over their traditional upright or squatting position.

For an example of how old and new birthing practices in Rhodes clash, see M. P. Lefkarites, "The Sociocultural Implications of Modernizing Childbirth among Greek Women on the Island of Rhodes," *Medical Anthropology* 13 (1992): 385–314. For studies assessing different maternal birthing positions see M. Biancuzzo, "Six Myths of Maternal Posture during Labor," *American Journal of Maternal and Child Nursing* 18 (1993): 264–269; C. Racinet, P. Eymery, L. Philibert, and C. Lucas, "Labor in the Squatting Position," *Journal of Gynecol. Obstet. Biol. Reprod.* 28 (1999): 263–270; N. Johnson, V. A. Johnson, and J. K. Gupta, "Maternal Positions during Labor," *Obstet. Gynecol. Surv.* 46 (1991): 428–434; and J. Golay, S. Vedam, and L. Sorger, "The Squatting Position for the Second Stage of Labor: Effects on Labor and on Maternal and Fetal Well Being," *Birth* 20 (1993): 73–78.

A number of books describe and portray an impressive array of upright birth postures, including G. Engelmann, *Labor among Primitive Peoples* (St. Louis: J. H. Chambers, 1882); J. Jarcho, *Posture and Practices during Labor among Primitive Peoples* (New York: Paul B. Hoeber, 1934); and more recently Liselotte Kuntner's *Die Gebärhaltung der Frau* (The Birthing Position of Women) (München: Hans Marseille Verlag, 1988). See also articles by A. J. Gibson, "Obstetrical Customs among Savage and Barbarous Peoples," *Medical Journal of Australia* 2 (1929): 222–228; H. Kirchhoff, "The Woman's Posture during Childbirth," *Organorama* 14 (1977): 111–119; P. Argenti, "Childbirth in the Greek Island of Chios in the 6th Century BC, 1780 and 1914," *London Journal of Obstetrics and Gynecology* 51 (1944): 344–349.

For books that critique the American way of birth including birthing position see D. Haire, "The Cultural Warping of Childbirth," *Environmental Child Health*, Special Issue, monograph no. 27 (1973): 171–191; G. Dick-Read, *Childbirth without Fear* (New York: Harper and Row, 1944); S. Arms, *Immaculate Deception* (Boston: Houghton Mifflin, 1975); R. W. Wertz and D. C. Wertz, *Lying-In: A History of Childbirth in America* (New York: Free Press, 1977); M. Edwards and M. Waldorf, *Reclaiming Birth: History and Heroines of American Childbirth Reform* (Trumansburg: Crossing Press, 1984); and J. Mitford, *The American Way of Birth*, (New York: Dutton, 1992).

The Evolution of Maternal Birthing Position 3

LAUREN DUNDES

Introduction

THE BIRTH OF A CHILD is one of the most significant events in a woman's life. Practices associated with the birthing process are, therefore, important to the woman's health and well-being as well as the successful outcome of her pregnancy. Included among these practices is the horizontal birthing position that has been the subject of a great deal of controversy.[1-14] This position has been widely used in Western cultures only for the last 200 years. Prior to this time, the recorded history of birthing indicates upright birth postures were used extensively.

Both the dorsal position, where the parturient is flat on her back, and the lithotomy position, where she lies on her back with her legs up in stirrups, have been challenged in the last 100 years.[1-5] Since the decline in the use of scopolamine and morphine "twilight sleep," there has been a trend encouraging parturients to utilize lateral, dorsal, and reclining positions to give birth, but such practices are far from universal.[5]

This paper will explore the historical roots of the dorsal and lithotomy birthing positions now practiced in most hospitals in the United States. Although various explanations for the change in position have been proposed, including facilitation of forceps usage, promotion of men's power over women (both midwives and parturients), and requirements with the use of anesthesia, none adequately explains the confluence of events that led to the shift away from the upright to the horizontal maternal birth position. Conflict between midwives and surgeons and interaction of the disciplines of obstetric surgery and lithotomy surgery that emerged 300 years ago appear to have contributed to this change. The transition was greatly influenced by the French who were at that time considered the leaders in obstetrical practice.

Worldwide Practices

Most cultures throughout the world either use, or have used, such birthing positions as kneeling, squatting, sitting, and standing for labor and delivery. [15-18] Earliest records of maternal birth positions show the parturient in an upright posture, usually squatting or kneeling. A bas-relief at the Temple of Esneh in Egypt depicts Cleopatra (69?–30 B.C.) in a kneeling position, surrounded by five women attendants, one of whom delivers the child.[5] The birthing chair dates back to the Babylonian culture, 2000 B.C. It then spread to many parts of the world.[19] In some parts of the world, various traditional birthing chairs are still used, while a modern version is now available in some Western hospitals.[20]

In a 1961 survey of 76 traditional cultures, Naroll et al. found that in only 14 (18 percent) did the women assume either a prone or dorsal birthing position.[17] The findings and conclusions of this cross-cultural survey are in accord with extensive work done earlier by Engelmann (1882) and Jarcho (1934).[7,15] Currently in many developing countries, traditional birth attendants (usually women) attend parturients. The birth position they use differs from that suggested by physicians and by trained midwives who have been taught the Western practice of horizontal labor and delivery positions.[21,22]

Interprofessional Rivalry

In Europe until about 1550, midwives were the only attendants at births.[23] When Paré, the famous surgeon-obstetrician, practiced medicine (1517?–1590), barber-surgeons began to compete with midwives for obstetric cases.[24] Initially, these surgeons were poorly trained; their social rank remained on a par with that of carpenters, shoemakers, and other members of guilds, known collectively as the "arts and trades" until the 18th century.[25] As time progressed, they sought recognition for the obstetric skills they had acquired in delivering women whose lives were threatened as a result of obstetric complications. Achieving recognition for their skills was made difficult, due to their status and because exposure of women's bodies to men was considered indecent. Physicians, granted special privileges and accorded higher status than surgeons, were not eager for this advancing profession to encroach on any of their territory. Neither did midwives, many of whom had received formal training, welcome the surgeons' intrusion as it represented a threat to their livelihood and recognized area of expertise.

Mauriceau (1637–1709), a prominent French physician at this time, recorded the climate of the times and the coexistence of the intense interprofessional rivalry:

> There are many Midwives, who are so afraid that the Chirurgeons should take away their practice, or to appear ignorant before them that they chuse rather to put all to adventure, then to send for them in necessity: others believe themselves as capable as the Chirurgeons to undertake all . . . and some do maliciously put such a terror and apprehension of the Chirurgeons in the poor women (for the most part undeservedly), comparing them to Butchers and Hangmen, that they chuse rather to die in Travail with the Child in their Womb, than to put themselves into their hands.[26]

Although midwives continued to retain their longstanding position as the primary birth attendants, barber-surgeons were increasingly called in cases likely to result in fetal and/or maternal morbidity or mortality; often they practiced manual extraction of the fetus from the mother in order to save her life.[23] The practice of obstetrics offered surgeons a plausible entry into the medical field. Their attendance at traumatic cases helped them develop a disease orientation to childbirth, and they held a competitive advantage over midwives due to their skills or practice in dealing with complications. Derogated by the physicians and forced to compete with midwives, they had to make themselves marketable. If most women viewed pregnancy as a normal, natural event, then the surgeons' services would not be required. If, however, pregnancy was seen as an illness, then their presence might appear more appropriate. Midwives did at times promote their own services by proclaiming the need for intervention, although intervention within a disease orientation benefited the male accoucheurs.

Guillemeau (the pupil and son-in-law of Paré) had advocated reclining bed birthing in 1598, supposedly for women's comfort and to facilitate labor;[27] the techniques used by surgeons to handle difficult births 50 years later could also be best performed in a reclining position. This led to using the bed as the place to perform childbirth, and the reclining position developed into the one practiced for normal as well as complicated deliveries. Women at the Paris Hôtel Dieu (a large hospital with a maternity section) delivered in a special bed; by the end of the 17th century, bed delivery had become a common practice in France except among rural women.[28]

Although convenience is continuously pointed to in the literature as the primary reason for changing to the supine birth position, the experience varied by country. By the 17th century, when births began to occur in bed, many women, especially in England, lay on their sides, which differed from the reclining position used in France that accommodated the birth attendant.[29]

Influence of Mauriceau

Despite Guillemeau's earlier advocacy of the reclining position and the influence of the barber-surgeons, the person generally credited with greatly influencing the change in birth position is François Mauriceau.[8,30] He claimed that the reclining position would be both more comfortable for the parturient women as well as more convenient for the accoucheur. In his 1668 book, *The Diseases of Women with Child and in Child-Bed*, he recommended the change of position and offered the following recommended rationale for doing so:

> [A]ll Women are not accustomed to be delivered in the same posture; some will be on their Knees, as many in Country Villages; others standing upright leaning with the Elbows on a Pillow upon a Table, or on the side of a Bed . . . but the best and surest is to be delivered in their Bed, to shun the inconvenience and trouble of being carried thither afterwards;
>
> The Bed must be so made, that the Woman being ready to be delivered should lie on her Back upon it, having her Body in a convenient Figure, that is, her Head and Breast a little raised so that she be neither lying nor sitting; for in this manner she breaths best, and will have more strength to help her Pains than if she were otherwise, or sunk down in her Bed . . . and have her feet stayed against some firm thing.[26]

Mauriceau also was affected by prevailing views of pregnancy as an illness. His 1668 work on midwifery in which he claimed that pregnancy, properly construed, was a "tumor of the Belly" caused by an infant was among the first of many early references to medical problems during pregnancy and childbirth[31] that defined all births as inherently pathologic and abnormal, leaving no room for the midwife.[32] Change in position was a natural accompaniment of the shift in concept.

Role of King Louis XIV

Some scholars claim that the change in birthing position was a perverted caprice of King Louis XIV (1637–1709), a contemporary of Mauriceau (1637–1709).[30,33] Since Louis XIV reportedly enjoyed watching women giving birth, he became frustrated by the obscured view of birth when it occurred on a birthing stool, and promoted the new reclining position. He also insisted on male accoucheurs attending births. The influence of the king's policy is unknown, although the behavior of royalty must have affected the populace to some degree. Louis XIV's purported demand for change did coincide with the changing of the position and may well have been a contributing influence.

King Louis XIV not only promoted the use of the male accoucheur, but also granted favors to a well-known lithotomist, Frère Jacques (born Jacques Beaulieu in 1651).[34] For unknown reasons, the procedures of obstetrics and lithotomy were preoccupations of this head of state. The lithotomy surgery of the urinary bladder for removal of a stone had been performed since at least 200 B.C.,[35] and was used extensively in France in the 17th century. Paré (1517–1590), who has been called the father of modern obstetrics,[23] was also involved in lithotomy surgery. The interaction of the evolving sciences of lithotomy and obstetrics is not surprising since techniques used in obstetric surgery (e.g., cesarean section) had features in common with those used in lithotomy. The lithotomist, Frère Jacques, a name made famous by the French folksong,[34] was taught anatomy by Fagon, who served as a surgeon to Louis XIV.

At one point, Frère Jacques so impressed Louis XIV that the king gave instructions for him to be lodged with the royal valet and to be given the King's License to do lithotomy operations.[34,35] Frère Jacques performed the lithotomy operations at the same Hôtel Dieu during the time period in which the new birth position was instituted. Although a precise relation between the reclining birth position—the forerunner of the lithotomy position—and the lithotomy operation is difficult to establish, the adoption of the lithotomy position for birthing and extensive practice of the lithotomy operation occurred at the same time and place in France in the 17th century.

Forceps and Anesthesia

It has also been argued that the change in birthing position was instituted because it provided improved access to the perineum when forceps were used.[8,9] Forceps had been known in obstetrics since the third century[36] and were also used in lithotomy procedures by Paré in the mid-1500s.[35] Obstetric forceps fell into disuse, however, until 1588 when they were rediscovered by Chamberlen. To guard their secret, the Chamberlen family, French Huguenots who fled to England for safety, carried the forceps in a locked case, and used them under a sheet with the patient blindfolded.[37,38] Mauriceau, because of his prominence, was offered the secret of the forceps by a descendant of Chamberlen in 1670. He declined to buy the instrument (which he never actually saw)[24] because he had witnessed their unsuccessful use in the delivery of one of his patients.[6]

It is reported that forceps were not used by others outside of the Chamberlen family until 1700,[24,31,37] and that the secret of forceps construction emerged around 1720 at which time their utilization increased dramatically.[39] Forceps could not initially have played a major role in affecting the birth position, since the birthing position had been changed many years before forceps came into wide usage, although they may have been an important factor in the retention of the reclining and lithotomy positions.

A number of scholars believe that the advent of general anesthesia eliminated women's ability to participate at all in labor and delivery, requiring them to lie down to be delivered.[40] However, a relationship between general anesthesia and the change in birth position is unlikely, since anesthesia was not used until almost 200 years after the reign of Louis XIV. In Europe, Sir James Simpson of Edinburgh introduced the use of chloroform in 1847, and the use of general anesthesia in obstetrics increased after chloroform was administered to Queen Victoria in 1853.[39]

Flat Maternal Birth Position in U.S.

Neither the lithotomy position nor the flat horizontal position was recommended by Mauriceau in the mid-1600s. He advocated the reclining posture which may be more favorable physiologically and more comfortable for the woman. The controversial flat position[41] (in contrast to reclining) first began to be used in the United States.[42,43] This position differed from that used in European countries. In Cazeaux's 1884 obstetrics book, it is reported that women in the United States lie flat on their backs, French women lie back on an inclined plane, English women lie on their left side, and German women use the birthing chair.[42] Since European practices greatly influenced those of the United States, it is understandable that American accoucheurs would have emulated the European practice of birthing in bed. Exactly why the United States deviated from the European reclining posture is not clear, however.

The employment of the flat dorsal birth position (circa 1834) is attributed to William Potts Dewees, the third chairman of obstetrics at the University of Pennsylvania.[8,44] Dewees advocated the dorsal birth posture, although he recommended side-lying for labor. The site of implementing his recommendation is uncertain, since Dewees does not define the term "sick room."[43] His writings support the contentions that the United States had deviated from European practice, and that convenience of the accoucheur was crucial.

> The British practitioner almost invariably directs the patient to be placed upon her side . . . while the Continental accoucheur has her placed on her back. . . . the woman should be placed so as to give the least possible hindrance to the operations of the accoucheur—this is agreed upon by all; but there exist a diversity of opinion, what that position is. Some recommended the side; others the knees, and others the back. I coincide with the latter. . . . Therefore, when practicable, I would recommend she should be placed upon her back, both for convenience and safety.[43]

Since he "coincides" with an established position, evidently he was reflecting an existing opinion and the flat position had been advocated by others preceding him.

Links between Lithotomy and Obstetrics in U.S.

William Shippen, Jr., the first chairman of Obstetrics and Anatomy at the University of Pennsylvania, was an influential leader and teacher in obstetrics until his death in 1808. Writing of Shippen, one scholar stated: "Among colonial physicians specializing in midwifery, no one deserves a more prominent place."[45] Shippen established a lying-in hospital in Philadelphia in 1765.[46] Yet when Shippen is discussed in midwifery literature, his career as an esteemed lithotomist is not explored. In fact, according to the lithotomy literature, Shippen is considered one of the most influential bladder stone lithotomists although only a few of his writings are extant.[47] Another connection between the two specialties involves Hugh Hodge, who followed Dewees as the Chairman of Obstetrics at the University of Pennsylvania Medical School. Like Shippen, Hodge was a student of lithotomy. His mentor (Caspar Wistar) was a bladder stone lithotomist and a pupil of Shippen's. Thus we have an additional link between obstetrics and lithotomy in the United States during the late 18th century.[44]

From the mid-18th to the 20th centuries, obstetric practices were not standardized, and various forms of horizontal positioning prevailed. Moreover, there was almost no control of or examination for medical licensing, and medical schools enforced only minimal requirements.[48] Such circumstances would delay the spread of Shippen's influence on birth position, which was also undoubtedly greatly affected by accoucheur advantage of horizontal positioning.

Conclusions

The pros and cons of childbirth in the dorsal and lithotomy positions have been discussed at least since Engelmann's time (1882)[7]; however, little has been done until recently to encourage alternative birthing positions that may be better accepted by and more beneficial to the parturient woman, her child, and the birth attendant. The adoption and use of the lithotomy position was not based on sound scientific research. By exploring the circumstances that existed when the maternal birth position changed, we see that the position was altered as a result of interprofessional struggles of surgeons and midwives and by the development of obstetrics as affected by the practice of lithotomy. A position was implemented without verification of its appropriateness. Today, with more women and their families exercising their rights to actively participate in the birth experience and to make it a more personal and more physiologically and psychologically advantageous experience, the time is ripe for further scientific investigation of the lithotomy position. Unlike our historical precedent, where an important change seems to have been influenced by the reputation of prominent persons and the prevailing circumstances of the times, it is currently possible to design and plan studies that evaluate the different birthing positions—options that have an important bearing on the health and safety of the parturients and the newborns.

References

1. Dunn, P.: Obstetric delivery today—for better or for worse. Lancet 1976; I:7963, 790–793.

2. Kitzinger, S.: Experiences of obstetric practices in differing countries. In: Zander, L. (ed), Pregnancy Care for the 1980s. London: Royal Society of Medicine, and Macmillan Press, 1984.

3. Shaw, N.S.: Forced labor: Maternity Care in the United States. New York: Pergamon Press, 1974.

4. Leifer, M.: Psychological Effects of Motherhood: A Study of First Pregnancy. New York: Praeger Special Studies, 1980.

5. Carlson, J.M., Diebl, J.A., Sachtleben-Murray, M., et al.: Maternal position during parturition in normal labor. Obstet Gynecol 1986; 68:443–447.

6. Wertz, R.W., Wertz, D.C.: Lying-In, A History of Childbirth in America. New York: Free Press, 1977.

7. Engelmann, G.: Labor among Primitive Peoples. St. Louis: J. H. Chambers, 1882.

8. Caldeyro-Barcia, R.: The influence of maternal position on time of spontaneous rupture of the membranes, progress of labor and fetal head compression. Birth Fam J 1979; 6:7–16.

9. Carr, K. C.: Obstetric practices which protect against neonatal morbidity: focus on maternal position in labor and birth. Birth Fam J 1980; 7:249–254.

10. Haire, D.: The Cultural Warping of Childbirth. Milwaukee: International Childbirth Education Association (ICEA), 1972.

11. Fenwick, L.: Birthing. Perinatology/Neonatology 1984; 8:51–62.

12. Roberts, J., Mendez-Bauer, C., Wodell, D.A.: The effects of maternal position on uterine contractility and efficiency. Birth 1983; 10:243–249.

13. Stewart, P., Hillan, E., Calder, A. A.: A randomized trial to evaluate the use of a birthing chair for delivery. Lancet 1983: I:1296–1298.

14. Roberts, J.: Alternative positions for childbirth—Part I: first stage of labor. J Nurse–Midwifery 1980; 25:11–18.

15. Jarcho, J.: Posture and Practices during Labor among Primitive Peoples. New York: Paul B. Hoeber, 1934.

16. Russell, J.G.: The rationale of primitive delivery positions. Br J Obstet Gynecol 1982; 89:712–715.

17. Naroll, F., Naroll, R., Howard, F.H.: Position of women in childbirth. Am J Obstet Gynecol 1961; 82: 943–954.

18. Jordan, B.: Birth in Four Cultures. Montreal: Eden Press, 1983.

19. Lagercrantz, V. S.: Zur verbreitung des geburtsstuhles in Afrika. Mitteilungen der Anthropologischen Gesellschaft. Vienna, 1939.

20. Johnson, T.R.B., Repke, J. R., Paine, L.L.: Choosing a birthing bed to meet everyone's needs. Contemp Ob/Gyn 1987, 29:70–73.

21. Cosminsky, S.: Traditional midwifery and contraception. In: Traditional Medicine and Health Care Coverage. Geneva: World Health Organization, 1983.

22. Cosminsky, S.: Knowledge and body concept of Guatemalan midwives. In: Kay, M. A. (ed): Anthropology of Human Birth. Philadelphia: F. A. Davis, 1982.

23. Townsend, L.: Obstetrics through the ages. Med J Aust 1952; 1.558–565

24. Ackerknecht, E. H.: A Short History of Medicine. Baltimore: Johns Hopkins Press, 1982.

25. Gelfand, T.: From the guild to profession: the surgeons of France in the 18th century. Texas Rep Biol Med 1974; 32:121–132.

26. Mauriceau, F.: The Diseases of Women with Child and in Child-Bed. London: John Darby, 1683. (Translated by Hugh Chamberlen from the original work published in French in 1668).

27. Guillemeau, J.: Child-Birth or the Happy Delivery of Women. London: A. Hatfield. 1612.

28. Eccles, A.: Obstetrics and Gynecology in Tudor and Stuart England. Kent: Kent State University Press, 1982.

29. Shorter, E.: A History of Women's Bodies. New York: Basic Books, 1982.

30. Arms, S.: Immaculate Deception. Boston: Houghton Mifflin, 1975.

31. Wilbanks, E.: Historical Review of Obstetrical Practice. In: Aladjem, S. (ed) Obstetric Practice. St. Louis: C. V. Mosby. 1980.

32. Rothman, B.K.: Anatomy of a Compromise: Nurse-midwifery and the rise of the birth center. J Nurse-Midwifery 1983, 28:3–7.

33. Mendelsohn, R. S.: Male Malpractice: How Doctors Manipulate Women. Chicago: Contemporary Books. 1982.

34. Ellis, H.: A History of Bladder Stone. Oxford: Blackwell Scientific Publications, 1969.

35. Riches, E.: The history of lithotomy and lithotrity. Ann R Coll Surg Engl 1968; 43:185-199.

36. Speert, H.: Iconographia Gyniatrica: A Pictorial History of Gynecology and Obstetrics. Philadelphia: F. A. Davis, 1973.

37. Corea, G.: The Hidden Malpractice: How American Medicine Treats Women as Patients and Professionals. New York: Williams & Morrow. 1977.

38. Chaney, J.A.: Birthing in early America. J Nurse-Midwifery. 1980: 25:5–13.

39. Edwards, M., Waldorf, M.: Reclaiming Birth-History and Heroines of American Childbirth Reform. Trumansburg: Crossing Press. 1984.

40. Walton, V.E.: Have it Your Way. Toronto: Bantam Books. 1976.

41. McKay, S.: Maternal position during labor and birth: a reassessment. 1980: 9:5. 288–291.

42. Tarner, S.: Cazeaux's Theory and Practice of Obstetrics. Philadelphia: Blakiston Son and Co. 1884.

43. Dewees, W.P.: A Compendious System of Midwifery. Philadelphia: Crey, Lea, and Carey. 1828.

44. Baas, J.H.: Baas' History of Medicine (translated by H. E. Handerson). New York: J. H. Vail, 1889.

45. Donnegan, J.B.: Midwifery in America. 1760–1860: A Study in Medicine and Morality. (Dissertation for History Department, Syracuse University).

46. Hiestand, W.C.: Midwife to Nurse-Midwife: A History: The Development of Nurse-Midwifery Education in the Continental United States to 1965. (Dissertation for Education in Teachers College. Columbia University).

47. Bush, R.B.: Lithotomy. Its practice and Practitioners in Philadelphia during the Colonial and Early Republican Period: An Essay in the Transit of Culture. (Dissertation in the Department of History. New York University, 1976).

48. Rosenberg, C.: The practice of medicine in New York a century ago. Bull Hist Med 1967; 41:223–252.

Editor's Introduction

4

Cross-Cultural Perspectives on Midwifery

SHEILA COSMINSKY

SHEILA COSMINSKY, PROFESSOR OF ANTHROPOLOGY at Rutgers University, is an expert on medical and nutritional anthropology. Her research in countries such as Guatemala, Belize, Kenya, Zimbabwe, and Japan demonstrates her strong interest in cross-cultural study. Cosminsky has published a number of articles that relate to her essay (reprinted from Francis X. Grollig and Harold B. Haley, eds., *Medical Anthropology* [The Hague: Mouton, 1976], 229–248) in this volume (e.g., "Birth Rituals and Symbolism: A Quiche Maya–Black Carib Comparison," in *Ritual and Symbol in Native Central America*, edited by P. Young and J. Howe [University of Oregon Anthropological Papers No. 9, 1976], 105–123; "Changing Food and Medical Beliefs and Practices in a Guatemalan Community," *Ecology of Food and Nutrition* 4 [1975]: 183–191; "Knowledge and Body Concepts of Guatemalan Midwives," in *Anthropology of Human Birth*, edited by M. A. Kay [Philadelphia: F. A. Davis Company, 1982], 233–252; S. Cosminsky, M. Mhloyi, and D. Ewbank, "Child Feeding Practices in a Rural Area of Zimbabwe," *Social Science & Medicine* 36, no. 7 [1993]: 937–947; and "Childbirth and Change: A Guatemalan Study," in *Ethnography of Fertility and Birth*, 2nd ed., edited by C. P. MacCormack [Prospect Heights, Ill.: Waveland Press, 1994], pp. 195–219). Cosminsky also cowrote an annotated bibliography with I. E. Harrison, *Traditional Medicine: Implications for Ethnomedicine, Ethnopharmacology, Maternal and Child Health, Mental Health, and Public Health: An Annotated Bibliography of Africa, Latin America, and the Caribbean*, 2 vols. (New York: Garland Publishers, 1976–1984).

There is growing interest in employing midwives, partly because of disillusionment with the medical model of birthing in which pregnancy is treated more as an illness than a joyful state of being. In addition to offering a contrasting philosophy about birthing, midwives' techniques tend to be distinct from physicians' (e.g., less dependence on high technology equipment).

Midwives, for example, can turn the fetus in utero so that it will have a smoother exit (see N. M. Scaletta, "Childbirth: A Case History from West New Britain, Papua New Guinea," *Oceania* 57 [1986]: 33–52; B. Jordan, *Birth in Four Cultures*, 4th ed. [Prospect Heights, Ill.: Waveland Press, 1993]). The midwives' skill also helps prevent the common Western procedure, episiotomy, as well as tearing. Cutting of the perineal area to allow the baby's head to emerge in birth is avoided by massaging the pelvic area to encourage the pelvic bones to yield the emerging infant. Next, oil is applied to enhance the effect of the slippery vernix caseosa and digital stretching of the perineum simultaneous with the squeezing of the area near the rectum as the child emerges.

Amazingly, in one case, midwives, when queried, reported being engaged in birth control practices that involved manual manipulation of the fallopian tubes or uterine position through massage. (See A. J. Rubel, K. Weller-Fahy, and M. Trosdal, "Conception, Gestation, and Delivery According to Some Mananabang of Cebu," *Philippine Quarterly of Culture and Society* 3 [1975]: 131–145.)

Midwives also are reported to return the power of the process to the parturient (see J. Murphy-Lawless, "Piggy in the Middle: The Midwife's Role in Achieving Woman-Controlled Childbirth," *Irish Journal of Psychology* 12 [1991]: 198–215; K. Weibust, "Alternatives in Childbirth: Questions about Active Birth and Resources of the Birthgiving Woman," *Ethnologia Scandinavica* [1988]: 67–75; A. J. Rubel, K. Weller-Fahy, and M. Trosdal, "Conception, Gestation, and Delivery According to Some Mananabang of Cebu," *Philippine Quarterly of Culture and Society* 3 [1975]: 131–145).

There is voluminous work on the gender power dynamics of birth. Samples include S. Arms, *Immaculate Deception* (Boston: Houghton Mifflin, 1975); L. M. Baldwin, H. L. Hutchinson, and R. A. Rosenblatt, "Professional Relationships between Midwives and Physicians: Collaboration or Conflict?" *American Journal of Public Health* 82 (1992): 262–264; R. E. Davis-Floyd, "The Role of Obstetrical Rituals in the Resolution of Cultural Anomaly," *Social Science and Medicine* 31 (1990): 175–189; R. E. Davis-Floyd and C. Sargent, eds., *Childbirth and Authoritative Knowledge: Cross-Cultural Perspectives* (Berkeley: University of California Press, 1997); N. D. Schrom, "History of Childbirth in America," *Signs* 6 (1981): 97–108; W. P. Handwerker, ed., *Birth and Power: Social Change and the Politics of Reproduction*, (Boulder, Colo.: Westview Press, 1990); B. K. Rothman, *Recreating Motherhood: Ideology and Technology in Patriarchal Society* (New York: W. W. Norton, 1989); C. Sargent, *Maternity, Medicine and Power: Reproductive Decisions in Urban Benin* (Berkeley: University of California Press, 1989); P. Plappone, *Beyond Conception: The New Politics of Reproduction* (Granby, Mass.: Bergin and Garvey, 1989); S. Romalis, ed., *Childbirth: Alternatives to Medical Control* (Austin: University of Texas Press, 1981); and L. Hsia, "Midwives and the Empowerment of Women—An International Perspective," *Journal of Nurse-Midwifery* 36 (1991): 85–87.

In addition, there are many books about the art of midwifery, for example, S. A. Kitzinger, *The Midwife Challenge* (London: Pandora Press, 1988); M. Grabrucker, *Vom Abenteuer der Geburt: die letzten Landhebammen erzahlen* [Of the Adventure of Birth: The Last Rural Midwives Tell Their Stories] (Frankfurt am Main: Fischer Taschenbuch Verlag, 1989); and C. Laderman, *Wives and Midwives: Childbirth and Nutrition in Rural Malaysia* (Berkeley: University of California Press, 1983). For a comprehensive history of midwifery, see J. Gelis, *La sage-femme ou le médecin: une nouvelle conception de la vie* [The midwife or the doctor: A new conception of life]. (Paris: Fayard, 1988).

Cross-Cultural Perspectives on Midwifery 4

SHEILA COSMINSKY

A LL HUMAN SOCIETIES HAVE PATTERNED SETS OF BELIEFS and practices concerning pregnancy, delivery, and the puerperium. Some societies have a specialist who is primarily concerned with these matters. This specialist is referred to as a "midwife."

This paper examines the variations that exist in the status and role of the midwife, primarily in non-Western societies, and considers some of the changes occurring with the spread of Western or modern medicine. Specific aspects that are analyzed are recruitment, acquisition of skills and knowledge, training, status, the midwife's role in prenatal care, delivery, and postnatal care. See table 4.1 for Ethnographic and Medical Sources.

The United States has witnessed the decline of midwifery with the rise of the obstetrician and other medical specialists (Stern 1972). Today, however, a renewed interest and the beginning of a resurrection of the midwife, or nurse-midwife, seem to be gradually occurring. Another is the realization that the United States' infant mortality rate is higher than at least fourteen other countries. Haire (1972) has made a comparative study of obstetric techniques and procedures in these countries and suggests that highly trained midwives are an important source of obstetrical care for normal women in countries which have a lower rate of infant mortality, e.g. in Norway, 96 percent of deliveries are by midwives. The emotional support given to mothers during the prenatal and labor stages seems to be accompanied by a lessened need for obstetrical intervention and medication during labor. Questions are being raised about various obstetrical practices used in the United States, such as the value of the supine position for delivery, the separation of the mother from her family, pathologic effects of chemical stimulation of labor, use of forceps, and performing routine episiotomies. Some of the questions that are raised in this paper concern the implications of the spread of certain of these practices to other parts of the world.

Table 4.1. Ethnographic and Medical Sources

Area	Source
Africa	
Buganda	Billington, et al. 1963; Rosco 1911
Chaga	Raum 1940
Ghana (Accra)	Goodman 1951
Nigeria (Ile-Ife)	Long 1964; Turtell 1965
South Africa	
(Alexandra Township)	Stein and Susser 1959
General	Gelfand 1964
Sudan	Kendall 1953
Asia	
China	Lamson 1934
Iban	Jensen 1967
India	Briggs 1920; Fuchs 1939; Ghosh 1968; Gideon 1962; Gordon, Gideon, and Wyon 1964, 1965; Minturn and Hitchcock 1963; Mistry 1952; Sarker, Choudhuri, and Ray 1955; Singh 1947; Stevenson 1920
Japan	Standlee 1959
Philippines	Ewing 1960; Frake 1957; Hart 1965; Nydegger and Nydegger 1963; Rubel, et al. 1971
Thailand	Wales 1933; Anuman Rajadhon 1965
Vietnam	Coughlin 1965
Europe	
Greece	Blum and Blum 1965
North America	
American Indian	
Arikara	Gilmore 1930
Cherokee	Oldbrechts 1931
Navajo	Leighton and Kluckhohn 1947; Lockett 1939
Ojibwa	Landes 1937, 1938
Zuni	Leighton and Adair 1963
Appalachia	Osgood, Hochstrasser, and Deuschle 1966
Hutterites	Eaton 1958
Rural South	Mongeau, Smith, and Maney 1960
Latin America	
Guatemala	Bunzel 1959; Cosminsky 1972; Rodriguez Rouanet 1970; Reina 1966
Mexico	Beals 1946; Foster 1948; Gerdel 1949; Kelly 1965; Lewis 1960; Madsen 1965; McKay 1933; Redfield and Villa Rojas 1934; Romney and Romney 1963; Schendel 1968
Peru	Wellin 1956
Oceania	
New Guinea	van Amelsvoort 1964

Definitions

The use of the term "midwife" ranges from referring to anyone who assists at birth, whether a specialist or not, to that employed by the World Health Organization (W.H.O.), which stresses professional training and formal education. Qualified and trained, according to a committee report (W.H.O. 1966), means at least secondary school education and training in scientific medicine. W.H.O. considers indigenous midwives together with any birth attendant as a "traditional birth attendant," who "mostly have no training at all in midwifery, but are usually well versed in folklore relating to maternal and infant care and are likely to be among the most highly respected members of their communities" (1966: 16). W.H.O. is developing programs for bringing the traditional birth attendant into the cadre of health personnel. However, the amount of training and education that they recommend is not feasible in many parts of the world and thus the traditional attendant, including indigenous specialists, will never attain the status of midwife according to W.H.O. standards.

Many ethnographic reports also do not differentiate a specialized status of midwife from any birth attendant. It is often difficult to ascertain whether such a status even exists. One of the problems in doing a cross-cultural study is the comparability of these categories. For example, among the Navajo, Lockett (1939) says that the midwife was a special status referred to by a special name. Leighton and Kluckhohn (1947) say that any female, although usually a relative, may attend birth; sometimes a "semi-professional" person is summoned. What does "semi-professional" mean? Is this the same status to which Lockett refers? What are the qualifications and training of such a person that make him or her "semi-professional"?

The indigenous midwife (e.g. *partera, comadrona, bidan, dai*) is referred to in the literature by a variety of terms, such as "empirical midwife" (Kelly 1965) or "lay midwife" (Osgood, et al. 1966), to distinguish them from licensed midwives who have formal medical education or degrees. Various societies also use different terms to distinguish them. In Vietnam, *ba mu vuon*, the traditional midwife, is distinct from the *nu ho sinh*, the government licensed midwife (Coughlin 1965). In Ica, Peru, native midwives are called *parteras*, whereas hospital-trained and licensed midwives are known by rural women as *profesoras*, the general term for people who deal in book knowledge (Wellin 1956).

For purposes of this paper, the term midwife refers to a position which has been socially differentiated as a specialized status by the society. Such a person is usually regarded as a specialist and a professional in her own eyes and by her community.

The main emphasis in this paper is on general statements, problems, and trends concerning midwives in different societies, especially non-Western ones. Only a few selected ethnographic examples will be presented.

Characteristics, Recruitment, and Training

Ford (1945) found elderly women assisting at birth in fifty-eight cultures and not assisting in only two. Most midwives are females. A few cases of male midwives, however, have been reported (Mexico, Philippines, Appalachia).[1]

Midwives also tend to be elderly and/or to have had children of their own. The majority are past the childbearing age, which means they are freer to assume midwifery responsibilities. In contrast, the government midwifery programs tend to train younger people. This person may also be unmarried and have no children, which might negatively affect her status in the community, especially as an expert on childbirth (Blum and Blum 1965: 154). In areas where both types of midwives exist, the formally trained one may be put in a supervisory position (Greece, India). Where age confers respect, this can and does create problems.

Some programs have recommended an age limit for midwives, such as 65 (Lamson 1934), or 70 (Mongeau, et al. 1960). It is at this age, however, when the midwife is often at the peak of her career. She is also probably training a younger assistant. The average age of "granny" midwives in a rural southern U.S. community was 66 (Mongeau, et al. 1960) and in Appalachia it was 70 (Osgood, et al. 1966). This age restriction would effect another change in the pattern of the midwife's status. The implications of such changes in age characteristics should be investigated.

A person may become a midwife through supernatural calling, inheritance, or voluntarily by her own means. In societies where supernatural agents are important in the selection and training of midwives, they usually appear in dreams or visions (Guatemala, Ojibwa, Philippines, rural southern United States). In some cases, these visions are interpreted by a diviner as indicating the person should be a midwife. The midwife claims that her skills and knowledge are taught in a dream or vision. In Guatemala, a midwife has usually been sickly, and the shaman divines the cause as a warning from God to take up her calling or destiny as a midwife. If she refuses, she or her family will be punished more severely by God. Other signs of her calling include having been born with a caul and finding certain objects, such as oddly shaped stones and a knife or scissors. Hart (1965: 26) points out that the supernatural source and validation of the midwives' skills give them an increased sense of adequacy and protect them by minimizing their liability.

Supernatural training may be combined with a pattern of inheritance. In some parts of the Philippines, the visions bringing knowledge of midwifery come from third-generation relatives, such as one's parents' grandparents (Hart 1965). Inheritance is the primary means of recruitment and training in some societies (Sudan, Vietnam, Peru).

A special variation of the inheritance pattern occurs in India, where the position of midwife (*dai*) is relegated to the lowest castes or the untouchables, and caste membership is inherited.

The most common pattern of training and acquiring skills is apprenticeship or assistant status to another midwife, often a relative (Ojibwa, Peru, Mexico, Appalachia, rural southern U.S.). Even where the midwife claims to receive her knowledge from dreams or vision, she has also often been an apprentice to another midwife (Philippines, Ojibwa). In some societies, as in parts of the Philippines, various combinations of recruitment and training patterns occur (Rubel, et al. 1971).

W.H.O. reports that two-thirds of the babies in the world are delivered without a trained attendant (W.H.O. 1966). They do not consider apprenticeship as training.

Only formal Western medical training is acceptable. Much of the literature stresses the lack of any "professional" training of scientific knowledge. The bias in the use of the term "training" is reflected in the following comment by an Indian villager, who was visited by a government health visitor encouraging antenatal clinic visits. The health visitor said that the midwife was all right, "but she had no training." The villager was amazed "and asked how any person could be untrained if she had delivered babies all her life" (Gideon 1962).

Kelly (1956) has suggested that the main areas in which the traditional midwife needs training are: (1) basic principles of hygiene and asepsis, (2) prenatal and postnatal advice and care, and (3) recognition of cases beyond her capacities, which, if possible, should be referred to a doctor. However, the midwife, through extensive experience, is often skillful in calculating the month of pregnancy, gauging the position of the fetus (Kelly 1956), and in dealing with the anxieties of her clients. Landes (1938) says that the Ojibwa midwife is a "highly skilled occupation, depending on an extensive herbal knowledge, detailed knowledge of female anatomy and physiology, varied massage techniques, and a cool and resourceful intelligence." As Wellin has emphasized (1956), native midwives do not lack education but possess a certain kind of education and command certain kinds of knowledge and understanding, which are integrated into the whole fabric of social life.

Nevertheless, W.H.O. states that "it is recognized that, without a system for regular supervision, the traditional birth attendant CANNOT [emphasis added] maintain a level of ACCEPTABLE performance. For this reason, it is essential that provision for supervision and guidance be an integral part of any programme destined to train and utilize the traditional birth attendant" (1966: 16). Although it may be beneficial to have some guidance and supervision, such a statement is patronizing and condescending and should be questioned. When such attitudes are exhibited in attempted programs, they may lower the status and authority of the traditional birth attendant or midwife and make her doubt her own sense of adequacy, although the aim of the program may be to raise it. Mongeau, et al. (1960) point out in their study of the "granny" midwife that changes brought about by the government training program have made her overcautious. This brings approval from the Health Department, but increases anxiety on the part of the patient.

Status

The midwife usually occupies a respected position, although variation does exist in her status in different societies. With the influence of modern medical programs, her position often becomes an ambiguous one. Hospital personnel, medical practitioners, and the educated classes tend to assign her a low status, regarding her as superstitious, ignorant, and dangerous (Wellin 1956). Within her community, however, she is usually respected and enjoys considerable status. In some cases, her use of modern techniques and medicines increases her prestige.

Kelly (1956) reports that the midwife enjoys a moderately high status in some *mestizo* areas of Mexico, but in indigenous areas, she sometimes has little personal prestige and is selected for her alleged esoteric powers, rather than for her skills. The reverse is generally true in Guatemala. Ladinos express distrust and fear of midwives, pointing out that many women die during childbirth in the village and desire to go to the city hospital (Solien de Gonzalez 1963). On the other hand, in Indian communities, the midwife has comparatively high prestige and is respected for her skills, although supernatural sanctions may add to her status.

The position of the midwife has varied in the Western world, as shown by her decline in the United States and the present highly developed midwifery programs in England and several European countries. In the fifteenth, sixteenth, and seventeenth centuries, however, the midwife was criticized by the church and state, and frequently considered as a witch and condemned. The use of any spells or traditional rituals was interpreted as witchcraft. Midwives were accused of infanticide and giving unbaptized babies to the devil. Municipal ordinances were enacted to regulate the practice of midwifery and enforce training (Forbes 1966).

Times have not changed very much in this respect. In Peru, native midwives are classed with "native curers," "witches," or "sorcerers" as a species of empiricism or quackery and are outside the legal pale. On the local level, however, no one interferes with their practice (Wellin 1956). In a recent study of medical practices in Mexico, Schendel (1968: 145) writes: "The majority of quack-curers [his translation of *curanderos*]—many of them part-time street vendors or dirty old crones—function basically as midwives." Although he says only a small number of these "quacks" are self-styled witches or *brujos,* according to Public Health doctors and the Mexican Secretary of Public Health, Dr. Amezquita, "They are all witch doctors." However, for the sake of better public relations, these unlicensed practitioners are officially referred to not as quacks or witchdoctors, but as untrained midwives. Midwifery is after all, one of their most active roles. It is also probably the role in which they possess the greatest potentiality for harm (Schendel 1968: 169). The lumping together of curers, witches, and midwives for these Mexican societies not only goes against most anthropological evidence, which indicates these are highly specialized statuses, but is also very ethnocentric and should be avoided.

Mexico, nevertheless, recognizing the importance and influence of the midwife, has started several training centers. Both old midwives and young girls who want to enter the profession are given a free one-year training course, living on the premises and receiving free room and board. They are then certified to serve as auxiliary nurses. Kelly (1965) has made a proposal of an anthropological approach to midwifery programs in Mexico. When programs are run by the Public Health doctors and nurses who have the attitude that native midwives are all quacks and witches, one wonders to what degree the suggestions that Kelly made are being taken into account. To my knowledge, there have been no anthropological studies of these programs, and this is a vital area for future investigation.

The indigenous midwife in India (the *dai*) occupies a status at the low end of the scale. Due to the belief that birth is an unclean and polluting process, only a person of low caste or an untouchable is allowed to deliver the baby, cut the cord, dispose of the placenta, and change the bandages. Midwifery is the traditional occupation of the castes of Chamars or leatherworkers (Briggs 1920), sweepers (Minturn and Hitchcock 1963), and barbers (Ghosh 1968). The nurse midwife, who has had about eighteen months of hospital training in midwifery and nursing, usually belongs to one of the higher village castes, for example the Jat or a farmer caste. However, she will not dispose of the placenta or cut the cord. She either brings an untouchable woman to do that, or the family has to get one, so that it is necessary to pay another person. Consequently, the pregnant woman is reluctant to use the nurse-midwife (Ghosh 1968; Gordon, et al. 1964). There are an increasing number of indigenous midwives who have received some scientific training in midwifery programs and also perform the traditional duties because of their low caste.

One of the problems in the spread of Western medicine is exporting the same status consciousness which American obstetricians and physicians exhibit. Some examples were mentioned above. This problem is also illustrated by changes currently taking place in Japan, where various types of formal midwifery training have existed since A.D. 772, incorporating new medical knowledge when necessary. A law was passed in 1947 which will in time eliminate all practitioners who are not high-school and nursing-school graduates, and who have not taken a supplementary course in their specialty. The emphasis on midwifery reforms developed partly from criticism by the Occupation Forces of Japanese medical service qualifications. Standlee warns that these changes "may in time remove the nurse from the bedside care of the patient.... it is to be hoped that it will not create the unrest, dissatisfaction, and personnel poverty that followed the imposition of an academic caste system among nurses in the United States" (1959: 139). The enforced grafting of a Western doctrine on a midwifery pattern that has served a society satisfactorily for over a thousand years should be questioned.

Prenatal Care

The role of the midwife during the prenatal period may vary from a minimal one, as in the Punjab (Gordon, et al. 1964) where the midwife usually does little until labor begins, to a more active one, as in Mexico and Guatemala. There the midwife is selected between the fourth and seventh month and visits the woman weekly or monthly. Time and frequency of visits vary between villages and may depend on the health of the mother and whether she is a primapara or a multipara.

The most common prenatal practice is that of abdominal massage. Massage is thought to make birth easier and allows the midwife to determine the position of the fetus and change it if necessary. One Guatemalan midwife told the author that she massages the woman, "little by little, not forcefully. If you rub with force, she will die." In some areas, however, massaging is heavier, and Foster attributes many miscarriages in Tzintzuntzan, Mexico, to heavy massaging. Hart (1965) stresses that vigorous massage or extreme manual rotation performed less than six weeks before labor can cause premature separation of the placenta from the uterus.

In some African societies, during the last month, the midwives manually dilate the passages to prevent obstructed labor. Gelfand (1964) suggests that one possible advantage of manual dilation is the apparent rarity of peritoneal tears. He suggests that despite the increased risk of infection, childbed fever is rare amongst African mothers. Unfortunately Gelfand generalizes about African mothers without making it clear to which specific societies he is referring, and such generalizations are open to serious question. He may be referring primarily to the Shona, among whom he worked.

The midwife often administers medicines, usually herbal teas, and gives advice on proper diet and exercises. In many societies certain foods are proscribed because they will make the body "cold" or harm the fetus (Philippines, Vietnam, Mexico, Guatemala).

Pregnancy is regarded as normal and not a cause for anxiety in some societies; in others, it is regarded as a "sickness" or as a period of danger, both physically and supernaturally. In some cases, modern medical practitioners have increased this anxiety. A government midwife in a Greek town said only if women are afraid will they go to a doctor (Blum and Blum 1965). The Hutterites in the United States are non-anxious about pregnancy and have their own midwives. Thus there is no motivation for prenatal examinations by physicians. Certain doctors have tried to secure patient interest in regular obstetric care by impressing upon them the hazards of pregnancy. Eaton points out (1958) that this may function to prevent a few cases of infant mortality and maternal deaths, but is "paid" for in part by an increase in anxiety among Hutterite women. One can raise the question as to whether this anxiety contributes to a more difficult labor and causes other problems.

Antenatal clinics are increasingly being included in medical programs for health education and to prevent birth complications. People at first do not consider such clinics necessary (Turtell 1965; Kendall 1953; Ghosh 1968) but through the influence of successful patients, acceptance is gradually increased. In Accra, Ghana, Goodman (1951) reports that people regard the clinics as social gatherings with the opportunity of obtaining free or cheap medicines. Where attendance is sporadic, the medical effects on the patients are doubtful (van Amelsvoort 1964). Nevertheless, they provide the opportunity of treating anemias, chronic malaria, helminthiasis, and of detecting possible birth complications (Goodman 1951; Turtell 1965).

In some societies, midwives perform abortions (Mexico, India, Greece). These may be for unwanted pregnancies or as a method of birth control. Midwives are also called if a spontaneous abortion or miscarriage is feared and may administer herbal infusions or other treatments to prevent miscarriages. Midwives also administer various medicines and perform rituals believed to help barren women (Beals 1946).

Delivery

In many societies, the mother is secluded in either a special hut or a partitioned part of the house (Ford 1945). This isolation may be due to the belief that the mother is in a polluted state or that the mother and newborn are highly susceptible to physical and supernatural dangers. In some places, as in parts of India, birth is highly secretive: the house is shut, and the woman is not supposed to cry out (Gordon, et al. 1964). This is to protect her from spirits and people who might want to do her harm. In a few societies (Navajo, Iban) birth is a more communal and public affair, there is no seclusion, and relatives and neighbors may attend.

Labor and delivery usually occur in the same location. Generally, in the United States, however, the mother is moved to a delivery room separate from the one in which she was in labor. Doris Haire (1972), while visiting hospitals in different parts of the world, saw a tendency to increase moving. For example, in the Orient, new hospitals tend to have delivery rooms built separate from labor rooms so that the woman must be moved as she approaches birth. Experiments on mice have shown that subjection to environmental disturbances during labor caused significantly longer deliveries and the disturbed mice gave birth to 54 percent more dead pups than did the control group. The effect on humans of environmental disturbance has not been studied (Haire 1972).

One or more persons usually assist the midwife. These attendants are most frequently elderly females, although some societies require the husband to assist and support the parturient (Mexico). The presence of relatives as birth assistants gives emotional support to the woman.

Patterns of management of labor range from "laissez faire" to an extreme speeding up of labor (as in the United States). As with prenatal care, the most commonly reported pattern is abdominal massage and pressure, often rubbing on some type of oil or herbal mixture. The dangers of placental separation or ruptured uterus were mentioned above (Hart 1965). However, Norman Casserly,[2] a male midwife in the United States, points out that massage during delivery keeps the blood flowing and the pelvic musculature relaxed, and neither external nor internal tearing occurs. The hormone relaxin renders joints and muscles flexible, rubbery, and there is no need for episiotomy (*Prevention* 1972).

Haire (1972) has summarized the disadvantages of routine episiotomies as practiced in the United States and says that obstetricians and gynecologists in many countries tend to agree that a superficial first degree tear is less traumatic to the perineal tissue than an incision which requires several sutures for reconstruction. Such operations are rare in non-Western societies, but crude episiotomies are carried out by village midwives in the northern Sudan because of labor difficulties due to female circumcision (Jeliffe and Bennett 1962: 69).

A particular type of manipulation known as heeling is reported for the Punjab (Gideon 1962; Gordon, et al. 1965). The midwife exerts pressure and countertraction with each labor pain with her feet on either side of the birth canal. The midwife also lubricates the vaginal canal with clarified butter or oil.

Midwives can be important agents of change, through which various Western practices are spread. One such change that has been occurring in some places is the substitution of the supine position for delivery for the traditional one of kneeling, sitting, or squatting (Kelly 1965; Madsen 1965: 89–138). One Guatemalan ladino midwife said that she "has not been able to change the position of delivery and considers it very unbecoming for her, as a practical nurse, to follow the Indian pattern" of kneeling (Reina 1966). Although most American doctors advocate the flat supine position, research suggests that it makes spontaneous delivery more difficult, and thus increases the use of forceps, episiotomies, chemical induction of labor, and other forms of interference (Haire 1972; Mead and Newton 1967). Such substitutions may therefore be more harmful if they abolish a practice which actually may be a safer one.

Herbal and patent medicines are frequently used by midwives to ease labor pains and/or to speed up labor (Arikara, Cherokee, Buganda, Guatemala, Mexico). Some medical personnel feel that the use of herbs, some of which have been shown to have oxytocic effects, whether for normal or delayed labor is dangerous (Jeliffe and Bennett 1962; Billington, et al. 1963; Schendel 1968). An underlying assumption is that the midwife uses these herbs indiscriminately and ignorantly. However, in many cases, part of the midwives' special knowledge is the amounts of such herbs to be used for various purposes and the effects of these amounts. The condemnation of indigenous herbal medicines, while using other forms of oxytocic agents, analgesics, and anaesthetics, which have unknown effects and some of which research is showing are harmful to the mother and fetus (Haire 1972) is hypocritical, ethnocentric, and dangerous.

Attempts to induce gagging, vomiting, sneezing, blowing in a bottle in order to make the muscles contract are frequently used in cases of difficult or prolonged labor. The midwife may also employ techniques based on a sympathetic magical connection, such as unlocking bolts and locks, opening drawers and doors, untying the mother's hair, and using charms made from molts of animals. The midwife may also perform various rituals, say prayers, and listen to confession from the parturient. In some societies, difficult labor is regarded as a sign of marital infidelity and the mother is urged to confess (Gelfand 1964).

Abnormal presentations and multiple births usually present complications, which may result in infection or death. Some midwives manipulate the fetus externally (Mexico) or use techniques of oiling and attempting to extend the vagina and manipulate the fetus internally (India). Surgery seems to be rare. Where medical assistance is available, midwives are urged to either send for a doctor or send the patient to the hospital if they suspect complications. In some societies, the midwife performs infanticide, particularly in cases of multiple births or deformed babies.

In most societies, the midwives give encouragement, emotional support, relieve pain, and allay anxiety; in a few groups (Buganda), the opposite seems to be the case—midwives increase the pain and discomfort, especially in the attempt to speed up labor (Ford 1964). The effects of these activities are a matter on which little research has been done and should be pursued.

W.H.O. has reported that one of the outstanding developments in maternity care is the increase in the number of deliveries taking place in hospitals or maternity centers.

Where this has occurred, domiciliary deliveries have decreased and the midwife is used mostly for prenatal and postnatal care. Ghosh (1968) suggests that where this is the case, midwives be asked to take more active part in health education, family planning, and immunization programs. Van Amelsvoort (1964) raises the question of the extent to which hospital deliveries actually reduce mother and child mortality. In the Asmat region of New Guinea, he says they had no figures or estimates to show whether normal delivery in the village was an important cause of mortality or that hospital delivery actually reduced mortality. Figures from a nearby area indicate that home delivery is not the main cause of fatalities of mother and child.

In most parts of the world, there is a shortage of medical personnel and hospitals are overcrowded. An increase in normal hospital deliveries puts an additional drain on hospital personnel and budget (van Amelsvoort 1964). Several authorities advocate home deliveries in a familiar environment with trained midwives, improved antenatal work, and better cultural contact rather than routine hospital admissions. Hospital deliveries should be recommended only if there are indications of complications (Stein and Susser 1959; Roberts 1960; Killen 1960; van Amelsvoort 1964).

In areas where homes are scattered and transportation difficult, midwives may have difficulty practicing domiciliary midwifery. Another alternative is practiced by some "qualified" and "trained" Buganda midwives. They run private maternity centers in their own homes. Women come to stay in the midwife's house to await delivery, where they enjoy a homey atmosphere and help around the house. The mother usually stays with the midwife for about three days after delivery (Billington, et al. 1963).

The Placenta and Umbilical Cord

The placenta is usually expelled without manual assistance. In cases of delayed expulsion, many of the same techniques for delayed labor are used, e.g. massage or abdominal pressure, medication, rituals, attempts to make the woman gag, sneeze, or vomit.

In societies where the placenta is believed to affect the future life of the child, the disposal of the placenta and cord may be a cause of anxiety in hospital deliveries (Wellin 1956). A few hospitals in northern Mexico deliver the placenta to the family upon request. Kelly (1956) suggests that this practice could be adopted elsewhere.

In most non-Western societies, the placenta is expelled before the umbilical cord is cut. Occasionally, the midwife squeezes the blood in the cord toward the infant's navel before cutting (Cherokee, Guatemala). The cord is usually tied with thread, string, or plant fiber, at a specific length which varies widely in different societies. Where the cord is customarily not tied (Buganda), the danger of hemorrhage exists.

Traditional methods of cutting and dressing the cord have been criticized as possible factors causing tetanus neonatorum, either because the cutting instrument is not clean or the dressing material is contaminated. Cutting tools include bamboo, shell, broken glass, knife, scissors, shears, sickles, trowels, and razors. Coughlin (1965) reports that in Vietnam, considerable numbers of tetanus cases result, according to medical sources, from the use of bamboo or glass. Custom forbids the use of any metal instrument for cutting the cord, lest the child be mute. No statistics are given, however. What is the rate of tetanus? How does this compare to the rate when other methods are used? In parts of Mexico and Guatemala, the midwife cauterizes the cord with either a candle flame, a burning end of a stick, or a red-hot blade, and applies hot candle wax (McKay 1933; Gerdel 1949; Romney and Romney 1963; Solien de González and Béhar 1966).

A study made by Gordon, Gideon, and Wyon (1964, 1965) in the Punjab attempts to determine which specific techniques of cutting and dressing the cord, employed by the various categories of midwives (untrained midwives, trained midwives, and nurse-midwives), are statistically associated with neonatal deaths, especially from tetanus. In nine out of twelve cases of tetanus, the dressing was ash made from cow dung and earth. While ash itself has some aseptic properties, the cow dung may have unburned particles or chance contamination. The sickle was the cutting instrument associated with the highest death rate. This study is a model which should be followed to investigate the actual effects of various methods used by midwives, rather than the blanket condemnation of these practices without evidence of detrimental effects.

Treatment of the Newborn

The newborn is sometimes slapped on the buttocks, held upside down, or sprinkled with water to make it cry. Various rituals are also performed. The child may be cleaned with oil or washed in lukewarm water. Usually the midwife visits and cleans the baby several times during the first week or two. The midwife may clear the baby's throat and nose of mucus and blood with her fingers, which could be a source of infection. The baby's eyes may be wiped with a rag or cotton, treated with a drop of lemon juice, oil, onion, flowers of Castille and San Juan, boric acid, or patented eye drops. Medicines are often given to prevent illness (Buganda) and purgatives administered to clean the meconium (Philippines, Mexico, Peru, India).

Various amulets may be used and the midwife may perform various rituals to protect the baby from diseases such as the evil eye (India, Peru, Mexico). Curing such illnesses of the infant is often another function of the midwife (Guatemala, Mexico, Peru). Rituals may also be performed which symbolize the sex identity of the baby (Mexico). The midwife may read certain signs of the child's and mother's fate, such as caul births, position of birth, lines on the umbilical cord, and the time of birth (Mexico, Guatemala, Thailand, Philippines). Shaping of the baby's head, nose, and limbs is also a function of the midwife in some societies (Zulli, Chagga).

Postnatal Treatment of the Mother

Little information is available on the immediate treatment after birth, especially concerning treatment of wounds of the birth canal and the vaginal area. Alcohol, salt, and various herbs are sometimes used to prevent infection (Thailand, Vietnam).

One of the most widespread postnatal practices is the binding of the mother's abdomen (abdominal binders are also often used prenatally). Patent medicated plasters may also be applied (Guatemala). Medicines of various kinds are often taken to recover strength and decrease soreness and pains. In many areas, the midwife massages the abdomen and the uterus area to ease after-pains, and massages the breasts to stimulate the flow of milk. This pattern is often combined with the application of heat. In indigenous parts of Guatemala and Mexico, the sweatbath is used. Throughout Southeast Asia (Thailand, Vietnam, Philippines, Iban, India) heat is applied by "mother roasting" or "lying by the fire."

At the end of the convalescent period, various rituals may be held in which the midwife plays an important part. In addition to restoring the mother's relationships with relatives and friends, and marking the return of the mother to normal activities, these rituals usually mark the end of the midwife's duties (Guatemala, Philippines).

Conclusion

Maternal and child health programs and midwifery training programs should have as fundamental points of reference the local body of beliefs and practices associated with pregnancy, birth, and postnatal care and the role played by the indigenous or local specialists. Kelly (1965) says that the cultural background can be analyzed in terms of three interrelated areas: (1) avoidance of unnecessary conflict with existing culture patterns, (2) exploitation of elements of the local culture which are favorable or neutral, and (3) delineation of harmful practices, which should be combated. Jeliffe and Bennett (1962), along similar lines, suggest an unprejudiced analysis of these beliefs to physical and psychological health, on the basis of current scientific principles.

As I have tried to point out in this paper, these are programmatic statements that have yet to be followed, hopefully by an unprejudiced analysis. Most of the literature dealing with either proposed or developed programs condemn many of the traditional beliefs and practices concerning childbirth and blame infant and maternal mortality on the midwives. Few systematic studies have been made demonstrating the actual effects of specific practices, especially in terms of morbidity and mortality rates. Hardly any anthropological studies exist of midwifery training programs, or maternal and child health programs, their effects, and their relationship to traditional midwifery. An important need exists for anthropological research in planning, running, and evaluating such programs.

Notes

1. Since most midwives are females, although a few males do practice midwifery, the feminine pronoun will be used in this paper when referring to midwives.

2. Norman Casserly is a male midwife in the United States who practices the methods of natural childbirth. He has been barred from this practice on the grounds of practicing medicine without a license. He is appealing his case claiming that pregnancy is a normal condition, not a pathological one, and consequently he was not practicing medicine.

References

Anuman Rajadhon, P. 1965 "Customs connected with birth and the rearing of children," in *Southeast Asian birth customs*. Edited by D. Hart. New Haven: Human Relations Area Files Press.

Beals, R. 1946 *Cheran: a Sierra Tarascan village*. Smithsonian Institution, Institute of Social Anthropology, Publication 2.

Billington, W. R., H. F. Welbourn, K. C. Wandera 1963 Custom and child health in Buganda; III: Pregnancy and child-birth. *Tropical and Geographic Medicine* 15:134-137.

Blum, R., E. Blum 1965 *Health and healing in rural Greece*. Stanford: Stanford University Press.

Briggs, G. 1920 *The Chamars: the religious life of India*. Calcutta: Association Press.

Bunzel, R. 1959 *Chichicastenango: a Guatemalan village*. Seattle: University of Washington Press.

Cosminsky, S. 1972 "Decision-making and medical care in a Guatemalan Indian community." Unpublished Ph.D. dissertation, Brandeis University.

Coughlin, R. 1965 "Pregnancy and birth in Vietnam," in *Southeast Asian birth customs*. Edited by D. Hart. New Haven: Human Relations Area Files Press.

Eaton, J. 1958 "Folk obstetrics and pediatrics meet the M.D.," in *Patients, physicians, and illness*. Edited by G. Jaco, 207–221. Glencoe: Free Press.

Ewing, J. 1960 Birth customs of the Tawsug. *Anthropological Quarterly* 33:129–132.

Forbes, T. R. 1966 *The midwife and the witch*. New Haven: Yale University Press.

Ford, C. 1945 *A comparative study of human reproduction*. Yale University Publications in Anthropology 32. New Haven: Yale University Press.

1964 *Field guide to the study of human reproduction*. New Haven: Human Relations Area Files Press.

Foster, G. M. 1948 *Empire's children: the people of Tzintzuntzan*. Mexico City: Nuevo Mundo.

Frake, C. 1957 Post-natal care among the eastern Subanun. *Silliman Journal* 4:207–215.

Fuchs, S. 1939 Birth and childhood among the Balahis. *Primitive Man* 12:71–84.

Gelfand, M. 1964 *Medicine and custom in Africa*. London: E. and S. Livingston.

Gerdel, F. 1949 A case of delayed afterbirth among the Tzeltal. *American Anthropologist* 51:158–159.

Ghosh, B. N. 1968 An exploratory study on midwifery practice of the local indigenous dais in Pondicherry and utilization of domiciliary midwifery services of a health centre by a semi-urban slum community. *Indian Journal of Public Health* 12:159–164.

Gideon, H. 1962 A baby is born in the Punjab. *American Anthropologist* 64:1220–1234.

Gilmore, M. 1930 Notes on gynecology and obstetrics of the Arikara tribe of Indians. *Papers of the Michigan Academy of Science, Arts, and Letters* 24:71–82.

Goodman, L. 1951 Obstetrics in a primitive African community. *American Journal of Public Health* 41:56–64.

Gordon, J., H. Gideon, J. Wyon 1964 Childbirth in rural Punjab. *American Journal of Medical Science* 247:344–357.

1965 Midwifery practices in rural Punjab. *American Journal of Obstetrics and Gynecology* 93:734–742.

Haire, D. 1972 The cultural warping of childbirth. *ICEA News*. International Childbirth Association.

Hart, D. 1965 "From pregnancy through birth in a Bisayan Filipino village," in *Southeast Asian birth customs*. Edited by D. Hart. New Haven: Human Relations Area Files Press.

Jeliffe, D. B., F. J. Bennett 1962 Worldwide care of the mother and newborn child. *Clinical Obstetrics and Gynecology* 5:64–84.

Jensen, E. 1967 Iban birth. *Folk* 8–9:165–178.

Kelly, I. 1956 An anthropological approach to midwifery training in Mexico. *Journal of Tropical Pediatrics* 1:200–205.

1965 *Folk practices in north Mexico.* Austin: University of Texas Press.

Kendall, E. 1953 A short history of the training of midwives in the Sudan. *Sudan Notes and Records* 33:42–53.

Killen, O. 1960 Rural health centres in Kiambu. *East African Medical Journal* 37:204–215.

Lamson, H. 1934 *Social pathology in China.* Shanghai: The Commercial Press.

Landes, R. 1937 *Ojibwa sociology.* New York: Columbia University Press.

1938 *Ojibwa woman.* New York: Columbia University Press.

Leighton, D., J. Adair 1963 *People of the Middle Place.* Human Relations Area Files.

Leighton, D., C. Kluckhohn 1947 *Children of the people.* Cambridge: Harvard University Press.

Lewis, O. 1960 *Tepotzlán: village in Mexico.* New York: Holt, Rinehart and Winston.

Lockett, C. 1939 Midwives and childbirth among the Navajo. *Plateau* 12:15–17.

Long, L. D. 1964 Sociocultural practices relating to obstetrics and gynecology in a community of West Africa. *American Journal of Obstetrics and Gynecology* 89:470–475.

Madsen, C. 1965 *A study of change in Mexican folk medicine.* Middle American Research Institute, Publication 25.

McKay, K. 1933 "Mayan midwifery," in *The peninsula of Yucatan.* Edited by G. Shattuck, 64–65. Carnegie Institute of Washington, Publication 431.

Mead, M., N. Newton 1967 "Cultural patterning of perinatal behavior" in *Childbearing—its social and psychological aspects.* Edited by S. Richardson and A. Gutmacher. New York: Williams and Wilkens.

Minturn, L., J. Hitchcock 1963 *The Rajputs of Khalapur, India.* New York: John Wiley.

Mistry, J. E. 1952 "Indigenous midwifery," in *The economic development of India.* Edited by V. Anstey, Appendix A. London: Longmans Green.

Mongeau, G., H. Smith, A. Maney 1960 The "granny" midwife: changing role and functions of a folk practitioner. *American Journal of Sociology* 66:497–505.

Nydegger, W., C. Nydegger 1963 *Tarong: an Ilocos barrio in the Philippines.* New York: John Wiley.

Oldbrechts, F. M. 1931 Cherokee belief and practice with regard to childbirth. *Anthropos* 26:17–33.

Osgood, K., D. Hochstrasser, K. Deuschle 1966 Lay midwifery in southern Appalachia. *Archives of Environmental Health* 12:759–770.

Prevention 1972 Mister midwife of San Diego. *Prevention.*

Raum, O. 1940 *Chaga childhood.* London: Oxford University Press.

Redfield, R., A. Villa Rojas 1934 *Chan Kom.* Chicago: University of Chicago Press.

Reina, R. 1966 *The law of the Saints.* New York: Bobbs-Merrill.

Roberts, J. 1960 Rural health projects in North Nyanza. *East African Medical Journal* 37:186–203.

Rodriguez Rouanet, F. 1970 Prácticas médicas tradicionales de los indígenas de Guatemala. *Guatemala Indígena* 4:52–86.

Romney, K., R. Romney 1963 *The Mixtecans of Juxtlahuaca, Mexico.* New York: John Wiley.

Roscoe, J. 1911 *The Baganda.* London: Macmillan.

Rubel, A., W. Liu, M. Trosdal, V. Pato 1971 "The traditional birth attendant in metropolitan Cebu, the Philippines," in *Culture and population.* Edited by S. Polgar, 176–186. Chapel Hill: Carolina Population Center.

Sarker, A., N. Choudhuri, G. S. Ray 1955 Birth and pregnancy rites among the Oraons. *Man in India* 35: 46–51.

Schendel, G.1968 *Medicine in Mexico.* Austin: University of Texas Press.

Singh, M. 1947 *The depressed classes: their economic and social condition.* Bombay: Hind Kitab.

Solien de Gonzalez, N. 1963 Some aspects of childbearing and child-rearing in a Guatemalan ladino community. *Southwestern J. of Anthropology* 19:411–423.

Solien de Gonzalez, N., M. Behar 1966 Child-rearing practices, nutrition, and health status. *Milbank Memorial Fund Quarterly* 44:77–96.

Standlee, M. 1959 *The great pulse: Japanese midwifery and obstetrics through the ages.* Rutland, Vermont: Charles Tuttle.

Stein, A., M. Susser 1959 A study of obstetric results in an under-developed community. *Journal of Obstetrics and Gynecology of the British Empire* 65: 763–773; 66: 62–74.

Stern, C. A. 1972 Midwives, male-midwives, and nurse-midwives: an epitome of relationships and roles. *Obstetrics and Gynecology* 39:308–311.

Stevenson, M. 1920 *The rites of the twice-born.* London: Oxford University Press.

Turtell, B. M. 1965 Midwifery and midwife training in Nigeria. *Nursing Times* 61: 1664–1665.

Van Amelsvoort, V. 1964 *Culture, stone age and modern medicine.* Assen: Van Gorcum.

Wales, H. G. 1933 Siamese theory and ritual connected with pregnancy, birth, and infancy. *Journal of the Royal Anthropological Institute of Great Britain and Ireland* 63:441–451.

Wellin, E. 1956 Pregnancy, childbirth, and midwifery in the valley of Ica, Peru. *Health Information Digest for Hot Countries* 3.

World Health Organization 1966 *The midwife in maternity care. Report of a WHO expert committee.* WHO Technical Report Series 33.

Editor's Introduction
Imagery and Symbolism in the Birth Practices
of Traditional Cultures

BRIAN BATES AND ALLISON NEWMAN TURNER

CHILDBIRTH IS IN ITS ESSENCE A LITERAL, PHYSICAL PHENOMENON, but it also can serve as a key metaphor in most societies. In Western societies, for example, one speaks of being "pregnant" with meaning, and one of the major intellectual periods in Western history is commonly referred to as the "Renaissance" or "rebirth" of knowledge.

Metaphors can also be found in childbirth rituals as Brian Bates of the Psychology Department at the University of Sussex and Allison Newman Turner, a staff nurse at Leicestershire General Hospital, convincingly demonstrate. Such rituals frequently involve the literalization of a metaphor such that untying a knot is supposed to magically facilitate a difficult delivery, or placing an ax underneath the parturient's bed is supposed to "cut the pain" by half.

Bates and Turner explore in their contribution to this volume (taken from *Birth* 12 [1985]: 29–35) how images associated with childbirth can ease the experience. The focus in traditional cultures has been on making birth a dynamic, positive experience; whereas Western cultures, in contrast, have tended to adopt techniques designed to distance the parturient from a painful experience. Though these Western methods may well lessen the need for medical intervention, their emphasis on pain reduction may result in diverting the woman's attention away from the act of giving birth.

Natural childbirth innovator Grantly Dick-Read has advocated birth without discomfort by insisting that women about to deliver should rest and should receive support from a companion. Women were advised to attain physical fitness and learn proper techniques for breathing and relaxation in preparation for a pain-free delivery. In the first stage of labor, the key is to reduce fear and tension by focusing on relaxing rather than on the birth experience itself. In the second stage of labor, Dick-Read recommends inattentiveness: "She becomes oblivious to her surroundings and careless of her appearance, expression and speech" (p. 220). Only when the baby is actually born should the mother indulge in "exaltation" (G. Dick-Read, *Childbirth without Fear* [New

York: Harper and Row, 1944], 220). See also F. Lamaze, *Painless Childbirth: The Lamaze Method* (New York: Pocket Books, 1972); B. Jordan, "The Hut and the Hospital: Information, Power and Symbolism in the Artifacts of Birth," *Birth* (1987): 36–40.

Authors also have examined how childbirth is portrayed in literature, for example, B. Korte, "In Sorrow Thou Shalt Bring Forth Children—On Children in Literature," *Orbis Litterarum* 45 (1990): 30–48—whose focus is more on literary childbirth among English and American writers since the seventeenth century; and M. Braude, *Life Begins: Childbirth in Lore and in Literature* (Chicago: Argus Books, 1935), who presents a more cross-cultural perspective.

In addition, the literature on birthing includes fascinating selections on the folklore surrounding this event. See E. S. McCartney, "Sex Determination and Sex Control in Antiquity," *American Journal of Philology* 43 (1922): 62–70; J. H. Marcus, "Childbirth and Its Ancient Customs," *New York Medical Journal* 106 (1917): 1213–1216; Alan Dundes, "The Genesis of Couvade and Couvade in Genesis," in *Studies in Aggadah and Jewish Folklore*, edited by I. Ben-Ami and J. Dan (Jerusalem: Magnes Press, 1983), 35–53; C. Haffter, "The Changeling: History and Psychodynamics of Attitudes to Handicapped Children in European Folklore," *Journal of the History of the Behavioral Sciences* 4 (1968): 55–61; F. N. Suibhne, "'On the Straws' and Other Aspects of Pregnancy and Childbirth from the Oral Tradition of Women in Ulster," *Ulster Folklife* 38 (1992): 12–24; G. E. Okereke, "The Birth Song as a Medium for Communicating Woman's Maternal Destiny in the Traditional Community," *Research in African Literature* 25 (1994): 19–32; and C. H. Carpenter, "Tales Women Tell: The Function of Birth Experiences Narratives," *Canadian Folklore* 7 (1985): 21–34.

Imagery and Symbolism in the Birth Practices of Traditional Cultures   5

BRIAN BATES AND ALLISON NEWMAN TURNER

Introduction

THE PHYSIOLOGICAL PROCESS OF BIRTH is a universal phenomenon, uniting women across cultures and throughout history. Despite earlier beliefs that women in primitive cultures gave birth with less suffering, the evidence now suggests that the degree of childbirth pain experienced is universally constant and that differences lie rather in the expression than in the experience.[1,2,3] But the experience of childbirth is also conditioned by its cultural setting—by the values attached to it and the circumstances prescribed by a society for its occurrence. It is the rituals surrounding childbirth that take it beyond an individual experience, which give it a specific cultural context, impose upon it a specific cultural interpretation and which relate the individual experience to a wider cosmology. Different cultures have thus focused upon different aspects of the childbirth experience according to their orientation towards the world and towards the processes of life and death, as Sheila Kitzinger[4] suggests: "In any society the way a woman gives birth and the kind of care given to her and the baby points as sharply as an arrowhead to the key values of the culture."

Western industrial cultures have tended to concentrate upon the physiological aspects of childbirth and have focused upon the development of medical techniques to make birth a safer and more efficient process according to scientific knowledge and technology. However, although this has led to a decline in both infant and maternal mortality rates, and complications of birth no longer endanger the life of the mother and/or child as they did in the past, these benefits have often been achieved at the expense of any real consideration of the psychological and spiritual aspects of the childbirth experience.

This article considers aspects of the birth practices of traditional cultures in the belief that such technologically simple approaches to childbirth may yield insights into the assumptions and psychological parameters of our own system.

Childbirth Symbolism and Imagery

Anthropological data suggest that many traditional cultures actively employ environmental effects in relation to childbirth, in which the physical environment is specifically manipulated in order to aid the parturient woman and to ease the birth. In the majority of traditional societies the symbolic impact of the environment is considered more powerful psychologically than its physical aspects. Although many cultures arrange the birth setting to be secluded, protected, comfortable and familiar to the parturient woman, the majority of environmental manipulations performed during labor are of a symbolic nature. It is with these manipulations of the symbolic environment that we shall be concerned here. Many of the procedures described below sound bizarre and sometimes even alarming. We are less concerned, however, with the detailed techniques of the traditional cultures than with the ideas underlying them. Despite their "primitive" aura the birth practices we reviewed showed a psychological sophistication often lacking in the approach to childbirth current in our culture.

It is also important to point out that the anthropological information relating to traditional childbirth practices is incomplete. Since the majority of anthropologists have been male, and thus frequently excluded from the traditionally female preserve of the birth setting, their information may often be sparse or inaccurate.[4]

Unlike drugs or physical manipulations such as massage, symbols and images cannot be seen to have such a direct relation to the physiological process of labor.[5] Such manipulations are defined here as symbolic because they operate according to the symbolic meanings and associations of the objects involved, rather than their actual physical attributes as perceived in an everyday sense. In this context the term imagery is also employed for two reasons. Firstly, the manipulations performed may not always be within the perceptual field or even the presence of the parturient woman and must thus be assumed to transmit their impact through the stimulation of images in the woman's mind. Secondly, as mentioned above, even when the practices are within the woman's sight, processes beyond simple perception must be supposed since the normal perception of the objects involved would not elicit the desired physiological response. It is therefore suggested that the effects of the environmental manipulations are mediated through the induction of images encouraged by the specific context.

Sexual Imagery

A number of childbirth rituals found throughout the world appear to be of a sexual nature. The Burma mountain dwellers have a ritual which involves the young men of the village assuming naked and obscene postures before the laboring woman, supposedly to embarrass and frighten away any evil spirits.[6] Several cultures, such as the Mbuti pygmies of Central Africa[7] and the Arunta of Central Australia,[6] have practices for the promotion of labor which involve the father of the baby stripping naked and exposing his genitalia. In Jamaica labor is speeded up by giving the woman a man's sweaty shirt to smell,[4] and in rural Delhi painful and prolonged labor is treated by giving the woman water to drink in which her husband's loincloth has been washed.[8]

The rationale behind many of these practices appears to be the linking of the woman's suffering with its original cause, i.e., the sexual act or the man's penis, although in some cultures the rationale is given in religious or spiritual terms. Some cases, such as the posturing of naked men before the laboring woman, may not in fact constitute the use of imagery, but may function simply as sexual stimuli inducing a physiological action in the parturient woman. In other cases, however, such as the shirt and loincloth practices, there may well be the introduction of imagery through which the objectively neutral stimulus is associated with the physiological reaction. The stimuli used in such practices are symbolic of the man who fathered the child and, in particular, of his sexuality. They may thus inculcate some form of sexual imagery in the woman, albeit at the preconscious level, which then stimulates the physiological responses normally elicited by sexual stimuli—the release of hormones[9] and contractions of the uterus[10] which serve to aid the birth process. In this connection it should be noted that in Western cultures the initiation of labor by sexual stimulation is well known to midwives but is still relatively unexplored in the research literature.[11] Research on the similarities of perceptual and imaginary processes[12,13] has suggested that perceptions and images may function in a similar manner, and it seems likely that neurophysiological responses might be activated in analogous ways by both percepts and images. If this is so, then the use of sexual symbolism and imagery during childbirth may be a fairly straightforward procedure of physiological arousal.

Simulative Imagery

This type of imagery, concerned with release, opening up, and expulsion, is found in the childbirth practices of almost every part of the world. In the Philippine Islands, for example, it is customary to put a key (unlocking) and a comb (untangling) under the laboring woman's pillow; the moultings from snakes or other animals may be used to make a belt for the parturient woman; a clay pot may be chipped, the chippings mixed with water and given to the woman to drink; a house ladder may be turned upside down, knives unsheathed, recently made furniture unnailed, recently sewn seams ripped open and drawers, trunks and cupboards unlocked.[14]

The custom of opening and unlocking at the onset of labor is very widespread. In some Indochinese villages people not only unlock all doors, windows, cupboards and such, but they also take down anything hanging under the ceiling, remove any amulets which have a "closing-the-portal" charm, forbid anyone to pause in a doorway or on a staircase or even to utter words such as "stuck," "fastened" or "hung."[6] In Australian aboriginal tribes the father of the baby may empty out his pouches in the case of prolonged labor;[1] the Nootka of west Canada forbid pregnant women to pause in doorways (delayed delivery) or do any weaving (tangled umbilical cord) throughout pregnancy,[7] and in Delhi villages all knots in clothing, ropes and the woman's hair are loosened to relieve the pain of contractions.[8] Other cultures uncork bottles, let domestic animals out of their pens and open up jackknives.[6]

The Philippines even have a custom of giving dried horse manure ashes dissolved in water to the laboring woman to drink in the belief that it will incite the body to expel such filth rapidly and the baby along with it.[14] Indians in rural Delhi have a similar custom for the tardy delivery of the placenta and afterbirth.[8] In other parts of India it is customary to break a jar of grain in order for the woman to see the grains flowing out,[4] and in Vietnam birth is often referred to as "breaking the jar" or "breaking the dyke."[15]

Also in India, prolonged labor may be treated by the placing of a tightly furled flower beside the woman in the belief that as it unfurls so will the woman's cervix dilate.[4] The Vietnamese refer to birth in terms reflecting this: "the bud opens and the flower blooms."[15] The Maltese keep a flower in water in the delivery room saying that when the bud blooms the child will be born,[6] and in Philippine villages the midwife throws a handful of flowers at the woman in labor when she arrives at the house.[14]

These practices appear to function in a rather more complex fashion than those involving sexual imagery since they do not involve the arousal of a normal physiological response, but rather depend upon the stimulation of empathetic processes since the perception of an open door, or whatever, would not ordinarily lead to bodily functions of expulsion and release. It may be useful here to consider Neisser's suggestions of perception as a constructive act.[16,17] Neisser argues that perception is not the mere sensory registration of the visual field but is a selective, discriminatory, constructive process in which the individual's perception will be strongly influenced by expectations and predilections, as well as by experience and memory traces. In this context Neisser attributes an important role to images which he sees as located at the intersection of memory and perception. He regards them not only as mediators between stored information and the incoming sensory stimulation, but also as the result of constructive processes of their own:

> Imaging is constructive process in the sense that while it depends on information stored earlier it does not simply revive that information. Instead the subject carries out a new activity, perhaps forming a new representation, more or less consistent with what be did before.[17]

It is thus conceivable that the individual is able to emphasize certain aspects of a remembered object by imaging, as is shown by the work on cognitive set by Leff, Gordon and Ferguson.[18] Following Neisser's assertion that perception is a constructive process, these researchers argue that the individual thus has the potential to control perceptions. They suggest that this is effected through the formation of cognitive sets which influence perception in two ways, firstly by giving priority to certain aspects of a stimulus at the expense of others, secondly by determining the associations, meanings, interpretations, and transformations accorded to a preceptual construct.

> Thus in varying subtle ways cognitive sets have effects not only on the content of perception, but also on the significance, interpretation and emotional overtones of one's experienced surroundings.[18]

In their experiments they found that subjects perceived stimuli in markedly different ways according to the cognitive set with which they had been instructed. For instance, an "abstract sensory focusing" set prepared the subject to concentrate upon the sensory qualities rather than the object itself, which appeared to intensify the perceptual experience and even create a new mode of awareness.

If we apply this framework to the process of imagery we begin to create an understanding of how the use of simulative imagery in childbirth might function. The various rituals and practices serve to suggest images to the woman in labor, but these images are not direct representations of the objects involved, but rather constructions created by the woman. These constructions will be profoundly influenced by her cognitive set, which at that time will be concerned with her labor and the physiological processes of release and expulsion.

There is some evidence from western psychological research that such autosuggestion can operate on an unconscious level through the observation of a model. Hull[19] has shown that when unaware subjects are presented with a human model performing tasks which involve leaning backwards or forwards, the subject also tends to sway backward or forward to a considerable extent, although he himself is unaware of this. Hull concludes that:

> The bodies of most normal persons tend, under favorable circumstances, rather uniformly to execute without voluntary or conscious intent, acts observed attentively or merely thought.[19]

Indeed, he maintains that internal representation is ultimately more effective here than actual perception. It would seem reasonable to suppose, then, that the mother participating in symbolic childbirth rituals would create perceptual images emphasizing the releasing and expelling qualities of the environmental cues being presented to her. These would, in the manner described by Hull, intensify the physiological processes of release and expulsion.

Religious Imagery

Childbirth in virtually all traditional societies is structured according to the religious beliefs of that society concerning birth. There is widespread belief in the vulnerability of the woman to malevolent influences during pregnancy and especially during childbirth. Numerous customs and rituals have developed to ensure the safety of the woman during her time of weakness. These usually consist either of appeasing the appropriate spirits or attempting to distract them away from the laboring woman and are usually performed by the father or other relatives.[1,6,10]

The practice of the Cuna Indians of Panama was described in some detail by Levi-Strauss.[21] When a Cuna woman is having a difficult labor, the midwife calls a shaman or medicine man. The cause of the trouble is believed to be the spirit of the womb, Muu, who is holding onto the baby and not letting it out. The shaman sits beneath the laboring woman's hammock and sings to her in great, repetitive detail the story of how and why he has been called to attend her and subsequently the attack that he and his fellow spirits are launching upon Muu's possessiveness, in order to release the baby. He describes to the woman how they enter the vagina single file and make their way up to the uterus. They call upon the aid of the souls of the other organs of the body and those of the various animals to help in the "victorious combat" with Muu—the wood-boring insects are asked to cut through the tangled fibers; the burrowing insects are called upon to help the baby move down the birth canal. As the shaman and his fellow spirits leave the vagina, they march out in a row rather than single file, signifying that dilation is complete. Similar beliefs and practices are found among other shamanistic cultures such as the Siberian peoples and the Eskimos,[1] though none has been documented in such detail as the Cuna ritual.

It seems likely that religious imagery functions in a more diverse manner than either sexual or simulative imagery. The Cuna birth song is perhaps the most graphic example of one way in which religious imagery might function through the use of autosuggestion, as demonstrated in the West by Coue and his followers.[22] The images of the shaman and his aids entering the womb and freeing the child from the grasp of Muu may serve to aid the release and expulsion of the baby in much the same manner that Coue found that the imagining of an iron bar along it served to make the arm rigid and unbendable. The detail with which the shaman describes the whole adventure perhaps renders this process even more effective by concentrating the woman's mind upon each aspect of the physiological activity in turn. It might also be that the invocation of the spiritual world with which the woman is familiar may serve to increase her suggestibility by encouraging belief that the process is in the hands of this spirit world in which she has implicit faith. Attendant practices such as the burning of incense, the administration of herbal mixtures and the use of music and singing might further serve to induce a state of suggestibility.

At a slightly different level, religious imagery may also function in a less specific manner as suggested by Levi-Strauss[21] in his own analysis of the Cuna birth song. This, he believes, functions by enabling the woman to relate her individual experience and suffering to more cosmic conceptions of life and the order of the universe by breaking down the barriers between the individual-physiological and the universal-mythical through the use of recognized symbols. These symbols enable the woman to relate her individual experience to a culturally defined set of beliefs, thus giving her pains meaning and order:

> The shaman provides the sick woman with a language by means of which unexpressed and other inexpressible psychic states can be immediately expressed. And it is the transition to this verbal expression at the same time making it possible to undergo in an ordered and intelligent form a real experience that would otherwise be chaotic and inexpressible—which induces the release of physiological processes.[21]

By providing the woman with a symbolic context for her experience, her pains can "assume cosmic proportions." She is no longer laboring alone and in isolation but in harmony with the rest of her society which is also involved in daily relations with the spirit world. The song emphasizes her place within a cosmic order, which relates her both to nature and to her fellow beings.

This appears to be a crucial process in the childbirth practices of all cultures—the relating of the individual experience to the universal principles and relations of that culture. The Mbuti pygmies, for example, emphasize their association with and regard for the forest in their birth rites; the Adamnese (Pacific Islands) and the Ainu (Japan) their relation to sacred trees; the Nootka their valuing of technical skill and labor; and so on:

> In short the details of any rite of passage, including those of birth, reflect the special
> preoccupations and emphases of the culture concerned.[7]

These practices serve to influence the parturient woman's feelings about the birth as a positive and active experience through the realization of its wider significance—factors which have been found to be salient to the ease and satisfaction of the birth experience.[23,24,25]

Discussion

"Natural childbirth" techniques have arisen as a direct response to the medical approach to childbirth, attempting to circumvent the need for medical intervention and anesthesia by promoting psychological techniques for coping with childbirth. The Read[26] and psychoprophylactic methods[27] concentrate upon educating mothers to understand the processes of birth and teaching them methods of breathing that require such intense mental concentration that the woman's attention is diverted away from the pain of the contractions. Other methods developed have included hypnosis,[28] muscular relaxation,[29] and mental concentration.[30] These techniques have attempted to reduce the technological aspects of childbirth by encouraging the woman to assume fuller responsibility and consciousness during the birth, through their understanding of the psychological processes involved.

A closer consideration, however, suggests that there is a fundamental difference in emphasis between natural childbirth techniques and those employed in many traditional cultures, which reflects to some extent the difference between their cosmological orientations. The use of symbolism and imagery in traditional childbirth rituals takes as its focus the bodily functions involved in birth. The simulative and sexual imagery in particular serve to stimulate and encourage the physiological processes in which the laboring woman's body is engaged. That imagery as a cognitive process does not distract from this purpose, for mind and body are expected to work in harmony, as one unit, with the sole aim of expelling the child as rapidly and as safely as possible. The impact of the symbolic environment is to concentrate the whole of the woman's being, psychologically and physiologically, upon the task in hand.

In contrast to this, the emphasis of the psychological techniques employed in modern childbirth practices has been the control of pain rather than the expulsion of the child. Although engendered by physiological sensations, the experience of pain has strong psychological aspects.[31,32,33] It would appear that in the natural childbirth techniques described above, it is this psychological experience of pain that is seized upon and isolated. The various techniques all center upon an attempt to distract or disassociate the mind from the experience of the body. Both the Read and psychoprophylactic methods use breathing control techniques to concentrate the mind upon a phenomenon apart from the contractions and sensations of labor. Even hypnotic techniques can be seen to use the power of the mind over the body, rather than in conjunction with the body, in that they are used to enable the woman to avoid the pain, not to push the baby out.[28] The only account of the use of imagery in childbirth in the psychological literature (apart from in the use of hypnosis) is the report of a psychologist using emotive imagery (the description of calm and pleasurable scenes) during contractions to distract the laboring woman's attentions from her pains and focus them elsewhere.[34] Although the woman's consciousness of the birth may be greatly enhanced by using psychological pain control, as opposed to anesthesia or analgesic drugs (and awareness during the birth has been found to be of major importance in determining the quality of the experience),[24,23,35,36] it would also appear that in some cases the woman may feel almost as divorced from the birth as she would have been had she taken drugs, since she keeps her mind diverted elsewhere while the baby is delivered. Suzanne Arms writes that the psychoprophylactic method "has the unfortunate side-effect of greatly altering a woman's natural experience of the birth from one of deep involvement inside her body to controlled distraction. . . . separated and detached from the sensations, smells and sights of her body giving birth. She is too involved in . . . control."[37]

The use of symbolism and imagery in the childbirth practices of traditional cultures suggests then their espousal of a cosmology radically different from that of modern technological society, and one in which mind and body are perceived as working in harmony. It is this holistic approach to physiological and psychological experience that forms the basis of the difference between traditional and technological attitudes of childbirth. Of course it would be futile to transplant symbolism and imagery from one culture to another, for such phenomena both derive from and function in accordance with their culture of origin. Examination of the equivalent interaction in the hospital or home delivery room is essential if we are to discover means of improving the birth experience. The quality of the parturient woman's orientation toward the experience and the nature of the culturally shaped messages she is receiving from the birth environment both require consideration.

The existence of this relationship between internal and external states is well-illustrated by an investigation carried out into the psychological effects of the use of the fetal monitor during labor.[38] It was found that those women who had previously experienced the loss of a baby tended to react positively to the monitor, feeling it to be a reassuring presence, a substitute for the physician, an aid to communication. Those women who had not previously suffered difficult or traumatic births, however, tended to regard the monitor with hostility, as a distraction, a competitor. A holistic approach to childbirth would research and take account of such individual responses to the environmental setting of childbirth, for in a complex, rapidly changing culture such as ours there is no commonly accepted cosmology and shared symbols are fewer. But we can devise ways of ascertaining the symbolic world of the individual mother, particularly through research using interview techniques open-ended enough to allow women to define the parameters of the experience in their own terms.[39]

Research on imagery and symbolism in childbirth could help in the design of environmental settings for child delivery appropriate to the psychological needs of the individual mother, and develop imagery techniques which relate specifically to the physiological sensations of labor as constructive and positive communications from her body. Psychological techniques using imagery have been shown to have considerable potential in dealing with serious illnesses such as cancer,[40] and in other clinical settings.[41] It is an open question how much could be achieved by paying more attention to the relationship between psychological imagery and the physiological and experiential dynamics of labor.

Acknowledgement

We should like to express thanks to Martin Richards for his helpful comments on an earlier draft of this paper.

References

1. Spencer, R. F. Primitive obstetrics. CIBA Symposia. 1950. 2(3): 1155–88.

2. Landy D., ed: *Culture, Disease and Healing: Studies in Medical Anthropology*. London: Collier-Macmillan. 1977.

3. Wolff, B. B., and Lanley, S.: Cultural factors in response to pain. In: Landy, D., ed, *Culture, Disease and Healing*. London: Collier-Macmillan. 1977.

4. Kitzinger, S.: *Women as Mothers*. London: Fontana. 1978.

5. Rosengren, W. R : Some social psychological aspects of delivery room difficulties. J Nerv Ment Dis. 1961; 132(6): 515.

6. Rajadhan, P. A.: Customs connected with the birth and rearing of children. In: Hart, D. V., Rajadhan, P. A. and Coughlin, V., *Southeast Asian Birth Customs*. Behavior Science Monographs. Connecticut: Human Relations Area Files.

7. Coon, C. S.: *The Hunting Peoples*. New York: Atlantic. Little Brown. 1972.

8. Trivedi, H. R. and Malhotra, P.: Magical significance of perinatal beliefs and practices in rural Delhi. In J Soc Work. 1974; 35(1): 35–40.

9. Newton, N.: The trebly sensuous woman. Psychology Today. 1971; 5(2): 68.71.

10. Bardwick, J. M.: *Psychology of Women; A Study of Biocultural Conflict.* New York: Harper and Row. 1971.

11. Richards, W.P.M.: Personal communication, 1984.

12. Brooks, L. R..: The suppression of visualization by reading. J Exp Psychol. 1967; 19:289–99.

13. Segal, S. J., and Fusella, V.: Influence of imaged pictures and sounds on detection of visual and auditory signals. J Exp Psychol. 1970; 83: 458–64.

14. Hart, D. V.: From pregnancy through birth in a Bisayan Filipino village. In: Hart, D. V., Rajadhan, A., and Coughlin, R. I., eds, *Southeast Asian Birth Customs.* Behavior Science Monographs. Connecticut: Human Relations Area Files Press. 1965.

15. Coughlin, R. J.: Pregnancy and birth in Vietnam. In: Hart, D. V., Rajadhan, A., and Coughlin, R. I., *Southeast Asian Birth Customs.* Behavior Science Monographs. Connecticut: Human Area Relations File Press. 1965.

16. Neisser, V.: *Cognitive Psychology.* New York: Appleton Century Crofts. 1967.

17. Neisser, V.: Changing conceptions of imagery. In: Sheehan, P. W., ed, *The Function and Nature of Imagery.* Academic Press. 1972.

18. Leff, A. L., Gordon, A. R., and Ferguson, J. G.: Cognitive set and environmental awareness. Env Beh. 1974; 6(4): 395–448.

19. Hull, C. L.: *Hypnosis and Suggestibility: An Experimental Mental Approach.* New York: Appleton Century Crofts. 1961.

20. Mead, M., and Newton, N.: Cultural patterning of behavior. In: Richardson, S. A., and Guttmacher, A. F., eds, *Childbearing; Its Social and Psychological Aspects.* Williams and Wilkins. 1967.

21. Levi-Strauss, C.: *Structural Anthropology.* Harmondsworth: Penguin Books, 1967.

22. Baudoin, C.: *Suggestion and Autosuggestion.* London: Allen and Unwin. 1922.

23. Breen, D.: The mother and the hospital: An unfortunate fit between woman's internal world and some hospital procedures. In: Lipshitz, S., ed, *Tearing the Veil: Essays on Femininity.* Routledge and Kegan Paul. 1978.

24. Davenport-Slack, B., and Boylan, C. H.: Psychological correlates of childbirth pain. Psychosom Med. 1974; 36(3): 215–223.

25. Doering, S. G., and Entwistle, D. R.: Preparation during pregnancy and ability to cope with labor and delivery. J Am Orthopsych. 1975; 45(5): 825–36.

26. Dick-Read, G.: *Childbirth Without Fear: The Principles and Practice of Natural Childbirth.* New York: Harper and Row. 1944.

27. Chertok, L.: *Motherhood and Personality: The Psychosomatic Aspects of Childbirth.* London: Tavistock Publications. 1969.

28. Clark, R. N.: A training method for childbirth utilizing hypnosis. Am J Obstet Gynecol. 1956; 72(6): 1302–04.

29. Jacobson, E.: Muscular relaxation: A technique for the reduction of childbirth pain. Am J Obstet Gynecol. 1955; 67:1035.

30. Earn, A. A.: Mental concentration-A new and effective psychological tool for the abolition of suffering in childbirth. Am J Obstet Gynecol. 1962; 83(1): 29–36.

31. Bobey, M. J., and Davidson, P.O.: Psychological factors affecting pain tolerance. J Psychosom Res. 1970; 14: 371–76.

32. Murray, J. B.: Psychology of the pain experience. J Psychol. 1971; 78: 193–206.

33. Szasz, T. S.: *Pain and Pleasure: A Study of Bodily Feelings.* New York: Basic Books. 1975.

34. Horan, J. V.: 'In vivo' emotive imagery: A technique for reducing childbirth pain and discomfort. Psychol Rep. 1973; 32: 1328.

35. Zax, N., Sameroff, A. I., and Farnum, I. E.: Childbirth education, maternal attitudes and delivery. Am J Obstet Gynecol. 1975; 123(2): 185–90.

36. Ritson, E. B.: An investigation of the psychological factors underlying prolonged labour. J Obstet Gynecol Br Commonwth. 1966, 73:215–21.

37. Arms, S.: *Immaculate Deception.* Boston: Houghton Mifflin. 1975.

38. Starkman, M. N.: Psychological responses to the use of the fetal monitor during labor. Psychosom Med. 1976, 38(4): 269–77.

39. Richards, M.P.M.: The limits of randomized controlled trials. Birth. 1983; 10(3): 164–65.

40. Simonton, C., Simonton, S., and Creighton, J.: *Getting Well Again.* Los Angeles: J. P. Tarcher. 1978.

41. Jaffe, D. T., and Bresler, D. E.: The use of guided imagery as an adjunct to medical diagnosis and treatment. J Humanistic Psychol. 1980; 20(4): 45–59.

Editor's Introduction
The Cultural Anthropology of the Placenta

ELAINE JONES AND MARGARITA A. KAY

A S THE UNITED STATES CONTINUES TO ATTRACT LARGE NUMBERS of immigrants, intercultural understanding becomes increasingly important. Such understanding needs to include birth practices. Unlike many peoples of the world, Americans have little interest in what happens to the placenta of the infant after its birth. Yet as nurse Jones and anthropologist Kay describe in chapter 6 (taken from J. Patrick Lavery, ed., *The Human Placenta: Clinical Perspectives* [Rockville: Aspen Publishers, 1987], 11–23), among many cultures, the placenta is believed to possess magical attributes. Hence, the cavalier disposal of the afterbirth by American hospital staff can unwittingly create stress disruptive to the new mother and her family.

Anne Fadiman's book *The Spirit Catches You and You Fall Down* (New York: Farrar, Strauss and Giroux, 1997) provides an apt example of the need for awareness of other cultures' beliefs and practices connected with the placenta. She describes the customary ritual burial of the placenta among the Californian Hmong (an ethnic group from Laos that has sought refuge in the United States since 1975). The placenta of a girl should be buried under her parents' bed while a son's is interred under the home's central pillar. Even the placental position at burial is important. It must be placed smooth side up to prevent infant vomiting after nursing. The Hmong believe that after death, at the close of the journey in which they revisit each of the places they have lived, they must reclaim their placental jacket before they can join their celestial ancestors and be reborn as a newborn human infant. Accordingly, those who cannot find their placentas are doomed to endless, lonely wandering. Unaware of such cultural differences, some American doctors erroneously assume that Hmong requests to keep placentas indicate their intent to indulge in placentaphagia. In Burma, it is reported that human placentas are in fact consumed to remedy valvular heart disease (C. V. Foll, "Some Beliefs and Superstitions about Pregnancy, Parturition and Infant Health in Burma," *Journal of Tropical Pediatrics* 5 [1959]: 51–58). But the Hmong have no wish to ingest their baby's placenta. If hospital personnel avoided the common practice of incinerating placentas or selling them for use in cosmetic products in cases in which parents valued the placenta, for whatever reason, cross-cultural relations would undoubtedly improve. (For further discussion of the disposal of placentas, see C. E. Barry, "Where Do All the Placentas Go?" *Canadian Journal of Infection Control* 9 [1994]: 8–10 and J. U. Schneiderman, "Rituals of Placenta Disposal," *American Journal of Maternal and Child Nursing* 23 [1998]: 142–143.)

For a particularly thorough treatment of cross-cultural placenta rituals, see J. R. Davidson, "The Shadow of Life," *Culture, Medicine & Psychiatry* 9 (1985): 75–92. Relevant data can also be found in V. Elwin's "Conception, Pregnancy and Birth among the Tribesmen of the Maikal Hills," *Journal of the Royal Asiatic Society of Bengal* 9 (1943): 99–148, especially section 17.

Jones is an associate professor at the University of Arizona College of Nursing and a coauthor of a book on family nursing: Marilyn M. Friedman, Vicky Bowden, and Elaine Jones, *Family Nursing: Theory, Research & Practice*, 5th ed. (Upper Saddle River, N.J.: Prentice-Hall, 2002). Kay, professor emerita at the University of Arizona College of Nursing, is the editor of a well-known book on birthing, *Anthropology of Human Birth* (Philadelphia: F. A. Davis Company, 1982), and the author of an encyclopedia entry on childbirth in Helaine Selin, ed., *Encyclopedia of the History of Science, Technology, and Medicine in Non-Western Cultures* (Dordrecht, The Netherlands: Kluwer Academic, 1997), 187–191. Kay is also the author of many other articles as well as chapters, and three other books.

The Cultural Anthropology of the Placenta 6

ELAINE JONES AND MARGARITA A. KAY

THE PLACENTA, A VISIBLE PRODUCT OF BIOLOGICAL PROCESSES, is studied in this text from the viewpoint of the system that anthropologists call "biomedicine." It is treated according to the logic of the cultural system of belief of Western scientific medicine. Biomedicine, following the heuristics of the anthropologist who, after all, also participates in Western culture, may be thought of as a system of beliefs, roles, and materials. The beliefs are ideas that reflect the culture's cosmology or the beliefs about how events occur and their ultimate and immediate causes. These ideas require proof according to formalized replication rites. The ideas are used by persons occupying certain status roles. The important roles in biomedicine are those of scientist and clinician. The functions, purposes, chemical pathways and pathophysiology of body systems are considered by persons occupying the status of scientist, which in Western culture is a position analogous to a high priest in many preliterate societies, both in earlier times and at present. The high priests know and manipulate the secret of their worlds, and for this ability they are both respected and feared. It is thought that if they can cure illness, they can also inflict it. Finally, a medical system also contains various materials, a vast array in contemporary biomedicine. Like all other cultures, biomedicine is ethnocentric; not only believing that its ways are the best, but usually unaware that there are other ways of considering a palpable object or process.

The anthropologist finds many systems of belief, systems that spring from the history, social structure, economics, politics, and other aspects of the lives of people who live in a particular society, reflecting their culture. When more than a century ago, Tylor[1] gave his classical definition of culture, he was articulating the distinctive feature of anthropology, its holism: " . . . that complex whole which includes knowledge, belief, art, morals, law, custom and any other capabilities and habits acquired by man as a member of society." To study the meaning that the placenta holds for people who are not part of biomedicine, one must look not only at what people say and do with the placenta; how they perceive, interpret and respond to it; but also at other aspects of their culture. A goal of anthropological study is not only to describe but also to explain the variation.

We will consider the placenta in various cultural contexts, without evaluating the biological efficacy of this cultural knowledge. In some ways, anthropologists have given more attention to the placenta than to other events and objects in childbearing systems. This selective attention is believed to have occurred because previously most anthropologists and their informants were men.

Childbirth was a concern of women; men were excluded from observation and participation. Male informants knew and could tell the anthropologist only what women had told them about childbirth. However, the disposal of the placenta might be relegated to men. Thus many ethnographies (thick descriptions of cultures) that reported thoroughly certain aspects of lifestyles might have only the sketchiest information about pregnancy and childbirth, but minute detail about the placenta, especially about its disposal. However, placenta-related behavior separated from its cultural context may be meaningless. Thus the richness of data about the placenta would unfortunately be incomplete.

Ethnophysiological Concepts

Delivery of the placenta is a grave concern for all societies. The medical ethnobotany of any group dependent on herbal remedies always has a variety of available plant brews to give the woman whose placenta is slow to separate.[2] Renaissance herbals, the compendia of plant remedies then known to Western culture, were first printed in the 16th century, yet the newly popular herb books list many of the same plant remedies today. The cures include the roots, flowers, seeds, or leaves administered in teas, douches, or steam of lily, lepidium, mandrake, horehound, marigold, calendula, angelica, chervil, parsley, saxifrage, bay berries, saffron, feverfew, camomile, dittany, briony, hog's fennel, fraxinella, laburnum, pine, rosemary, and rue. According to humoral doctrine, the accepted pharmacology and pathophysiology for thousands of years, those herbs that acted on the uterus were categorized as "hot" and "dry."[3] A retained placenta is a most dreaded complication of birth. Contemporary ethnographers of childbirth, who are usually women, have observed the concern. For example, Sargent[4] quoted a Bariba midwife who stated that "anyone can deliver a baby but it is the placenta which kills"; Sargent also found a variety of procedures for a retained placenta. Jordan[5] noted that although Mayans were reported to smile happily at the newborn infant immediately after birth, participant observation showed a different course of events. When she actually filmed the delivery, Jordan saw that the immediate attention was fixed upon delivery of the placenta.

Placental Rituals in Cultural Context

Union of sperm and ovum starts not only a future infant, but also a placenta. Regard for the placenta is reflected in its ultimate disposal, which varies by culture. To study the placenta in cultural context, various aspects of the culture must be attended to.

While part of what happens in childbirth is purely instinctive and physiological, it also reflects social values, which vary with each society.[6] Placental disposal, a specific part of childbirth, is therefore likely to reflect wider cultural values regarding the roles of men and women in a particular society. "Gender preference" is one variable in different societies that attempts to explain diversity in placental disposal. Some systems of a culture are especially closely related, for example, belief systems. What people know and believe about their world should then be reflected in what they say and do with the placenta. Thus, the ways in which placental disposal is prescribed is either high ritual or low ritual. If attributions of magical capabilities of the placenta were evident in ethnographic data, the culture was considered high ritual. If no magical attributions were described or if the power was seen as polluting (e.g. as some cultures who see menstrual blood as polluting) the culture was categorized as low ritual. In some cases, the ethnographic data specifically refer to the meaning of the placenta that was held by the society practicing the disposal ritual. In other cases, the meaning was inferred, possibly incorrectly. It seemed likely that the meaning of the placenta to the culture would underlie the ritual dichotomy. Either the placenta is regarded for its power, and thus treated elaborately, or it is seen as disgusting and disposed of perfunctorily.

Placental power could be seen as "magical" from the ethnocentric viewpoint of biomedicine. Anthropological research today eschews the term *magic*, for faith to one culture is superstition to another. However, considerations of magic and ritual by early anthropologists continue to be instructive.

In his famous *Golden Bough*, Frazer[7] described two kinds of sympathetic magic: imitative and contagious. Imitative or homeopathic magic is premised upon the association of ideas by similarity, that "like produces like"; whereas contagious magic is activated with the underlying belief that things that were once in contact continue to have influence upon each other even after they are severed. Frazer used "the navel string and afterbirth, including the placenta" to illustrate contagious magic.

Malinowski[8] said that "the function of magic is to ritualize man's optimism, to enhance his faith in the victory of hope over fear." Humans use this magic when their body of empirical knowledge as to the behavior of nature and the means of controlling is inadequate.[8] The function of ritual therefore is to relieve anxiety. Radcliffe-Brown,[9] however, said that the existence of ritual created anxiety, for if incorrectly performed, "the psychological effect of the rite is to create . . . a sense of insecurity or danger."

If the placenta is invested with power, rituals in its disposal may demonstrate social values and may be functional for the culture, representing efforts to protect the group or the individual. As Malinowski[8] points out, people "resort to magic only where chance and circumstances are not fully controlled." In the preindustrial societies described by the early anthropologists, as well as in the third world countries today, the survival of the individual child, or of the entire group can be precarious.

Study Design

The Human Relations Area Files (HRAF) are a collection of primary source materials on selected preindustrial cultures or societies representing all major areas of the world. The files are organized into separate cultures that contain descriptive information on a single culture or on a group of closely related cultures. The sources are selected by culture or area experts on the basis of extensive bibliographic research.[10] Source material in each file is organized according to a comprehensive subject classification system with over 700 distinct subject categories.[11]

The major portion of the data was taken from the HRAF. Additional information regarding contemporary American placental practices was gathered from interviews with hospital nurses, lay midwives, and reviews of popular literature.

Representative cultures were selected from among 294 cultures through utilization of the HRAF probability sample of 60 world cultures.[10] The cultures included in the probability sample are listed by major world area in table 6.1.

We categorized the cultures as virifocal or femifocal, based on evidence of gender preference reported in ethnographic accounts in the HRAF. We devised the categories of virifocal and femifocal rather than use the standard terms used by

Table 6.1.   HRAF Probability Sample: 60 Cultural Units with OWC Codes

Asia	Middle East	Europe	North America
Koreans AA1	Kurd MA11	Serbs EF6	Tlingit NA12
Taiwan Hokkien AD5	Somali MO4	Lapps EP4	Copper Eskimo ND8
Central Thai AO7	Amhara MP5	Highland Scots ES10	Blackfoot NF6
Garo AR5	Hausa MS12		Ojibwa NG6
Khasi AR7	Kanuri MS14		Iroquois NM9
Santal AW42	Wolof MS30		Pawnee NQ18
Sinhalese AX4	Libyan Bedouin MT9		Klamath NR10
Andamans AZ2	Shluh MW11		Hopi NT9
			Tarahumara NU33
			Tzeltal NV9

Africa	Russia	South America	Oceania
Dogan FA16	Yakut RV2	Cuna SB5	Ifugao OA19
Twi (Ashanti) FE12	Chukchee RY2	Cagaba SC7	Iban OC6
Tiv FF57		Aymara SF5	Toradja OG11
Ganda FK7		Ona SH4	Aranda O18
Masai FL12		Mataco S17	Kapauku OJ29
Pygmies (Mbuti) FO4		Guarani (Cayua) SM4	Trobrianders OL6
Azande FO7		Bahia Brazilians SO11	Lau (Fijians) OQ6
Bemba FQ5		Bororo SP8	Truk OR19
Lozi FQ9		Yanoama SQ18	Tikopia OT11
		Tucano SQ19	
		Bush Negroes SR8	

Source: R.O. Lagace, *Nature and Use of the HRAF Files,* 1974.

anthropologists. In some cultures, higher valuing of males was consistent with patrilineal and patrilocal social organization. Other societies that focused on men had bilinear descent systems. Similarly, some cultures described as characterized by female superiority or equality had matrilineal inheritance systems, and others had bilinear inheritance rules. Therefore, apparent cultural gender preference was employed as the criterion for categorization.

Two hypotheses were formulated to test the relationship of gender preference and placental ritualization: (1) virifocal cultures will practice low-ritual disposal, consistent with lower valuing of feminine activities, and (2) femifocal cultures will practice high-ritual placental disposal, reflecting a view of the female as a powerful force (table 6.2).

Thus each culture was categorized according to study criteria as virifocal or femifocal and as either high or low on placental ritualization, or as "no mention" if there was no information in available ethnographies on placental disposal (table 6.3).

A chi-square of 0.94 was calculated for the relationship between cultures' gender preference and placental ritualization, indicating a statistically nonsignificant relationship (table 6.4).

Cross-cultural comparisons are complex for many reasons, including intracultural variations in belief systems and practices and dependence on the descriptions provided by ethnographers. Data from many cultures were consistent regarding high placental ritualization in femifocal societies and low placental ritualization in virifocal societies. For example, among the Khasi people, descent is counted from the mother only, and Gurdon[12] writes that "in some villages a newly married man is spoken of by the bride's family as 'someone else's son.'" The father of a child is involved in placental disposal:

> When the naming ceremony is over the father takes the placenta, sprinkles rice meal on it and swings it three times over the head of the child. Thereupon he leaves the house and fastens the jar including the contents to a tree near the hut. When the father returns his feet are sprinkled with water so that the child may stay healthy.[13]

The high value of women parallels an elaborate ritual with a product of the mother's body, the placenta, to insure the health of the newborn.

Santal culture was virifocal and had low placental ritualization. The Santal wife "[had] no legal status in the eye of tribal jurisprudence; she was simply bought and belongs to the husband's family as a chattel."[14] Consistent with the low status of

Table 6.2.   Childbirth Practices in Cultural Context

Social Organization	Placental Ritualization
Gender preference	
Virifocal	Low ritual
Femifocal	High ritual

Table 6.3. Categorization of Population Sample According to Placental Ritualization and Gender Preference

	Placental Ritualization	
No Mention	High Ritual Virifocal	Low Ritual
N = 11	N = 15	N = 20
Lapps	Korean	Taiwan Hokkien
Highland Scots	Central Thai	Santal
Lozi	Serbs	Andamans
Yakut	Dogan	Masai
Bahia Brazilians	Tiv	Pygmies (Mbuti)
Tucano	Ganda	Azande
Somali	Chukchee	Guarani
Libyan Bedouin	Cagaba	Yanoama
Shluh	Aymara	Bush Negroes
Iroquois	Pawnee	Kurd
Sinhalese	Klamath	Amhara
	Tzeltal	Hausa
	Trobrianders	Kanuri
	Truk	Wolof
	Tikopia	Blackfoot
		Ojibwa
		Ofugao
		Arando
		Kapauka
		Lau (Fijians)
	Femifocal	
N = 2	N = 4	N = 8
Bemba	Khasi	Garo
Tlingit	Copper Eskimo	Twi (Ashanti)
	Hopi	Cuna
	Toradja	Ona
		Mataco
		Bororo
		Tarahumara
		Iban

N = 60

Table 6.4. Frequency of Placental Ritualization by Gender Preference in 60 Cultures

	Placental Ritualization			
Gender Preference	No Mention	High Ritual	Low Ritual	Total
Virifocal	11	15	20	46
Femifocal	2	4	8	14
Total	N = 13	N = 19	N = 28	N = 60

$X^2 = 0.94$, N5

women, "the afterbirth [was] buried in a pit in one corner of the courtyard of the house"; there was no mention of magic associated with it.[15]

Failure to demonstrate similar relationships between gender preference and placental ritualization in other cultures may have been a result of intracultural variations, incomplete information in available ethnographies, and insufficiently complex conceptualization of variations in relationships between men and women. Korean culture was categorized as a high-ritual, virifocal society, since correct disposal of the placenta was considered necessary to prevent harm from coming to the mother,[16] and the "theoretical position of the male is outstandingly dominant."[17] Although Korean society was reported to be patriarchal, "If a woman can make a thing as quickly and as well as a man she will receive the same wages as he."[18]

An example of possible miscategorization resulting from incomplete ethnographic information was suggested in Garo culture, which was labeled low ritual/femifocal. The culture is indeed matrilineal, and the steps in placental disposal were quite detailed.[19] There was, however, no apparent consequence attached to nonadherence to the prescribed ritual, hence it did not meet criteria for high-ritual classification. Nevertheless it seems unlikely that a people would conform to a detailed, specific method of disposal if there were no belief system regarding consequences of nonadherence. It may be that the ethnographer did not know, or did not record the meaning, and the culture was consequently miscategorized.

The description of the relationship of men and women in Central Thailand is qualitatively much different from the reports of Santal men and women, yet both cultures were categorized as virifocal.

Refinement in conceptualization of placental rituals and belief systems involved in overall gender preferences would contribute to better understanding of the meanings inherent in specific cross-cultural and intracultural practices.

Cross-Cultural Variation

Disposal Rituals

Practices surrounding the human placenta and its disposal provide an example of rich culture diversity in childbirth practices. Nineteen cultural units were categorized as high ritual, and 28 as low ritual. Sources from only 13 of the 60 cultural units contained no mention of the placenta. Distinctive features of some high-ritual cultures related to belief in the spiritual nature of placenta and definite consequence related to placental disposal. Low-ritual cultures differed not only in terms of magical attributions but also in a common view of the placenta as unclean rather than spiritual. Shades of the cross-cultural differences between high- and low-ritual practices can be found intraculturally in America, as well: Lotus birth parallels high-ritual practices, and common methods of placental disposals in standard biomedical hospitals are definitely low ritual.

High Placental Ritual Cultures

A culture was categorized as high placental ritual if the placenta was imbued with magical capabilities in causing or preventing a specific event. In cultures with high placental rituals, it was considered important to dispose of the placenta properly, or some undesirable consequence would ensue. The consequence might be as minor as pimples on the baby[20] or as major as death of the child.[21] The consequences might be fairly immediate, or sometime in the distant future. For example, incorrect disposal could result in a difficult delivery in a subsequent pregnancy;[22] correct disposal could facilitate a child learning to talk at an early age.[23]

The particular rituals varied in terms of who was involved in the ritual and whether there was distinction made in disposal according to the sex of the baby. Many of the practices in high-ritual cultures were based on a belief in a sympathetic relationship. Cultures classified as high ritual are particularly distinctive in terms of belief in the spiritual nature of the placenta and consequences related to placental disposal.

Spiritual Nature of the Placenta

Explicit descriptions of the spiritual nature of the placenta were found in geographically distant cultures. Ethnographies from Ganda in Africa, Toradja and Tikopia Islands of Oceania, and Pawnee of North America provided detailed descriptions of beliefs in the spiritual nature of the placenta.

Roscoe[21] reported that in Ganda the afterbirth was placed at the root of a plantain tree, and "if the child was a boy, it was put at the root of a plantain tree from which beer was made. If it was a girl, at the root of a plantain and used as a vegetable . . . it was guarded by old ladies who prevented anyone from going near it; they tied ropes . . . from tree to tree to isolate it . . . when the fruit was ripe it was cut by the lady in charge. If it was the plantain used for beer, she had to brew it and . . . if it was the kind used for food it was cooked." The afterbirth was called the second child, and was believed to have a spirit, which became at once a ghost. It was on account of this ghost that they guarded the plantain by which the afterbirth was placed because the person who partook of the beer made from this plantain or of food cooked from it took the ghost from its clan, and the living child would then die in order to follow its twin ghost.

People of Tikopia in Oceania identified the particular part of the placenta that contained the spiritual component and viewed it in a very negative light, at least as far as female infants were concerned: The afterbirths of male children were buried at once outside the eave on the nonsacred side of the house, but the placentas of female children were left until the morning. In the morning certain objects were observed in the afterbirth, sometimes two, sometimes three or even four. They were described as sometimes being pale, but more often black, and "moving and crawling within the placenta."[24] The objects were removed and buried separately. They were described as "umuru atua," manifestations of a supernatural being, Feke—the Octopus Deity. If the objects were buried with the afterbirth, they would affect the health of the child, who would either die or become insane. The precaution applied only to girl children because Feke was noted for his lubricity. Firth[24] noted that the theme of heterosexual intercourse with supernatural beings resulting in the illness of mortals ran through many Tikopia customs.

The personification of the placenta is evident in accounts of Pawnee midwives' ritual of disposal. Dorsey and Murie[25] wrote that the midwife disposed of the after-birth by "placing it on a bunch of grass, and wrapping it in a piece of tanned buffalo hide; she [then] carried it outside into the woods. There she put it on a tree saying: 'I place this afterbirth upon you, that the animals may not eat it nor the birds. You stand here firmly, let this child that I have attended grow up without sickness to be a man (or woman).' Next she said to the afterbirth 'I place you securely upon this tree, so that nothing will touch you, and so that you will turn into dust. If the mother who is sick yonder should give birth to another, make the delivery easy.'" The midwife then re-turned to the lodge.[25]

Addressing the tree and the placenta in the first person may have reflected cultural beliefs about the relationship of living things to one another, as well as specific beliefs about the nature of the placenta and wish for the child's health.

Talking directly to the placenta was also a part of Toradja rituals.[26] Adriani and Kruyt[26] wrote that "sometimes the afterbirth is addressed, before it is left behind: 'You, afterbirth, do not say that I do not love you; we love you. Do not tickle the soles of the feet of your little brother/sister and do not pinch his stomach.'"

The Toradja believed that there was a soul that accompanied a person during his or her lifetime, called a "navel soul." It lived with the placenta or originated from it. For this reason, the afterbirth must be handled with care for if there was anything lacking in this, it would be noticeable in the child who would cry a great deal and be troublesome.[26]

Although explicit discussion of the placenta as having a separate spiritual identity was absent in descriptions of some of the cultures called "high ritual," personification was implied in the assumptions regarding consequences of incorrect placental disposal.

Cosminsky[27] found in Guatemala that the placenta is thought to have a special re-lationship to the child, and that it is referred to as the second child, thus requiring careful disposal. However, this consisted only of burning the placenta and burying the ashes, i.e., low ritual. In some cases, the contagious magical relationship may be trans-ferred to the place where the placenta is disposed of. For example, Henderson and Henderson[28] reported that the Onitsha Ibo buried the placenta with a banana, palm, or sago stem. The tree that grew up later would be named after the child and would always belong to that infant.

Laderman[29] describing Malaysian placental beliefs, which she finds are similar to beliefs of other Southeast Asian cultures such as the Philippine and Indonesian groups, states that the placenta is the fetus's semihuman sibling, which develops during the second month of pregnancy. After delivery, the midwife washes the afterbirth in water into which lime juice has been squeezed and prepares it as if for a traditional human burial, including salt, tamarind, a small piece of absorbent cotton, and a bit of white cloth.

Consequences Related to Placental Disposal

Consequences of not conforming to prescribed rituals in disposal of the placenta varied from rather minor to the most severe, i.e., death of the child. There were multiple effects from different parts of the disposal rituals in some cultures. Most consequences related to the infant or the mother's health, though some ethnographers recorded effects on other people as well.

Expected consequences were rather general in some ethnographic accounts, such as when the placenta was considered "good luck" by Serb peasant women who dried it and kept it wrapped in a scarf with other personal effects. Other descriptions were more specific, such as the belief of some Aymaran that if the placenta were burned (rather than buried) the child would have a black face, and if a dog ate it, the mother would get sick.[30]

Tikopian Islanders ultimately buried the placenta in the path or in some well-trodden place, which must not be exposed to the sun. If the child was heard to hiccough, then someone went out and trod on the place where the afterbirth was buried, to cure the hiccoughs.[24]

The warnings regarding correct placental disposal speak of a belief in a magical relationship between infant and placenta, after birth and into adulthood.

Ritual acts related to the child's adult role were also seen in other cultures. Copper Eskimos sometimes set the baby's course at birth toward a career as a shaman: "A wouldbe shaman must be made suitable right after birth. Even as soon as the afterbirth has been extruded the infant is lifted up and allowed to look through it, a ceremony that gives the child second sight."[31]

The Aymaran might cover the placenta with flowers and bury it in the shade, accompanied by miniature farm implements if the child were a boy or cooking utensils if it were a girl.[32] In addition, the Aymaran midwife floated a piece of the placenta in a basin of water to divine by its movement the child's future.[32]

In the following cases the placenta was seen as a part of the mother, continuing to act on her even after it separated from her body. Villa Roja[33] reported that in Tzeltal culture "the placenta can be burned, thrown to the dogs, or deeply buried in case the mother does not want another pregnancy soon." In contrast, Klamath women could throw their afterbirths carelessly away if they wished to prevent further pregnancies.[34]

There were a few instances where the placenta was thought to affect people other than the baby and mother. For example, it was regarded as good medicine by Toradjan people who were bothered by cracks in the soles of their feet; they were advised to step on the placenta.[26]

A second example comes from the Oraibi Hopi: The Hopi father took the placenta and other items from the birth, and threw them on the placenta pile, a special place on the edge of the village. This was done so that "no person would step upon them and cause his feet to become sore, and chapped, his eyes yellow, and his urine thick."[35]

High Placental Ritual in America

Cultures described as high ritual have a common belief in the placenta's role in causing and preventing certain events, usually related to the health of the infant or mother. These beliefs reflect a certain mystical view of birth, either explicitly or implicitly. Only a few American practices in placental disposal explicitly recognize the spirituality of birth and the placenta. One example is lotus birth, described by Baker.[36]

Lotus birth is the maintenance of connection with the afterbirth, which is allowed to wither and fall off by itself, usually in 2.5 to 7 days. Baker[36] says that "generally once [the placenta] is washed and dried, it is placed in a bowl at bedside." Baker[36] described her decision to adopt a lotus birth: "I have chosen to follow this ritual birth process because of a primary understanding of the incredibly vital link which exists between mother and baby. Lotus birth is a demonstration that all attachments to placenta, to mother, to earth will eventually cease of their own accord."

A second, less explicit but somewhat spiritual practice is consumption of the placenta. One woman described the experience this way: "I felt myself filling up, taking back what I had created for baby's use while in the womb. I felt very natural, like a mama cat."[37] An accompanying article[38] gave a number of recipes for preparing the placenta for consumption, such as placenta stew and placenta pizza.

The placenta has been included within the context of Taoism when a lay midwife remarked that she would not recommend eating the placenta in most cases because it was "too much yang so soon after birth." Rather, she considered yin foods more beneficial to a woman immediately following delivery.

Low Placental Ritual Cultures

Cultures categorized as low ritual did not evidence any magical attributions to the placenta, though methods of disposal were sometimes performed according to detailed specifications. Most of the low ritual cultures, however, had perfunctory disposal methods, such as unceremonial burial; the only attribution made to the placenta was uncleanliness or contamination.

One of the ethnographers of Garo detailed disposal procedures that incorporated a view of the placenta as unclean and without any presumed magical characteristics:

> After the baby is born, the midwife catches the afterbirth in a special little bamboo basket that the men have made and ties it up. The midwife carries the basket containing the afterbirth into the jungle where she places it in the fork of a tree, along with the leaves on which the baby first lay. . . . She should return by way of a stream where

she can wash off any dirt and blood that she has accumulated during the delivery. When she returns to the house the man who has sacrificed (some animal), he shouts for the pollution to leave and the midwife calls back that it has left.[19]

Among the Taiwan Hokkien, "the umbilical cord and afterbirth are wrapped in a rag and buried in the river bottom"; anything related to the birth, especially if it has been in contact with the woman's blood, is considered unclean."[39]

Similarly, Messing[40] reported on Amharan viewpoint of the placenta as "dirty":

> It is believed that both embryo and placenta consist of menstrual blood that has not come out and become coagulated like buttermilk; fermented with the male semen, like yeast. The placenta (named with a word that means discharged dirty part) is buried out of sight.

Methods of placental disposal in low-ritual cultures fell into four categories: burial, burning, hanging in trees, and tossing into a trash pile or a river. Burial is the most common disposal method. The site of burial varied but was consistently unceremonial.

The Kanuri buried the placenta in the compound, while the new baby was being nursed.[41] Andamans buried the placenta in the jungle or in the floor of the dwelling.[42] Santal husbands dug a hole in the floor with a ploughshare and buried the placenta there but not directly under a rafter.[43] A Santal does not refer to his birthplace, rather he refers to "the village where my afterbirth was buried."[43] The Kurd also buried the afterbirth, but did so at some distance from the house[44]; whereas the Hausa buried it behind the house.[45]

Methods of placental disposal changed over time in some cultures, such as the Southern Ojibwa. Ojibwan informants agreed that in the very early days the placenta was always hung in the crotch of a tree formed by the main bunk and a branch at such a height that no dogs or other animals could reach it; burial was taboo. In later days it was buried, and informants thought that the whites introduced the custom of burial.[46]

Other cultures had more than one acceptable method of disposal. Playfair remarked that the Garo might either bury the afterbirth or place it in a gourd and hang in on a tree.[47] Arandans either burned or buried it.[48] The Iban deposited the afterbirth in a plaited bag and hung it on a tree in their cemetery or in their *tembawai*, the site of their former house.[49] A variation on hanging the placenta in a tree was included in a description of Kapauku practices: "The afterbirth is placed by the mother on leaves and deposited on some branches and made into a bundle supported by two forked poles, standing about 5 feet high. This structure is erected in the bush near the house by which the delivery occurred."[50]

The Twi-Ashanti disposed of the placenta very simply—they threw it away in the village kitchen midden.[51] Merker remarked on a similar placental disposal by Masai people: "The afterbirth which is not the object of superstitious customs, is tossed into the livestock kraul by the midwife in some districts" or buried there at night in others.[52] Blackfoot were said to "throw away" the afterbirth,[53] and Kahn writes that Bush Negroes threw it into the river.[54]

Low Placental Ritual in America

Two common methods of placental disposal in Tucson, Arizona, are the discarding practiced in hospital settings and the less common disposal via burial, with a tree planted on the burial site (thus providing nutriment to the tree). These disposal methods reflect the belief that body exuviae are perhaps not actually polluting but at least dirty.

An informal survey of five Tucson hospitals indicated fairly consistent methods of disposal. Three hospitals sent the placenta to pathology for analysis before it was trashed or incinerated. It was immediately put in the garbage disposal at a fourth hospital, unless there were twins or a "bad baby"; at the fifth hospital the placenta was stored in the nursery refrigerator so it would be easily available to the neonatologist "in case something came up with the baby."

Placentas may also be used in manufacturing cosmetics. Balaskas and Balaskas[55] remarked that "hospitals usually donate placentas to cosmetic factories," which use the hormones to make their products. Some local hair stylists regularly ask customers if they want their hair "placentaed." Hydrolyzed animal protein is listed among the ingredients of one vial of "Placenta," a hair rinse manufactured by CBN Laboratories of Phoenix, Arizona.

"Purified water, lactic acid, quaternium 18, placental extract, hydrolyzed animal protein, benzalkonimn chloride, quaternium 15, mica and titanium dioxide, coumarin, fragrance, FD & C Yellow No. 6." Directions for use say that the consumer should towel dry the hair, work in entire contents of the 3/4 oz. vial, not rinse it out, and style as usual.

Summary and Conclusions

This overview was an effort to describe the wide variety of customs for disposing of the placenta. A probability sample of 60 cultural units drawn from the Human Relations Area Files was used to learn if placental disposal could be related to the usual anthropological categories such as social organization, descent, religion, or subsistence patterns. Dissatisfied with these, we created new labels of social structure: virifocal and femifocal. Placental disposal was dichotomized into high ritual and low ritual. The gender preference of a society was cross-tabulated with its placental ritual.

We appreciated anew the anthropological truism that to separate any behavior from its cultural context is to do analytic damage. High-ritual or elaborate placental disposal could mean respect for the placenta as a spiritual entity or fear of the power of the placenta. Low-ritual disposal could mean disgust, as simply too bloody for the squeamish, or also fear that the placenta could be dangerous, with power to pollute. The large amount of cultural data on the placenta proved to be a confusing abundance, since the reasons for a particular custom were not always clear. Both the collection and interpretation of data by the ethnographer depended upon his or her anthropological theory. One could not be sure of the meaning of the placental disposal to the people practicing the ritual. Their informants were rarely queried. Scholars have reminded us not to take a people's rationales at face value. Radcliffe-Brown[9] stated that although the reasons given by members of a community for customs they observe are important data, one should not suppose that they give a valid explanation of the custom. It is also wrong, he said, that when the anthropologist "cannot get from the people themselves a reason for their behavior to attribute to them some purpose of reason on the basis of his own preconceptions about human experiences."

The definitions of the placenta and prescriptions for its disposal are determined by the logic of the culture, which is a sufficient, although tautological, explanation. Nevertheless, in the existing variation there is an important message. The same entity, event, or object is variously defined according to the meaning it holds. These beliefs are subject to change, as other aspects of the culture change. Perceptions of the placenta ranged from it being viewed as inert, nonliving material to living material. Thus there is great variety in what is considered living, and what is believed to be its beginning, power, and end. These differences should be respected. The beliefs of biomedical culture at one particular time should not be imposed upon another culture.

References

1. Tylor, E. B.: Primitive Culture. London, Murray, 1871.

2. Kay, M., Yoder, M.: Hot and cold in women's ethnotherapeutics: The American Mexican West. Presented at 11th International Congress of Anthropological and Ethnological Sciences, Vancouver, Canada, September 1923, 1983.

3. Gerard, J.: The Herbal, Johnson (ed, 1633). New York, Dover Press, 1975.

4. Sargent, C.: Solitary confinement: Birth practices among the Bariba of the People's Republic of Benin, in Kay, M. A. (ed): Anthropology of Human Birth. Philadelphia, F. A. Davis, 1982, pp 193–210.

5. Jordan, B.: Studying childbirth: The experience and methods of a woman anthropologist, in Romalis S (ed): Childbirth: Alternatives to Medical Control. Austin, Tex, University of Texas Press, 1981, pp 181–216.

6. Kitzinger, S.: Women as Mothers. New York, Vintage Books, 1978.

7. Frazer, J. G.: Sympathetic magic, in The Golden Bough. New York, Macmillan, 1922.

8. Malinowski, B.: The Sexual Life of Savages in Northwestern Melanesia, I II. New York, Horace Liveright, 1929. Malinowski, B.: Magic, Science and Religion. Garden City, NY, Doubleday & Company, 1954.

9. Radcliffe-Brown, A. R.: Structure and Function in Primitive Society. London, Cohen & West, 1952.

10. Lagace, R. O.: Nature and Use of the HRAF Files. New Haven, Conn., Human Relations Area Files, Inc, 1974.

11. Murdock, G. P., Clellan, S. F., Hudson, A. K., et al: Outline of Cultural Materials, 4th edition. New Haven, Conn, Human Relations Area Files Inc, 1971.

12. Gurdon, P.R.T.: The Khasis, with an introduction by Sir Charles Lyall. London, David Nutt, 1907.

13. Stegmiller, P. F.: Aus Dem Religiösen Leben der Khasi (The Religious Life of the Khasi). Anthropos, Salzburg, Leo Gesellschaft; 1921, vol. XVL pp 407–441.

14. Mukherjee, C.: The Santals, 2nd edition. Calcutta, A Mukherjee & Co Ltd, 1962.

15. Biswas, P. C.: Santals of the Santal Parganas. New Delhi, Bharatiya Adimjati Sevak Sangh, 1956.

16. Knez, E. I.: Sam Jong Dong: A South Korean Village, thesis. Maxwell Graduate School, Syracuse University, Syracuse, NY, 1959.

17. Osgood, C.: The Koreans and Their Culture. New York, Ronald Press CD, 1951.

18. Hulbert, H. B.: The Passing of Korea. New York, Doubleday, 1906.

19. Burling, R., Regsanggri: Family and Kinship in a Garo Village. Philadelphia, University of Pennsylvania Press, 1963.

20. Hanks, J. R.: Maternity and Its Ritual in Bang Chan, data paper No. 51. Cornell University, Department of Asian Studies, Southeast Asia Program, Ithaca, NY, 1963.

21. Roscoe, J.: The Banganda: An Account of Their Native Customs and Beliefs. London, Macmillan & Co, 1911.

22. Fischer, A.: Reproduction in Truk, Ethnology, Pittsburgh, University of Pittsburgh Press, 1963, vol. 2, pp 526–540.

23. Reichel-Dolmatoff, G.: The Kogi: A Tribe of the Sierra Nevada de Santa Marta, Colombia, II (Spanish). Bogota, Colombia, Editorial Iqueima, 1951.

24. Firth, R.: Ceremonies for Children and Social Frequency in Tikopia. Sydney, Australia, Oceania, 1956, vol. 27, pp 12–55.

25. Dorsey, G. A., Murie, J. A.: Notes on Skidi Pawnee Society. Field Museum of Natural History, Anthropological Series, Chicago, Field Museum Press, 1940, vol. 27, no. 2, pp 65–119.

26. Adriani, N., Kruyt, A. C.: The Bare'e-Speaking Toradja of Central Celebes (The East Toradja), II, Karding Moulton J (trans). Amsterdam, Noord-Hollandsche Uitgevers Maatschappij, 1951.

27. Cosminsky, S.: Knowledge and body concepts of Guatemalan midwives, in Kay, M. (ed): Anthropology of Human Birth. Philadelphia, F. A. Davis, pp 233–252.

28. Henderson, H., Henderson, R.: Traditional Onitsha Ibo maternity beliefs and practices, in Kay M (ed): Anthropology of Human Birth Philadelphia, F. A. Davis, 1982, pp 175–192.

29. Laderman, C.: Wives and Midwives. Berkeley, CA: University of California Press, 1983.

30. Hickman, J. M.: The Aymara of Chinchera. Peru: Persistence and Change in a Bicultural Context, dissertation. Cornell University, Ithaca, NY, 1963. University Microfilms Publications, No. 64-3641. Ann Arbor, University Microfilms 1964 (1971).

31. Rasmussen, B.: Intellectual Culture of the Copper Eskimos: Report of the Fifth Thule Expedition. Copenhagen, 1932, vol. 9, pp 1921–1924.

32. Tschopik, H. Jr.: The Aymara. Bureau of American Ethnology, Bulletin No. 143. Washington, DC, Smithsonian Institution, 1946, vol. 2, pp 501–573.

33. Villa Roja, A.: The Tzeltal, in Wauchope, R. (ed): Handbook of Middle American Indians. Austin, University of Texas Press, 1969, vol. 7, pp 195–225.

34. Pearsall, M.: Klamath Childhood and Education. California University Anthropological Records, 9 (1950) 3:339–351. Berkeley and Los Angeles, University of California Press, 1950.

35. Talayesva, D. C.: Sun Chief: The Autobiography of a Hopi Indian. Simmons, L. W. (ed). New Haven, Conn.: Yale University Press, 1942.

36. Baker, I. P.: Lotus birth. Mothering 1983; 28: 75.

37. April, E.: Coffee tea or me, the story of how I ate my placenta. Mothering 1983, 28: 76.

38. Robbins, R.: Placenta recipes. Mothering 1983; 28: 76.

39. Gallin, B.: Hsin Hsing. Taiwan. A Chinese Village in Change. Berkeley and Los Angeles, University of California Press, 1966.

40. Messing, S. D.: The Highland-Plateau Amhara of Ethiopia. dissertation. Philadelphia, PA: University of Pennsylvania, 1957.

41. Smith, M. F.: Baba of Karo. A Woman of the Muslim Hausa. London, Faber & Faber Ltd, 1954.

42. Radcliffe-Brown, A. R.: The Andamen Islanders: A Study in Social Anthropology. Cambridge University Press, 1922.

43. Culshaw, W. J.: Tribal Heritage: A Study of the Santals. London, Butterworths Press 1949.

44. Masters, W. M., Rowanduz: A Kurdish Administrative and Mercantile Center. Dissertation, University of Michigan, Ann Arbor, Michigan, 1953.

45. Hassan, M., Naibi, M. S.: A Chronicle of Abuja Health FL (trans). Ibadan, Abuja Native Administration and Ibadan University Press 1952.

46. Hilger, M. I.: Chippewa Child Life and Its Cultural Background, Bureau of American Ethnology, Bulletin 146. Washington, DC, 1908–1910; Smithsonian Institution, 1951.

47. Playfair, A.: The Garos. Introduction by Sir J. Bampfylde Fuller. London, David Nutt, 1909.

48. Basedow, H.: The Australian Aboriginal. Adelaide, Australia, FW Preece & Sons, 1925.

49. Howell, W.: The Sea Dyak. The Sarawak Gazette, 38–40. Kuching, Sarawak: 1908–1910.

50. Pospisil, L.: Kapuaka Papuans and Their Law. Yale University Publications in Anthropology, No. 54. New Haven, Conn.: Yale University and Yale University Press, 1958.

51. Rattray, R. S.: Religion and Art in Ashanti. Oxford, England. Clarendon Press, 1927.

52. Merker, M.: The Masai: Ethnographic Monograph of an East African Semite People. 2nd edition. Berlin, Dietrich Reimer (Ernst Vohsen), 1910.

53. Wissler, C.: The Social Life of the Blackfoot Indians. American Museum of Natural History, Anthropology Papers, 7, Part I. New York, American Museum of Natural History, 1911.

54. Kahn, M.C.D.: The Bush Negroes of Dutch Guiana. New York, Viking Press, 1931.

55. Balaskas, J., Balaskas, A.: Active Birth. New York, McGraw-Hill, 1983.

Editor's Introduction
The Social History of the Caul

THOMAS R. FORBES

THE CAUL IS A THIN, TRANSLUCENT TISSUE, a fragment of the amniotic membrane that may cover the head of some newborns. It is quickly removed so that the newborn's breathing is not impeded. Its name varies by culture but commonly includes such terms as cap, helmet, mask, and veil. Charles Dickens's title character in *David Copperfield* (1850) is born with a caul. Mention of this fetal membrane is generally omitted from literature on birthing, possibly because of its infrequent occurrence. Yet the variety in perceptions of the caul demonstrates the broad array of cultural contexts that can frame a biological phenomenon.

It is only the more extensive detailed accounts of birthing that include mention of the caul such as in the neglected yet excellent article by Verrier Elwin (1902–1964), "Conception, Pregnancy and Birth among the Tribesmen of the Maikal Hills," *Journal of the Royal Asiatic Society of Bengal* 9 (1943): 99–148. Elwin, who began his work as a missionary in India (but later resigned his holy orders to author some 40 books and 400 articles on anthropological topics), relates how infants born with a caul reflect their wish to hide their and their mothers' shame resulting from their mothers' misdeeds. Thus in this culture described by Elwin, the caul signals unlucky status and/or punishment. The membrane was buried with the placenta and umbilical cord. In contrast to the negative associations in India described by Elwin, Forbes comments in chapter 7 (taken from *Yale Journal of Biology and Medicine* 25 [1953]: 495–508) that cauls were of such value that they were sold to sailors in eighteenth- and nineteenth-century England because of their purported ability to protect those in their possession from drowning—a fact corroborated by Foll, who notes that the British believe that a boy born with a caul will never drown (C. V. Foll, "Some Beliefs and Superstitions about Pregnancy, Parturition and Infant Health in Burma," *Journal of Tropical Pediatrics* 5 [1959]: 51–58). Foll also reports that the caul is propitious in Burma as well; those born with it are bound for success and likely to be public figures, accomplishments they will allegedly achieve on their own.

For other essays on folk medicine by Forbes, who was a professor at the Yale University School of Medicine, see "Verbal Charms in British Folk Medicine," *Proceedings of the American Philosophical Society* 115 (1971): 293–316; his discussions of lithotherapy, "*Lapis Bufonis:* The Growth and Decline of a Medical Superstition," *Yale Journal of Biology and Medicine* 45 (1972): 139–149; and "The Madstone," in *American Folk Medicine: A Symposium,* edited by Wayland D. Hand (Berkeley: University of California Press, 1976), 11–19; and especially his further research on birthing, *The Midwife and the Witch* (New Haven: Yale University Press, 1966). For details of Elwin's remarkable career, see *Tribal World of Verrier Elwin: An Autobiography* (New York: Oxford University Press, 1964); Bhabagrahi Misra, *Verrier Elwin: A Pioneer Indian Anthropologist* (New York: Asia Publishing House, 1973); and Ramachandra Guha, *Savaging the Civilized: Verrier Elwin, His Tribals, and India* (Chicago: University of Chicago Press, 1999).

The Social History of the Caul   7

THOMAS R. FORBES

L'imagination engendre la superstition, la raison engendre la science.[15]

THE HISTORY OF OBSTETRICS, perhaps more than that of many sciences, includes a large measure of superstition. In earlier centuries the normal phenomena of pregnancy and labor were understood, if at all, incompletely; related abnormalities were even more puzzling. Before adequate scientific explanations were available, speculation had to suffice, and superstition was often a result.

Infrequently, in past ages as now, a baby is born with a thin, translucent tissue, a fragment of the amniotic membrane, covering its head. The remnant is known as a *caul*.[5] The modern obstetrician quickly removes the membrane (it may be interfering with the infant's efforts to begin respiration) and discards it. His professional predecessors, the physicians and midwives of earlier centuries, would have been more interested, for strong magic and strange beliefs were once related to the caul.

In countries all over the world it was expected that the membrane would bring fame and fortune to its owner.[9,34,41,50,67,80,107] Aelius Lampridius, a classical historian, related that the emperor Antonius Diadumenianus or Diadematus (born 19 September 208 A.D.) was so called because at birth his head was encircled with a fillet (*diadema*), twisted like a bowstring and so strong it could not be broken.[33,35,63,69,86] One supposes that the caul in this case had been rolled into a band. Although the possession of the fillet was expected to bring him good luck, Diadumenianus was assassinated while

From the Departments of Anatomy and the History of Medicine, Yale University School of Medicine. Read 17 October 1952 before the Beaumont Medical Club. The author is indebted to Professor G. Lincoln Hendrickson of Yale University for translating two passages and to the reference staffs of the Medical Library and Sterling Library for assistance in locating much material.

Thomas R. Forbes was Secretary-Treasurer, The Beaumont Medical Club, 1950–. (The Beaumont Club had only three Secretary-Treasurers. Dr. Samuel Harvey served from 1921–33 and Dr. Thoms, one of the founders, from 1933–50.)

a youth.[106] Caul superstitions were recorded again after the Dark Ages. Cornelius Gemma, a sixteenth-century physician, scorned belief in the powers of the caul.[39] He described it quaintly as being "nothing other than the remnant of another membrane, much softer than the amnion, but nevertheless more solid, bound with a purple border or fringe, and wrapped around the whole head down to the umbilicus, not without great danger to the baby unless the membrane was removed as quickly as possible; thus I myself have observed it in my first-born son who came helmeted [*galeatus*] into the world." Van der Spiegel, a Belgian anatomist, explained how the amniotic membrane may in childbirth "be draped partly or completely around the head, so that in the male it may be called a helmet [*galea*] by the German obstetricians, or in the female, as the Italians put it, a fillet [*vitta*] or shirt" [*indusium, camisia*].[89] He suggested that it is ridiculous to attach supernatural significance to a phenomenon which can be readily explained.

Charles Drelincourt (1633–1697), another physician, wrote *De Foetum Pileolo Sive Galea* [On the Little Cap or Helmet of Fetuses].[33] Unfortunately, his rather extended discussion consisted largely of harsh sarcasm directed at the ideas of some of his colleagues regarding the caul. Drelincourt made it clear that he too rejected any idea of the membrane's power to bring good fortune.

In the following century, Thiers, in his interesting *Traité des superstitions*,[95] quoted the French proverb that the happy man was born with a veil (*est né cöeffé*) and expressed the opinion that any advantage coming to one who wears the caul as a charm could only be with the help of the Devil. Haller, the Swiss physiologist, made passing reference in his *Physiologie*[43] to the caul as a supposed sign of good luck. Thomas Bartholin scoffed at the superstitions because, he said, he had known unlucky children who were born with cauls and lucky children who were born without them.[12] Spindler,[90] another physician of the period, said that he had never heard of a caul worn as a charm bringing good luck, but then told of a male patient who ascribed his impotence to the fact that his wife wore such a charm, i.e., the caul could have an evil influence. In Hungary it was darkly prophesied that he "who is born in the cloak [*Hulle*] dies in the rope."[50]

The beneficent effect of the caul was sometimes regarded as extending to the offspring of the original owner, but, according to a superstition of the Middle Ages and later, this effect would be lost if the caul were given away or sold outside the family.[4,50] On 20 May 1658 the will of "Sir John Offley, Knight of Madely Manor, Staffordshire" was probated. The document includes the following bequest: "Item, I will and devise one Jewell done all in Gold enammelled, wherein there is a Caul that covered my face and shoulders when I first came into the world, the use thereof to my loving Daughter the Lady Elizabeth Jenny, as long as she shall live."[22] It was directed that the caul be passed on to the males of succeeding generations and that "the same Jewell be not concealed nor sold by any of them." One notes that the bequest refers not only to the possession but also to the "use" of this curious heirloom.

Lemnius discussed the caul in his *De Miraculis Naturae*, first published in 1559. A 1658 edition, in English, of this work[60] includes the chapter heading: "Of the Helmets of

Children newly born, or of the thin and soft caul, wherewith the face is covered as with a vizard, or covering, when they come first into the world." He quotes "old Wives . . . who do but dote, and know not what they say" to the effect that a black caul presages accidents, misfortunes, and haunting by evil spirits unless the caul "be broken and given in drink, which against my will many have done to the great hurt of the child." But if the caul is red or clings to the crown of the head, the child is expected later to achieve great success.[60] Such interpretations were examples of *amniomancy*, the practice of foretelling the future by inspection of the caul.[57,88] If the caul were "white" (i.e., colorless) or red, it would bring good fortune; if black or lead-colored, the child would be unlucky.[57,80,88] In Herzegovinia, a part of Jugoslavia, it was thought that a baby born with a black caul would grow up to become a witch or sorcerer unless, on the first night after the birth, a woman carried the caul to the roof top and announced that "A child was born at our house in a bloody shirt" [*Hemde*]. Elsewhere in Jugoslavia the midwife carried the newborn baby itself to the threshold and announced three times that a real baby had been born, and not a witch or sorcerer.[80] Whether these procedures were regarded as charms or simply as attempts to prevent superstitious rumors among the neighbors is not reported.

Reference to the caul as a "shirt" (see above) illustrates the curious terminology that was developed for the membrane in various countries. Andrews[3] and others have called attention to the fact that semantic changes often involve a shift in meaning from the general to the specific. Certainly several terms which originally identified the entire amnion came later to signify only the *caul*, e.g., *membrana agnina* and *amiculum* (Latin), *coëffe* and *coiffe* (French) and *Schafhäutlein* and *Kinderbälglein* (German). The word *caul* itself, on the other hand, was sometimes used as a synonym of *amnion*. (*Caul*, in addition, could mean a net, the web of a spider, the base of a wig, a woman's cap, and any of several anatomical investing layers.)[71]

One finds further that the same ideas suggested themselves repeatedly in different lands in the fanciful names appropriated to identify the caul. Examples are *membrana agnina* (Latin, lamb's skin), membrane *agnelette* (French, lamb's skin), and *Schafhäutlein* (German, little lamb's skin); *galea* (Latin, helmet) and *Helm* and *Knabenhelm* (German, Dutch, helmet, boy's helmet) ; *pileus, pileolus* (Latin, a close fitting cap like a skull cap); *calotte* (French, skull cap); *Haube, Häublein, Glückshaube, Wasserhaube, Wehmutter-häublein* (German, cap, little cap, lucky cap, water cap, midwife's cap); *silly hood, silly how, sely how, haly how* (English, Scottish, lucky or holy cap); *coiffe, coëffe* (French, veil); *veil* (English); *involucrum* (Latin, covering, wrapper); *Kinderbälglein* (German, child's covering); *súpot* (Tagalog, bag, paper bag); *amiculum* (Latin, dear friend, cloak); *sigurkuft* (Icelandic, lucky coat or cape). Other terms which imaginatively described the caul include *pellis secundina, indumentum* (Latin, second skin, mask), *mask* (English), and *Muttergottestüchlein* and *Kindesnetzlein* (German, Virgin's handkerchief, child's little net).[1,8,9,20,28,37,38,42,44,46,50,51, 60, 61,70,71,74,76,83,89,101,105] The resemblance of the caul to a close-fitting shirt or under-garment is suggested repeatedly: *indusium* (Latin, shirt), *camicia della Madonna* (Italian, Virgin's shift), and *Hemd, Hemdlein, Westerhemd*, and *Muttergotteshemdlein* (German, shirt, little shirt, vest-like shirt, Virgin's shift).[44,50,51,89,101,103]

As would be expected, literary references to the caul are not uncommon. The *Oxford Dictionary* gives examples dated as early as 1547.[71] *Kell*, a variant of the term, had appeared in print by 1530. Subsequently, the caul was alluded to in English plays,[32,71] poetry,[49] and elsewhere, including the familiar introduction ("I was born with a caul") in *David Copperfield*.[31]

Because of the pronunciation and meaning of *cowl*, it has been suggested that this word is cognate with *caul* and the related Scottish *kell*.[14,71,98] A fancied similarity of the monk's cowl to the caul is also said to be the basis of the belief that a child born with a caul was destined by Providence for the monastery or convent.[19,106] In Austria it was expected that a boy would become an archbishop if he carried his caul in his clothes.[50] *Notes and Queries*, that extraordinary repository of antiquarian and other information, offers a quotation from a British newspaper, the Leeds *Mercury*, for 14 September 1889.[70] A laborer's wife bore a son on whose head was a caul. "The veil was placed on one side, and no notice was taken of it until some hours after the child's birth. When examined, however, it was found that the words 'British and Foreign Bible Society' were deeply impressed upon the veil. When this discovery was made the greatest excitement prevailed in the neighbourhood, some of the women declaring that nothing short of a miracle had been enacted. The doctor, who inquired into the matter, however, soon explained the affair. The veil, whilst in a pliable condition, had been placed upon a Bible, on the cover of which the words 'British and Foreign Bible Society' were deeply indented. The words were in this way transferred to the veil; but some of the inhabitants still ascribe the affair to supernatural influence."

Elsewhere in England it was believed that, for as long as he kept his caul, the individual born with it would be a wanderer.[83] In Iceland, in the islands near New Guinea, in the Kentucky mountains, and elsewhere one born with a caul was thought to be clairvoyant.[9,36,40,57,96] The Dutch and the Negroes of North America and the West Indies believed that he could see and talk with ghosts.[7,41,47,57] The caul was also a protection against sorcery, evil spirits, and demons.[9,57] In Germany the owner carried his caul when he was conscripted, with the hope that this charm would speed his release from military service.[78] Finally, the appearance of the caul gave an indication of the present health of the owner, even if he were absent; a dry, white, crisp caul meant good health, while a damp, black, limp caul betokened illness.[47,57,93]

It was regarded as important that the caul either be preserved or disposed of carefully at childbirth. The basis for this idea was very likely the widespread belief that in the caul resided the child's guardian spirit or "life token."[9,41,47,50,57,78] In Iceland the caul was buried by the midwife under the threshold over which the mother would later pass.[41,50] Hastings[47] suggests that this may have been done so that if the child died, its spirit could return to the mother and be born again. In Belgium it was thought that the child would be lucky if the caul were buried in a field, unlucky if the membrane were burned or thrown on the trash heap.[41,50,78,107] The owner would have great misfortune[47] or even die if the caul were lost[93] or torn.[57]

There is a curious report that when a child was christened, the caul was secretly baptized.[50] It was frequently worn in the clothes or carried in an amulet as a protective agent.[41,47,50,76,80,103] The caul might even be eaten by the owner in an egg dish, according to Hovorka and Kronfeld.[50] In the islands near New Guinea, a child washed with water in which the caul had been steeped and later fed the powdered caul would be freed of the power of clairvoyance,[36] which evidently was not always regarded as an asset. On the other hand, in Pomerania it was believed that if the caul were burned to a powder and then given to the baby with its milk, the child would become a vampire.[103]

In Germany and elsewhere in Europe the midwife sometimes stole the caul, according to report, to give it to another child,[50,107] perhaps her own,[78] or to sell it to a witch.[34,48] The latter were reported to prize cauls highly as potent aids in their evil doing. Vesalius[101] makes passing reference in the *Fabrica* to preservation of the caul by ignorant people of some races, adding that both the midwives and the "secret philosophers" greatly coveted this membrane. It is quite clear, however, that Vesalius spurned the superstition.

The *Journal de L 'Estoile pour le Regne de Henri IV*,[59] a colorful account of daily events in Paris in the sixteenth century, tells how two priests who were also practitioners of witchcraft battled for a caul in a church on 21 October 1596. It seems that one, *le sorcier*, forgot to take his caul with him when he left the altar. The other, finding the caul, refused to return it, whereupon a noisy quarrel followed *avec grande scandale de tout le peuple*. The finder of the caul succeeded in retaining it, but was promptly accused of sorcery and thrown into prison. He subsequently escaped with the help of his friends and proceeded to take his revenge on his colleague. That possession of a caul was thought to be worth such a scandalous episode clearly illustrates the strength of the superstition at that time.

Twenty-one years later Louise Bourgeois, famed midwife to the court of France, in a textbook of obstetrics (intended for her daughter), spoke her mind on the ethics of midwifery.[18,40] Mme. Bourgeois issued a specific warning about the caul (206): "*Ne retenes jamais la membrane amnios (dit la coiffe de l'enfant, de laquelle aucuns enfans viennent couverts la teste & les epaules) d' autant que les sourciers s' en servent*"—that is, never preserve the caul, as it may be used by sorcerers. One such use is suggested in Burton's *Anatomy of Melancholy*;[30] a list of ingredients for love potions or "philtres" includes dust of a dove's heart, rope with which a man was hanged, tongues of vipers, and "the cloak with which infants are wrapped when they are born" (498). Brissaud [19] tells how girls would ask the women assisting in a delivery to save the caul, "believing that if this powder were given to a man, he would at once fall in love with a maiden." In Germany a young man might carry his caul with him to aid him in winning the affection of a girl.[78] In the southern Slavic countries a girl wore her caul as a love charm; if she then touched the skin of a man, he would instantly be attracted to her.[50] Lean (1903)[58] reports that in Scotland there is the expression, *rowed in his mother's sark-tail*, that is, wrapped in his mother's shift, as well as the belief that an adult who as a baby had been so protected would be successful in his love affairs. It is suggested that all this related to the superstition about the caul as a love charm.

According to *The Golden Bough*, on the island of Timor the owner of a caul may use it as a charm to save a failing rice crop.[36]

The caul was frequently believed to confer eloquence on its owner. Several sources report that St. John Chrysostom (347?–407 A.D.), one of the Fathers of the Church, inveighed against the superstitious use of the caul as an aid to persuasive speech, but a rather extensive search of his writings has not disclosed the passage. However, Theodorus Balsamo,[8,69] a twelfth century canonist who likewise criticized employment of the caul as a charm, tells of a prefect who "was arrested while evidently carrying in his bosom a caul [*indumentum*] of a newborn infant, and said this had been given to him by a certain woman for the purpose of turning away and stopping up the mouths of those who tried to speak against him." Whence he was the subject of condemnation Aelius Lampridius[33,35,63,69,86] tells how the Roman midwives made off with cauls, which could be sold to credulous lawyers. The latter believed that possession of the membrane would help them to plead their cases successfully. The same superstition appeared also in Iceland, Denmark, England, and elsewhere in Europe.[9,50,107]

The caul was considered valuable as a remedy, both general and specific. From Norse mythology came the belief that if the caul had been dedicated to the Norns, giant goddesses who held men's fates in their hands, childbirth would be easy.[79] In Denmark it was thought that if a woman crept under a foal's caul stretched on sticks she would have a painless labor, but as a penalty her sons would become were-wolves and her daughters nighthags.[68] Ambroise Paré refers[73] to the belief that birth with a caul confers happiness. He adds the clinical suggestion that in a difficult birth the amnion would always be stripped away from the infant, just as "the Snake or Adder when she should cast her skin thereby to renew her skin, creepeth through some strait or narrow passage."[52] Mauriceau, in his textbook of obstetrics,[65] rejects the superstition and dryly remarks that children with cauls "may be said to be fortunate, for having been born so easily; and the Mother also for having been so speedily delivered; for the difficult Labours, Children are never born with such Caps, because being tormented and pressed in the Passage, these Membranes are broken and remain there" (cf. Paré's comment, above).

Sir Thomas Browne[20] recognized the caul superstitions of his period: "Great conceits are raised of the involution or membranous covering, commonly called the Silly-how, that sometimes is found upon the heads of children upon their birth; and is therefore preserved with great care, not only as medical in diseases, but effectual in success, concerning the Infant and others; which is surely no more than a continued superstition." According to Thomas Bartholin,[10,12] the caul could be made into a medicine and hand lotion for mother and child. He adds a matter-of-fact commentary on the state of professional ethics: if the midwife preparing such a concoction used a substitute for the caul, she could be arrested!

Hovorka and Kronfeld[50] have described an old remedy for malaria. Its remarkable ingredients include snails, egg white, laurel berries, powder from a burned piece of shirt, rust from a coffin nail, a pinch of burned and powdered human bones, *and* a powdered caul. Unfortunately, the rationale for this masterpiece is not stated. In Dalmatia, the caul was placed under the owner's head when he lay on his deathbed so that his passing would be easy.[80]

If the caul could bring good health, it could also ward off disaster and danger. There is a relatively recent report of an English farmer who ascribed his own good health and that of his two sons, then fighting in World War I, to the fact that each of them carried the caul of a lamb born in the farmer's flock.[102] This would seem to be simply an extension of the idea of the protective influence of the human caul. (One recalls that both the human amnion and the caul proper were sometimes described in terms comparing them to lambskin.)

Coal miners carried cauls to prevent the explosion of fire damp.[19]

One of the most widespread of all the caul superstitions was that it would protect against drowning.[19,53,54] Perhaps the most impressive support for this idea is a perfectly serious statement quoted in *Notes and Queries*[54] regarding a baby born with a caul so effective "that when his mother tried to bathe him he sat on the surface of the water, and if forced down, came up again like a cork." McKenzie,[66] Fairfax-Blakeborough,[34] and others have suggested that the belief in the caul's ability to preserve its owner from drowning is assumed from the membrane's investment of the fetus while it is immersed in the amniotic fluid. Naturally the caul had a particular appeal to sailors. Thomas Hood, the humorous poet, told[49] of a "jolly mariner" who defied a storm because "in his pouch, confidingly, He wore a baby's caul." However, the charm did not prevent disaster in a great storm:

Heaven never heard his cry, nor did
The ocean heed his caul.

Cauls were formerly offered for sale near the London and Liverpool docks,[4] and advertisements for this commodity appeared in British newspapers until at least the First World War:[91] in the *Daily Advertiser* for July 1790, in the *London Times* for 20 February 1813 and 8 May 1848, in the *Bristol Times and Mirror* for 30 September 1874 ("TO SEA CAPTAINS: For sale, a Child's Caul in perfect condition. £5."), in the *Globe* for 24 July 1903 ("Large Male Caul for sale; no reasonable offer refused.), etc.[48,55,64]

The prices asked for cauls, while perhaps little influenced by the supply, which must have been reasonably constant, certainly fluctuated with demand. The latter seems to have been regulated largely by the degree of hazard of the sailor's life and his consequent concern for his safety. Thus, one reads that in 1779 as much as 400 marks was paid for a caul. By 1799 the price paid by British sailors reached 30 guineas. (These were the days of Lord Nelson and great sea battles.) By 1815 the price was down to 12 guineas, and by 1848 a caul was advertised for sale in *The London Times* for 6 guineas. The advertisement states that the caul, "for which fifteen pounds was originally paid, was afloat with its late owner thirty years in all perils of a seaman's life, and the owner died at last in the place of his birth." In 1874 a caul was offered "TO SEA CAPTAINS" for £5. In 1895 a newspaper advertised a price of £5 "or offers"; a week later another advertisement (apparently by another owner) had cut the price to £1 "or offers." A still lower point was reached in the last years before the First World War, when cauls could be purchased for a few shillings. Superstition, however, had not died; when later the deadly submarine campaign was taking its toll, worried sailors and their friends paid as much as £3 to £5 for the protective membrane.[23,34,64,68,91,103]

The longevity of some superstitions is surprising until one realizes that the basic phenomenon is often the desire to believe. Fear of the future, worry over personal safety, uncertainty as to a favorable outcome—all these are facets of man's terror of the unknown. One battles the terror in various ways. The educated man is deprived by his very education of most of his ability to believe blindly, and sophistication usually cloaks the lingering remnants of his credulity. (We have seen that belief in the protective value of the caul was rejected by the physician.) Hence he is likely to seek through a reasoned approach some relief from his fear of the future. On the other hand, every age, every culture has provided an abundance of superstition for those who would accept it. The good health, success, and safety offered by the caul beliefs are tempting enough. It is small wonder that these superstitions have persisted. It is likely that they will continue to survive.

Mention must now be made of a group of related beliefs. Witkowski[106] says that the *hippomane*, a potion of the ancients, contained as one of its ingredients the fleshy membrane covering the head of a foal at birth. Classical writers applied the term *hippomanes* to a fleshy mass said to be found on the head of a newborn foal. It appears that the hippomanes and the equine equivalent of the caul, although different structures, have been confused. Both are unusual remnants of the fetal membranes, and the relevant superstitions have much in common.

In ancient times and down through the Middle Ages, *hippomanes* (Latin, Greek; French, *hippomane*; German, *Fullengift, Fohlenmilz, Fohlenbrot,* etc.) might signify a poison, a love potion or ingredient thereof, a plant which produces estrus in the mare, estrus itself, the estrous secretion, or particularly a bit of dark flesh said to lie on the forehead of the newborn foal.[6,26,27,56,71,72,82,94,97,100,106] According to recent interpretations the hippomanes is the result of a local accumulation of the secretion from the glands of the pregnant uterus. The enlarging mass causes in the horse the progressive invagination of the overlying area of chorio-allantoic membrane into the allantoic cavity or, in the lemur, into the yolk sac.[45,94] When fully formed the hippomanes consists of a small round or elongate mass of viscous material invested with chorio-allantoic or chorion-yolk sac membrane; the membrane also provides the pedicle connecting the structure to the inner surface of the allantois or yolk sac proper. Thieke states[94] that the hippomanes may even become detached and lie free in the allantoic cavity between the embryo and its membranes.

One can imagine that a foal might be born with either a folded amniotic fragment (the equivalent of the human caul) or a true chorio-allantoic hippomanes adhering to its head; presumably such an occurrence inspired the inaccurate classical concept. Aristotle describes[6] the growth as black, round, and smaller than a dried fig. The mare, he says, promptly bites off and swallows the hippomanes; if someone steals it (as a love charm), its smell makes the mare frantic. The mass was highly prized as the ingredient of potions. Vergil tells[99] how Dido, desperate because Aeneas was going to leave her, asked a witch to cast magic spells. The witch invoked the deities of darkness, and scattered herbs and water from Lake Avernus:

quaeritur et nascentis equi de fronte revulsus et matri praereptus amor.
—"and the hippomanes [*amor*, literally, the love], snatched from the forehead of a horse at birth, forestalling the mother, is sought."

In the first century A.D., Lucan, discussing love potions, mentions[62] the hippomanes as a powerful agent. Juvenal and Suetonius both tell[56,92] how the Empress Caesonia prepared a love potion from the hippomanes for her husband Caligula; the philtre, however, drove him mad.

Pliny, writing in the first century,[77] Aelian[2] and Solinus[87] in the third century, and Photius in the ninth century[75] followed Aristotle closely in their descriptions of the hippomanes. Aelian added that the mare's rage when the *caruncula* is stolen is due to her jealousy of the sorcerers who would make use of the mass in potions for human beings.

After Europe emerged from the Dark Ages, references to the hippomanes again appeared. Porta mentioned it in his *Magiae naturalis*[81] in connection with love potions, as did Wierus in a chapter entitled *De Veneficis.*[104] (It is noteworthy that *Veneficis* signified both sorcerers and poisoners, just as *veneficium* meant both witchcraft and poisoning.) Ruini's fascinating book on the horse[84] told, as Thieke has pointed out,[94] of a structure which certainly must be the hippomanes, although Ruini did not give it a name. In a horn of the uterus of the pregnant mare, he says, there has been found an unattached mass which is usually lead-colored, egg-shaped, "and about a half-finger thick if the mare has not carried it for long." Ruini believed that this mass was the poisonous residue of the semen. Clauder remarked[25] that "What the hippomanes actually is, and what its proper use may be, has exercised the wits of physicians and philosophers in many ages." He rejected the superstitions, including the idea that prompt removal of the mass ensured that the foal would become a swift racer and the belief of a colleague that the administration of 10 grains of dry hippomanes would protect a child against epilepsy.

Bayle's great dictionary discussed[13] the hippomanes superstitions in some detail, but did not imply their current acceptance. A few years later, in 1755 and 1756, Daubenton[28,29] published what appear to be the first attempts to investigate the hippomanes in scientific fashion. As a comparative anatomist particularly interested in the horse, he dissected many pregnant mares and repeatedly found gelatinous masses in the uterus between, he says, the allantois and the amnion. He concluded: "*Cette expéri-ence prouve clairement que l'hippomanes est un sédiment de la liqueur contenue entre l'allantoïde & l'amnios. . . .*" He also suggested[28] that very rarely a colt might be born with a hippomanes bound to its forehead by an amniotic remnant or *calotte,* like the infants "*qui nais-sent coëffés, selon l'expression vulgaire. . . .*" He reported[29] finding the hippomanes of the donkey, cow, deer, goat, and ewe.

Buffon in his *Histoire naturelle*[21] and Bourgelat in a volume on veterinary medicine[17] both discussed the hippomanes with considerable understanding. Sind, in another vet-erinary text,[85] supported the incorrect idea that the hippomanes is a piece of fetal membrane. Nineteenth century works on comparative anatomy described the struc-ture less erroneously and in more detail.[16,24] It remained for Thieke[94] and Hamlett,[45] however, to dispel misunderstanding of the phenomenon by explaining it. The term *hippomanes,* horse madness, itself survives, testimony to a superstition of the days when biology was born.

References

1. Adelmann, H. B.: *The embryological treatises of Hieronymus Fabricius Aqua pendente.* Ithaca, N.Y., Cornell University Press, 1942. pp. 248, 270, 747, 765.

2. Aelianus, Claudius: *De natura animalium . . .* London, Gulielmus Bowyer, 1744. Lib. III, cap. XVII; Lib. XIV, cap. XVIII.

3. Andrews, Edmund: *A history of scientific English.* New York, R. R. Smith, 1947. p. 39.

4. Anon.: Cauls. Lancet, 1899, I, 137.

5. Arey, L. B.: *Developmental anatomy.* Philadelphia and London, W. B. Saunders, 1945. p. 105.

6. Aristotle: *Historia animalium.* Translated by D. W. Thompson. Oxford, Clarendon Press, 1910. Book VI, 18, 572a; Book VI, 22, 577a; Book VIII, 24, 605a.

7. Babcock. W. H.: Folk-tales and folklore collected in and near Washington, D. C. Folk-lore J., 1888, 6, 85.

8. Balsamo, Theodorus: *Canones sallctorum patrum qui in Trullo . . . convenerunt.* In: Migné, J. P., *Patrologiae cursus completus . . . Series graeca,* Paris. 1865, 137, columns 722-723.

9. Bartels, Max: Isländischer und Volksglaube in Bezug auf die Nachkommenschaft. Ztschr. f. Ethnologie, 1900, 32, 52.

10. Bartholinus, Thomas: *De insolitis partus humani viis. . . .* Hafnia, Matthia Godicchenius, 1664. pp. 158–159.

11. Bartholin. Thomas: *Antiquitatum veteris puerperii synopsis.* Amstelodami, Henricus Wetsten, 1676. pp. 111–112.

12. Bartholin, Thomas: *Neu-verbesserte Künstliche Zerlegung des Menschlichen Leibes.* Nürnberg, Jo-hann Hofmann, 1677. pp. 321–322.

13. Bayle, Pierre: A general dictionary historical and critical. Translated by J. P. Bernard, Thomas Birch, John Lockman, and others. London, James Bettenham, 1741. Vol. X. pp. 356–364.

14. B. B.: Derivation of "caul." Notes and Queries, 1852, ser. I, 5, 557.

15. Beauvois: Les superstitions médicales du Bas-Berry. France méd., 1902, 49, 40.

16. Blumlenbach, J. F.: *A manual* of *comparative anatomy.* Translated by William Lawrence. Re-vised by William Coulson. London, W. Simpkin and R Marshall, 1827. p. 361.

17. Bourgelat, M.: *Éléments de l'art vétérinaire.* Paris, 1769. (Cited by Thieke, 1911.)

18. Bourgeois, Louise: *Observations diverses, sur la stérilité, perte de fruict, foecondité, accouchements, et Maladies des femmes et enfants nouveaux nais:* Paris, A. Saugrain, 1617. Book II, p. 206.

19. Brissaud, Edouard: *Histoire des expressions populaires rélatives a l'anatomie, à la physiologie et à la médecine.* Paris, G. Masson, 1892. pp. 320–321.

20. Browne, Sir Thomas: *Pseudodoxia epidemica.* London, printed by T. H. for Edward Dod, 1646. Book V, Chap. 22, Section 17.

21. Buffon: *Histoire naturelle.* Paris, Imprimerie Royale, 1753. Vol. 4, p. 214.

22. Cestriensis: Family caul-child's caul. Notes and Queries, 1853, ser. 1,7,546.

23. Chanter, H. P.: Folk-lore: cauls. Notes and Queries, 1923, ser. 12,12,58.

24. Chauveau, A.: *The comparative anatomy of the domesticated animals.* Translated and edited by George Fleming. New York, W. R. Jenkins, 1873. pp. 897–899.

25. Clauderus, D. Gabr.: *De hippomane.* In: *Miscellanea curiosa sive ephemeridum . . . Norimbergae, 1685.* Decuriae II, Annus tertius, Observatio LXIII, pp. 165–166.

26. Collin de Plancy: *Dictionnaire infernal.* Paris, P. Mongie, 1826. Vol. III, p. 249.

27. Collumella, L. Junius Moderatus: *Of husbandry.* Translated. London, A. Miller, 1745. Book VI, Chap. 27.

28. Daubenton: *Mémoire sur l'Hippomanès. Histoire de l'Acad. roy. des sci., année 1751.* 1755, pp. 293–300.

29. Daubenton: *Observation sur la liqueur de l'Allantoïde. Histoire de l'Acad. roy. des. sci., année 1752.* 1756, pp. 392–398.

30. Democritus Junior [Robert Burton]: *The anatomy of melancholy.* Oxford, Henry Cripps, 1638. p. 498.

31. Dickens, Charles: *The personal history of David Copperfield.* London, Bradbury & Evans, 1850. p. 1.

32. Digby, George: *Elvira, or the worst not always true.* 1667. In: *A select collection of old Plays.* London, Septimus Prowett, 1827. Vol. XII, Act V.

33. Drelincurtius, Carolus: *Opuscula medica. Hague comitum, apud Gosse & Neaulme, 1727.* pp. 507–515.

34. Fairfax-Blakeborough, J.: Folk-lore: cauls. Notes and Queries, 1923, ser. 12, 12,9.

35. F.C.H.: A child's caul. Notes & Queries, 1857, ser. 2, 3, 397.

36. Frazer, Sir J. G.: *The magic art and the evolution of kings.* In: *The golden bough.* New York, Macmillan, 1935. Vol. I, pp. 187–188, 190–191.

37. Galen, Claudius: *De usu partium corporis humani.* Lyon, G. Rouille, 1550. p. 836.

38. Galien, Claude: *De fusage des parties du corps humain.* Lyon, Guillaume Rouille, 1566. p. 886.

39. Gemma, Cornelius: *De natura divinis characterismis Antverpia, Christophorus Plantinus, 1575.* Lib. I, Cap. VI, pp. 88–89.

40. Graham, Harvey: *Eternal Eve.* Altrincham, Wm. Heinemann, 1950. p. 13.

41. Grimm, Jacob: *Teutonic mythology.* Translated from the fourth edition by James Steven Stallybrass. London, George Bell, 1883. Vol. II, pp. 874–875.

42. Grimm, Jacob, and Grimm, Wilhelm: *Deutsches Worterbuch.* Leipzig, S. Hirzel, 1873.

43. Haller, Albrecht von: *La generation . . . Traduite de la Physiologie de M. de Haller.* Paris, Des Ventes de la Doue, 1774. Vol. II, p. 23.

44. Haller, Albrecht von: *Onomatologia medico-chirurgica completa, oder Medizinisches Lexicon.* Frankfurt and Leipzig, Stettin, 1775. Columns 31, 622.

45. Hamlett, G. W. D.: The occurrence of hippomanes within the yolk sac of lemurs. Anat. Rec., 1935, 62, 279.

46. Hansemann, D. von: *Der Aberglaube in der Medizin und seine Gefahr für Gesundheit und Leben.* Leipzig and Berlin, Teubner, 1914. pp. 27–28.

47. Hastings, James, ed.: *Encyclopaedia of religion and ethics.* New York, Scribner, 1910. Vol. II, pp. 639, 663; Vol. VIII, pp. 44–45.

48. Hazlitt, W. C., ed.: *Popular antiquities of Great Britain.* Edited from the materials collected by John Brand, F.S.A. London, John Russell Smith, 1870. pp. 139–142.

49. Hood, Thomas: *The sea-spell.* In: *The Poetical works of Thomas Hood.* Edited by Epes Sargent. Boston, Phillips, Sampson, 1857.

50. Hovorka, O. von, and Kronfeld, A.: *Vergleichende Volksmedizin.* Stuttgart, Strecker & Schroder, 1908. Vol. I, p. 188; Vol. II, pp. 327, 593–594.

51. Hyrtl, Joseph: *Die alten deutschen Kunsworte der Anatomie.* Wien, Wilhelm Braumüller, 1884. pp. 81–82.

52. Johnson, Th.: *The works of the famous chirurgeon. Ambrose Paré, Translated out of Latin and compared with the French.* London Mary Clark, 1678. p. 545.

53. Jones, W. H., and Kropf, L. L., translators and editors: *The folk-tales of the Magyars.* London, Stock, 1889. pp. 120, 378.

54. J. T. F.: A child's caul. Notes and Queries, 1899, ser. 9, 3, 26.

55. J. T. F.: Caul. Notes and Queries, 1904, ser. 10,1,26.

56. Juvenal: *Satires.* Translated by G. G. Ramsay. London, Wm. Heinemann; New York, G. P. Putnam, 1928. Satire VI, lines 614–617.

57. Leach, Maria, ed.: *Funk & Wagnalls' Standard dictionary of folklore, mythology and legend.* New York, Funk & Wagnalls, 1949.

58. Lean, V. S.: *Lean's collectanea.* Bristol, J. W. Arrowsmith. 1903. Vol. II, Part I, p. 99.

59. Lefèvre, Louis-Raymond: *Journal de L'Etoile pour le Règne de Henri IV.* Paris, Gallimard, 1948. Vol. I, entry for 21 Oct. 1596.

60. Lemnius, Laevius: *The secret miracles of nature.* London, Jo. Streater, 1658. p. 105.

61. Lewis, C. T. and Short, Charles, eds.: *A New Latin dictionary.* New York, American Book Co., 1907.

62. Lucanus, M. Annaeus: *De bello civili.* Translated by J. D. Duff. London, Wm. Heinemann, 1928. Book VI, lines 454–456.

63. Magie, David: *The Scriptores historiae Augustae.* London, Wm. Heinemann; New York, G. P. Putnam, 1924. Vol. II, section 4.

64. Malins, Edward: Note on obstetric superstition. Obstet. J. Great Britain and Ireland, 1874, 2, 9.

65. Mauriceau, Francis: *The diseases of women with child mid child-bed.* Translated from the French by Hugh Chamberlen. London, R. Ware et al., 1755. p. 132.

66. McKenzie, Dan: *The infancy of medicine.* London, Macmillan, 1927. p. 327.

67. Melton, John: *Astrologaster, or, the figure-caster.* London, Barnard Alsop, 1620. pp. 45–46.

68. M. G. W. P.: The caul, silly-how, or silly-hood. Notes and Queries, 1897, ser.8, 11, 234.

69. Migné, L' Abbé: *Encyclopédie théologique.* Tome vingtième: *Dictionnaire des Superstitions, erreurs, préjugés, etc.* Paris, J. P. Migné, 1856. Columns 225-226.

70. M. P.: Folk-lore: caul Notes and Queries, 1889, ser. 7, 8, 284.

71. Murray, J. A. H.. ed.: *A new English dictionary on historical principles.* Oxford, Clarendon Press, 1893.

72. Ovidius Naso, P.: *Amores.* Translation by Grant Showerman. Cambridge, Mass. Harvard University Press; London, Wm. Heinemann, 1947. I, viii.

73. Pareus, Ambrosius: *Opera.* Paris, J. Dupuys, 1582. p. 686.

74. Pettigrew, T. J.: *On superstitions connected with the history and practice of medicine and surgery.* Philadelphia, Barrington and Haswell, 1844. pp. 115–116.

75. Photius: *Myriobiblion, sive Bibliotheca librorum quos Photius Patriarcha Constantinopolitanus legit & censuit* Antwerp, Andreas Schott, 1621. pp. 1574-1575.

76. Pitkin, F. H.: Ancient superstitions that still flourish. Practitioner, 1909, 83, 848.

77. Plinius Secundus, C.: *The histoire of the World.* Translated into English by Philemon Holland. London, Adam Islip, 1601. Tome I, Book 8, Chap. 42, p. 222; Tome II, Book 28, Chap. II, pp. 326–327.

78. Ploss, H.: Die Glückshaube und der Nabelschnurrest: ihre Bedeutung im Volksglauben. Ztschr. f. Ethnologie, 1872, 4, 186.

79. Ploss, H.: *Das Kind in Brauch und Sitte der Völker.* Leipzig. Th. Grieben, 1884. p. 13.

80. Ploss, Heinrich, and Bartels, Max and Paul: Das *Weib in der Natur- und Völkerkunde.* Berlin, Neufeld und Henius, 1927. Vol. II, pp. 861–864.

81. Porta, I. B.: *Magiae naturalis, sine de miraculis rerum naturalium.* Antverpia, Christophorus Plantinus, 1560. Lib. II, Cap. XXVII.

82. Propertius. Sextus: *Elegiac.* Translated by H. E. Butler. London, Wm. Heinemann, 1929. Book IV, Section V, lines 17–18.

83. Ratcliffe, Thos.: A child's caul. Notes and Queries, 1899, ser. 9, 3, 175.

84. Ruinus, Carolus: *Anatomia et medicina equorum noua.* Frankfurt am Mayn, Matthias Becker, 1603. Book 4, p. 169.

85. Sind, J. B. von: *Vollständige Unterricht in den Wissenschaften eines Stallmeisters.* Göttingen and Gotha, 1770. [Cited by Thieke, 1911.]

86. Smith, William, ed.: *Dictionary of Greek and Roman biography and mythology.* Boston, Little and Brown, 1849. Vol. I, p. 996.

87. Solinus, Gaius Julius: *Polyhistory.* Poitiers, Enguilbert Marnes, 1554. p. 122.

88. Spence, Lewis: *An encyclopaedia of occultism.* London, George Routledge, 1920.

89. Spigelius, Adrianus: *De formato foetu.* Patauii, de Martinis & Pasquatum, 1626. p. 10.

90. Spindler, Paul: *Observationum medicinalium centuria.* Francofurti ad Moenum, Philippus Fievetus, 1691. p. 121.

91. St. Swithin: A child's caul. Notes and Queries, 1899, ser. 9, 3, 26.

92. Suetonius Tranquillus, Gaius: *Gaus Caligula.* In: *The lives of the Caesars.* Translated by J. C. Rolfe. London, Wm. Heinemann; New York, G. P. Putnam, 1930. Book IV, Section L.

93. Sykes, W.: Child's caul. Notes and Queries, 1886, ser. 7, 2, 145.

94. Thieke, Arthur: *Die Hippomanes des Pferdes Inaug.* -Diss. Jena, Gustav Fischer, 1911. Also in: Anat. Anz., 1911, 38, 454, 464.

95. Thiers, J.B.: *Traité des superstitions qui regardent les sacremens.* Paris, Compagnie des Libraires, 1741. Vol. I, p. 367.

96. Thomas, D. L., and Thomas, L. B.: *Kentucky superstitions.* Princeton, Princeton University Press, 1920. p. 10.

97. Tibullus. Albius: *Carmina.* Lipsiae, Caroli Tauchnitii, 1829. Liber II, Elegia IV, line 58.

98. Timbs, John: *Doctors and patients.* London, Richard Bentley & Sons, 1873. p. 149.

99. Vergilius Maro, P.: *Aeneidos.* Translated by H. R. Fairclough. Cambridge, Mass., Harvard University Press; London, Wm. Heinemann, 1938. Book IV, lines 509–516.

100. Vergilius Maro, P.: *Georgica.* Lib. III, ver. 280. [Cited by Bayle, 1741.]

101. Vesalius, Andreas: *De humani corporis fabrica.* Basileae, Ioannis Oporinus, 1543. p. 543.

102. Weeks, W. S.: Folk-lore: cauls. Notes and Queries. 1923, ser. 12,22,75.

103. Weissbart, Max: Der Aberglaube im Geschlechtsleben der Frau. Mutter und Kind, 1906, 2, 172, 182, 198, 212, 227.

104. Wierus, Ioannes: *De prae stigiis daemonum, & incantationibus ac ueneficiis Librifex . . . Basileae, ex officina Oporiniana,* 1577. p. 382.

105. Wirsung, Christophorum: *Arzney Buch.* Heydelberg, J. Mayer, 1568. p. 452.

106. Witkowski, G. J.: *Histoire des accouchements chez tous les peuples.* Paris, G. Steinhil, 1887. p. 196.

107. Wuttke, Adolf: *Der deutsche Volksaberglaube der Gegenwart.* Berlin, Wiegandt & Grieben, 1900. p. 381.

Editor's Introduction   8
Roasting, Smoking, and Dieting in Response to Birth: Malay Confinement in Cross-Cultural Perspective

LENORE MANDERSON

IN CHAPTER 8 (taken from *Social Science & Medicine* 15B [1981]: 509–520), Manderson describes the usual forty-day Malaysian period of confinement that helps women compensate for their body's change from the so-called hot state of pregnancy to a cold state believed to be caused by parturition. The confinement involves behavioral and dietary rules that purportedly reestablish the mother's equilibrium. It is viewed as an indispensable respite from the everyday demands of life and is reputed to prevent postpartum depression as well as to ensure good health later in life.

In contrast, in the United States, parturients usually have few formal rituals that acknowledge their new status as mothers. American women long ago dismissed the advice of Dr. John Whitridge Williams (1866–1931), of the famous *Williams' Obstetrics* text, who advised women to stay in bed for three weeks, and then remain in their rooms to adjust to movement out of bed for an additional week (see H. Speert, *Obstetrics and Gynecology in America: A History* [Baltimore: Waverly Press, 1980]). Similarly, a well-known nineteenth-century obstetrician, Dr. Hugh L. Hodge, recommended that women remain recumbent in bed almost constantly for one month lest premature exertion damage the recovering body or cause ailments later in life (H. L. Hodge, *The Principles and Practices of Obstetrics* [Philadelphia: Blanchard and Lea, 1864]).

Some American organizations decry the modern lack of recuperative period for parturients. Both the American College of Obstetricians and Gynecologists and the American Medical Association have protested insurance company–induced shorter lengths of postpartum stay, commonly just twelve to fifteen hours. Problems of premature hospital discharge go beyond women's ability to recover physically and bond with their babies; heavy bleeding and infections can occur in mothers. In addition, jaundice in infants usually does not appear until twenty-four to thirty-six hours after birth. Although easy to treat with special ultraviolet lights, untreated jaundice can cause brain damage after only a few days. Experts in the field are considering whether home visits can fill the void, particularly in Western culture where extended family may not be available to assist and to help identify danger signs.

There are several excellent accounts of the period of confinement found in other cultures. J. R. Hanks, "The Birth of a Child in Bang Chan, Thailand," in her *Maternity and Its Rituals in Bang Chan*, Cornell Thailand Project Interim Reports Series 6 (Ithaca: Department of Asian Studies, Cornell University, 1963), 41–57, describes a Thai birth that focuses on a two-week period of "roasting." In the postpartum roasting (lying by a hot fire), heating and drying are believed to make a woman strong by drying out the womb and restoring her health, firmly establishing her role as a mother. This practice lasts anywhere from a few to about forty days depending on the culture (forty is a ritual number in Islamic culture). Diet also follows rules of hot and cold wherein the new mother eats only foods considered "hot" (e.g., salted rice, dried fish, and baked bananas). Such food restrictions continue until a child is weaned (i.e., for up to about two years). The dietary prohibitions are taken seriously, as indicated by the following admonition, "Drink no cold water, or you will die" (p. 55). For additional discussion of the notions of hot and cold derived from Chinese humoral medicine, see B.L.K. Pillsbury, "'Doing the Month': Confinement and Convalescence of Chinese Women after Childbirth," *Social Science and Medicine* 12 (1978): 11-22; E. Jensen, "Iban Birth," *Folk* 8–9 (1966–67): 165–178; C. Frake, "Post-Natal Care among the Eastern Subanun," *Silliman Journal* 4 (1957): 207–215; D. Sich, "Traditional Concepts and Customs on Pregnancy: Birth and Post-Partum Period in Rural Korea," *Social Science & Medicine* 15B (1981): 65–69; and C. V. Foll, "Some Beliefs and Superstitions about Pregnancy, Parturition and Infant Health in Burma," *Journal of Tropical Pediatrics* 5 (1959): 51–58. Incidentally, Foll reports one of the most bizarre customs surrounding conception and birth—the Burmese veneration of a mummified and calcified fetus, believed to bestow wealth and good luck on the parents. For this reason, women carrying dead fetuses are loath to have them removed. Also strange is the consumption of human placentas for prevention of valvular heart disease. While Westerners may dismiss such nutritional customs on the grounds that they lack scientific support, critics have questioned the validity of some of Americans' deeply entrenched parturition-related dietary prohibitions that commenced in the 1940s. Prior to the 1940s, doctors assumed women needed energy for the arduous task of labor (see L. M. Ludka and C. C. Roberts, "Eating and Drinking in Labor: A Literature Review," *Journal of Nurse Midwifery* 38 [1993]: 199–207; J. Broach and N. Newton, "Food and Beverages in Labor. Part I: Cross-Cultural and Historical Practices. Part II: The Effects of Cessation of Oral Intake during Labor," *Birth* 15 [1988]: 81–85; M. Matthews and L. Manderson, "Vietnamese Behavioral and Dietary Precautions during Confinement," *Ecology of Food and Nutrition* 11 [1981]: 9–16; L. Minturn and A. W. Weiher, "The Influence of Diet on Morning Sickness: A Cross-Cultural Study," *Medical Anthropology* 8 [1984]: 71–75; and G. Hochstein, "Pica: A Study in Medical and Anthropological Explanation," *Essays on Medical Anthropology*, edited by T. Weaver [Athens: University of Georgia Press, 1968]).

Americans might assume that the ban on food and drink in labor is based on science, not custom. Yet such safeguards are in place for potential cesarean sections, even though most who undergo this procedure are *not* given general anesthesia (which necessitates fasting). Furthermore, while most physicians assume that there is a risk of aspirating vomit (in which the resulting blockage of the trachea impedes breathing and aspirated stomach acid can damage the lungs and/or result in infection), there is some question about whether consumption of food and drink during labor actually increases this risk. Since the stomach is never totally empty, and great care should always be exercised with general anesthesia, the ban on eating and drinking may not be warranted and may actually adversely affect pain suffered and the length of labor (Ludka and Roberts, 1993). In any case, there is a lack of evidence that demonstrates the need for the food and drink ban. Recent studies suggest that the risk from such consumption may have been overestimated.

In addition, American women also have had various food prescriptions and proscriptions postpartum such as obstetrician Hodge's recommendation that a woman's diet "should always be 'low,' that is, of simply farinaceous articles, neither too hot nor cold, as the former might prove too exciting, while cold drinks might cause intestinal or uterine pain" (Hodge, p. 208). Recommendations for the amount of weight gain during pregnancy also have varied, including when doctors told women to limit weight gain, advice now rejected in order to protect the unborn child. Yet even today, we might compare other cultures' strict, seemingly oppressive dietary regulation to Americans' contrasting lack of regulation that for some includes consumption of cigarettes, caffeine, alcohol, junk food, and drugs (legal and illegal), which probably have more significant repercussions on the fetus than dietary rules such as those followed in some nonindustrial countries.

For further reading on Malaysian births, see P.C.Y. Chen, "An Analysis of Customs Related to Childbirth in Rural Malay Culture," *Tropical and Geographical Medicine* 25 (1973): 197–204; C. S. Wilson, "Food Taboos of Childbirth: The Malay Example," *Ecology of Food and Nutrition* 2 (1973): 267–274; and C. Laderman, "Giving Birth in a Malay Village," in *Anthropology of Human Birth*, edited by M. A. Kay (Philadelphia: F. A. Davis Company, 1982), 81–100.

Lenore Manderson, a fellow of the Academy of Social Sciences in Australia, is a medical anthropologist and social historian, and professor of women's health at the University of Melbourne. She has published numerous articles and a number of books including *New Motherhood* (with Mira Crouch; New York: Routledge, 1993), which explores women's perceptions of childbearing, as well as *Global Health Policy, Local Realities: The Fallacy of the Level Playing Field: Directions in Applied Anthropology* coedited with Linda M. Whiteford (Boulder, Colo.: Lynne Rienner Publishers, 2000) and *Violence against Women in Asian Societies*, coedited with Linda Rae Bennett (New York: Routledge Curzon, 2003).

Roasting, Smoking, and Dieting in Response to Birth: Malay Confinement in Cross-Cultural Perspective

8

LENORE MANDERSON

ACCORDING TO HUMORAL MEDICAL THEORY, food and body states may be classified as "hot" or "cold." During periods of physical vulnerability, behavioral and dietary precautions may be invoked for therapeutic and prophylactic purposes following the humoral medical principle of the treatment of opposites. Childbirth in particular affects humoral balance, and in confinement precautions are observed to replace heat lost during parturition and to protect the mother against cold and wind. Women in Asia and Latin America especially share several postpartum precautions, including physical confinement, restrictions on bathing, the prescription of hot and proscription of cold foods; for many women these precautions are supplemented with the direct application of heat, including by "mother roasting," steaming, or smoking. The postpartum precautions, as detailed for Malay women, provide a framework for the management of birth and the ritual and social assumption of motherhood.

Introduction

Women in traditional or less industrialized societies are perhaps more familiar than Western women with birth as a personal and social experience. However, few women in any culture actually witness or participate in delivery until they have delivered their own first child, and birth loses none of its mystery either with the education of women concerning the physiological changes or pregnancy or with the medicalization of delivery.[1] Thus, regardless of its formalization birth remains subject to mystical interpretation and magical intervention. Women in modern industrialized societies no less than in small-scale communities follow dietary and behavioral precautions to ensure a healthy pregnancy, safe delivery and rapid recovery, acting upon their own and others' beliefs regarding both physical changes and metaphysical and ritual vulnerability.

As Dana Raphael points out, giving birth does not automatically make a mother out of a woman.[2] In some cultures, a woman is a mother from the time of the detection of pregnancy; in others, the status of motherhood is conferred only after the delivery of an infant of the "right" (usually male) sex, or after the infant is already several months old.[3] Pregnancy, parturition and the puerperium are all stages in the process of mother-becoming, a *rite de passage* which Raphael has termed "matrescence." In Western societies particularly, this critical process is overlooked and woman are considered to have become mothers with delivery. Socially this is not the case however. Women who deliver in hospitals in effect become mothers on discharge, at which time they are given "ownership" and full responsibility for their newborn.[4] The ritualized handing over of infant from mothercraft nurse to biological mother serves poorly to prepare the mother for the years of mothering ahead and little recognizes the importance to her of becoming a mother; this contrasts sharply with the ritual provisions in other cultures wherein pregnancy-parturition-confinement constitute a continuum interrupted and punctuated by the actual birth of the child.

In particular, those cultures with a history of humoral medical theory have an especially rich scripting for the management of childbirth and the preparation of the woman as a new mother. This preparation includes dietary and behavioral prescriptions that operate throughout the pregnancy and for an extended period postpartum. In accordance with humoral medicine and concepts of hot and cold, women may avoid excessively "hot" foods during pregnancy; after birth, they avoid "cold" foods, may be confined to a particular area of the house, wear warm clothing and may "roast," or "steam" as a further measure for recovery.

In this paper, we shall examine humoral medical tradition and childbirth practices in Malay society, focusing on the therapeutic and prophylactic measures invoked for postpartum women. The substantive data presented in the paper are based on fieldwork undertaken by the author in peninsular Malaysia in June–July 1978 and from November 1978 to May 1979, when information relating to childbirth and food habits was collected from extensive open-ended interviews with key informants and from a questionnaire completed by 278 women from five states.[5] Following discussion of humoral medical theory and the treatment of pregnant and puerperal women, and the presentation of the empirical data, we shall then consider these measures cross-culturally to explore and move towards understanding the basis of these beliefs and practices.

Humoral Medicine and the Theory of Hot and Cold

Humoral medical theory spans all continents. Medical and ethnographic records attest its survival in the cultures of Africa, Asia, and the Americas; dispersed fragments of the theory continue in folk tradition from Europe to Australia.[6]

For many cultures, humoral theory is assumed to derive from the classical traditions of Hippocrates and Galen. Accordingly, the body is composed of four elements (earth, fire, air and water) corresponding to four humors (black bile, yellow bile, blood and phlegm) which are characterized by varying combinations of the four natural properties (hot, cold, wet and dry): earth and black bile are cold and dry; fire and yellow bile are hot and dry; air and blood hot and wet; water and phlegm cold and wet.[7] This theory was borrowed into Arabic medical tradition during the early Islamic period; into Anglo-Saxon culture in the eleventh and twelfth centuries: into Iberia culture with the occupation of the peninsula by the Moors; and was taken by adventurers and conquerors to the New World: humoral beliefs and practices there diffused to folk culture and/or integrated with indigenous concepts of hot and cold.

Humoral pathology occurs also with some variation in the Ayurvedic tradition of Indian medicine, although in this case there are only three prime fluids or *dosa* (wind, gale and mucus).[8] The influence of Greek humoral theory on Indian medicine and of Ayurvedic theory on Greek nosology remains debatable; the extent of cross-cultural borrowing between the Arabs and Indians is no less clear. Again there are certain remarkable similarities between classical humoral theory and Chinese medicine although any direct relationship between the two remains in question[9]: according to Chinese traditional medicine, the body has two vital forces or ch'i of opposing qualities of yin (cold) and yang (hot) and is subject to the laws of the five elements (earth, fire, water, wood and metal).

The incorporation of humoral pathology into indigenous medical and folk beliefs in Southeast Asia reflects the dominant politico-cultural influences of the region and reinforces theories of acculturation from a foreign "great tradition" into local "little traditions." Humoral medicine observed in Burma, Thailand, Laos, and Kampuchea derives largely from Ayurvedic tradition brought with the Sanskritization of mainland Southeast Asia. Vietnamese traditional medicine suggests some Indian influence but derives predominantly from Chinese tradition. In the Philippines, as Hart has argued,[10] humoral medicine was introduced by Spanish colonists. In the Malayo-Indonesian world, Muslim traders and missionaries were probably the major bearers of the tradition, but political and cultural links with Hindu and Buddhist India and trade links with China suggest origins possibly more diffuse.[11] Again, there remains the possibility of the indigenous origin of these beliefs.

In popular form and as observed today, the critical element of the tradition is the classification of the body and foods as hot and cold, with a lesser emphasis also on the effect of wind or air. The ranking of hot and cold by degree, and the parallel classical differentiation of wet and dry, have largely disappeared in all cultures where humoral medical theories have existed and where a simple hot-cold dichotomy continues.[12]

According to humoral medical theory, health is maintained through equilibrium. Disease disrupts the hot-cold balance of the body and in diagnosis the body is said to have an excess of hot over cold, or an excess of cold over hot. Treatment involves adjustment of the diet to redress the imbalance: illness diagnosed as hot is therefore treated with cold food and/or medicine; cold illness is treated with hot food and medicine. Physiological changes, including pregnancy and confinement, youth and old age, also alter humoral balance and thus, for example, the elderly should avoid excessively cold foods. The overindulgence of hot or cold foods can similarly disrupt internal equilibrium; again, health may be restored by the dietary treatment of opposites. The classification of foodstuffs and medicines generally relates neither to the temperature of the item, nor to its spiciness or raw or cooked state, but to the reputed effect of the food on the body.[13] Thus a "hot" food is said to heal the body; a "cold" food cools the body. Whilst the classification of food and medicine is variable, essentially individual, and at times arbitrary both across and within cultures, in general most fruits and vegetables are classified as cold whilst meat, fried foods and condiments are considered to be hot.[14]

Hot and Cold in Pregnancy and the Puerperium

As noted above, physiological changes including pregnancy and confinement alter the humoral balance of the body and behavioral and dietary precautions may be invoked to protect the woman's health in a state of physical as well as magical vulnerability.

The diagnosis of pregnancy in accordance with humoral pathology varies across cultures. Malays regard pregnancy as a hot state and appropriate dietary precautions operate for all three trimesters: with the recognition of conception, to prevent miscarriage; in later months, to prevent the birth of a large infant and thus to avoid a difficult and prolonged labor.[15] Topley, however, reports that Cantonese traditionally consider that the pregnant mother is polarized in the direction of cold and the fetus in the direction of hot; hence expectant mothers avoid foods either definitely hot or cold which might cause further polarization, generating "wind" and condensing "poison" in the womb.[16] Vietnamese women consider the expectant mother and fetus to be in a cold and "non-tonic" state during the first trimester, a neutral state in the second trimester and a hot and "tonic" state in the third trimester: thus the consumption of hot and cold, tonic and non-tonic foods are adjusted during the course of pregnancy, whilst the consumption of excessively hot and cold foods are avoided throughout.[17] Amongst the northern Thai pregnant women should avoid becoming physically warm through contact with heat or fire, but this prescription appears to relate to fear of retention of the afterbirth rather than to the diagnosis of pregnancy as a hot state.[18] In other cultures with a tradition of humoral medicine, there is further variation relating to the diagnosis of pregnancy and the prescription foods.[19] Exact classification of pregnancy is therefore problematic.

Women from several cultures consider that hot food (or medicine) taken in the first trimester will act as an abortifacient and thus restrict their intake of foods thus classified.[20] However, the majority of food taboos during pregnancy appear to be invoked for magical rather than (humoral) medical reasons and are in the interest not of the mother but of the health of the unborn child and its appearance at birth. Moreover, in Malay society and in many other cultures, pregnancy is not considered an overly vulnerable state, traditional behavioral and dietary precautions are frequently ignored and prenatal care is not a major concern.

Parturition brings about an abrupt change to the woman's ritual and physical state and in most societies with a humoral medical tradition strict behavioral and dietary restrictions apply. The management of birthing, including the nature of decision-making, the involvement of others, the position of the parturient during labor, and the response to the newborn and the newly delivered mother, are all culturally determined and vary considerably. But near universally in cultures with a humoral medical tradition, parturition is believed to deplete the woman of heat and to place her in a state of especial vulnerability to cold.[21] Postpartum practices aiming to protect the woman from cold and wind and to restore her to health bear remarkable similarity cross-culturally.

Childbirth, then, depletes the mother of heat, blood and "air" or vital breath, and renders her vulnerable to cold, wind, magic, and disease.[22] Coldness may prevent the circulation of blood, inhibit the discharge of lochia, delay the woman's recovery, or cause illness and even death either immediately or at a much later date. Protective restrictions for the newly delivered mother are therefore taken seriously. The woman is confined to her home and often to a well-sealed room for from 4–6 weeks. During this time, she dresses in warm clothing. Frequently her bathing is restricted or her bath water especially prepared with hot herbs and spices for her protection. Her diet is strictly prescribed to include only foods, beverages, medicines and herbs that are classified as manifestly hot. Frequently too the additional precaution of mother roasting or smoking is undertaken to provide heat externally to dry out the womb. This latter practice is notable in Southeast Asia but is not unknown in other societies with a tradition of humoral medicine. Below, we shall consider in detail the puerperal restrictions as they apply to Malay women in peninsular Malaysia, then examine the evidence of similar restrictions in other cultures.

Postpartum Confinement in Malay Society

As already noted, in Southeast Asia the application of hot and cold properties to foods, disease and body states is part of and a remnant from an extensive humoral medical tradition. Hart's monograph is perhaps the best known study of humoral pathology in the region and provides a comprehensive analysis of hot and cold food classifications and beliefs.[23] His work amongst Malays, however, has several antecedents: Newbold (1839), Maxwell (1883), Skeat (1900) and Gimlette (1913) provide us with early studies of Malay culture, magic and medicine with reference to humoral pathology of assumed Islamic origin.[24] In 1958 and 1959 Margaret McArthur undertook a pioneer study in two Malay *kampungs* (villages) in the west coast states of Melaka and Perak: her unpublished study offers extensive information of anthropological and nutritional interest.[25] Christine Wilson's doctoral dissertation provides further information regarding food habits and beliefs for a Trengganu Malay village (east coast);[26] recently Carol Laderman has also undertaken research in Trengganu on humoral beliefs, nutritional status, medicine and magic.[27] Wilson, Siti Hasmah, Chen, Fraser and

Millis describe variations of the traditional lying-in period of postpartum women, during which time dietary restrictions are but one of a number of precautions taken to prevent the new mother catching cold and to replace lost heat.[28]

The following section of this paper draws from and builds on the above works. As indicated above, the substantive data are drawn from fieldwork in Malaysia in 1978 and 1979, which included a lengthy questionnaire delivered to 278 Malay, Chinese, Tamil and Thai women who presented at maternal and child health clinics in five states: Negri Sembilan and Melake to the southwest of the peninsula, Penang and Kedah in the northwest and Trengganu on the east coast. The descriptive material included below is taken from interviews with a number of key informants, all middle aged multiparous Malay women who are identified with pseudonyms. One of the women, "Mak Enjar," was a practicing traditional midwife (*bidan*) in Singapore; she, like other *bidan* in the peninsula, supervises the majority of births and confinements in rural areas.

As discussed above, in accordance with humoral pathology Malay women believe that pregnancy is a hot state, that with parturition heat is lost and the woman moves to a state of excess cold, and that during the postpartum period of 40–44 days, care should be taken to restore the woman to a state of equilibrium. Her diet and behavior is prescribed to this effect. The most dramatic of these precautions is the custom of "mother roasting" which, as noted above, is common throughout Southeast Asia.

A number of variations of puerperal roasting and smoking exist within Malay society. Christine Wilson describes one of the most complete methods of roasting, one that she observed in the east coast state of Trengganu in 1968–9.[29] According to her account, women, confined in the home, sleep and lie much of the day on a wooden platform or roasting bed (*salin*), beneath which a fire is burnt, to shrink swollen tissues, dry up the blood and prevent hemorrhage. Traditionally, the *bersalin* is observed for 40 days, although in both confinements witnessed by Wilson, roasting ceased after one month. In one of these cases, the woman spent less than two hours a day on the platform and was fairly active during her confinement; in the other, the woman spent some five hours daily lying over the fire. Chen similarly reports the practice of roasting by lying over a fire for one or two hours at a time, two or three times a day, during a 44-day confinement.[30] Throughout this period the woman is usually heavily dressed, notwithstanding often oppressively warm weather, with cardigans and stockings or socks, to provide further protection against cold and wind. Chen notes too the use of a large heated stone (*tungku*), wrapped with herbs, applied to the woman's abdomen when she was not lying over the fire, and the massage of the limbs, neck, back and chest with special "hot" herbs for the first three days postpartum.[31]

Lying on a platform over a fire is but one variation of "mother roasting" observed by Malays and is only part of a variety of puerperal practices designed to "dry out the womb" and restore the new mother to health. The variation described by Wilson and Chen is still observed on the east coast of the Malay Peninsula and hospitals in

Trengganu report several cases of third-degree burns amongst newly delivered women each year.[32] By contrast, Fraser reports that in his study community in South Thailand, women lie beside, not over, the fire for a 40-day period.[33] And Asmah, one of my informants from the northwest state of Kedah, reported the following *berdiang* observed from the third or fourth day postpartum to the 44th day:

> Mustard and other seeds are thrown on a charcoal burner so the smoke is spicy. You sit (naked) virtually over the burner, a blanket over you and the burner as a tent, and you sweat in the spicy smoke. Then you have a bath with certain leaves. After the oath, the stomach is oiled then covered with (powdered) lime (*kapur sireh*, used in chewing betel) and lime juice (limau nipis). The four or five yards of bengkung, a very thick strong cloth, are wound from under the bust to the knees: this forces you to take little steps so your muscles are not stretched. At the end of the 44 days, you feel fresh and firm, with no stretch marks.

Asmah elaborated that during pregnancy the woman's pores opened and she absorbed air, and was thus vulnerable to unhealthy and evil elements. Parturition increased her vulnerability by depriving her of heat and by placing her in a polluted state that attracted evil spirits.

Safiah, another Kedah informant, observed the *berdiang* after bathing under the supervision of a traditional midwife, but only for half an hour a day and only from the 39th to 44th day of her confinement. She used mustard seeds, fenugreek and the leaves and dried roots from *tutup bumi* (*Elephantopus*) to spice the smoke: she explained that the smoking cleansed the body of "dirt" including smell and caused the vagina to shrink. Whilst she observed the roasting for a protracted period only, she applied an iron (tungku) to her abdomen for the full 44-day period from 7:00 to 8:30 in the morning, after bathing and from 5:00 to 6:30 each evening. Safiah explained that the iron was heated for about two hours on charcoal first, then placed on leaves such as *daun gelanggang* or Cassia leaves, *daun kankung laut* or *Ipomoea digitata* and *daun tahi ayam* or *Ageratum conyzoides* and wrapped in cloth; the weight of the iron varied according to the individual. Safiah bathed daily in the morning in warm water with lemon grass, Pandanus leaves and camphor plant leaves (*Blumea balsamifera*), then rinsed with flower water bought from a Chinese shop and dusted herself with powder, including sandalwood to smell nice. Heated lime and lime juice was then applied to the abdomen, and the binding wrapped: Safiah, though, used alcohol spirit and wore a Western corset instead.[34]

Adibah, a Singapore Malay, also reported smoking or *ganggang*. In her detail of puerperal custom, mustard seed, fenugreek and coriander are tied in a bag of cloth and boiled in bath water, then guava leaves are thrown in. This spicy water used for bathing serves to keep out the "wind" and helps to heal the woman internally. After the morning bath, the woman undergoes the *berganggang*, with benzoin and mustard seeds being thrown on the charcoal to smoke the birth canal. The sweat from the smoking is then rubbed off. Next green coconut oil is applied to the abdomen to prevent irritation, after which the lime and lime juice is applied before binding. A small 12-inch-deep cloth is used for the first two or three days postpartum; thereafter the wider *bengkung* is used. In addition, fresh cloves are boiled in water until the water is thickly spiced; this water is to be used by the confined woman to wash her crotch after urination. According to Adibah, bathing should be avoided on wet and cool days, but the smoking and binding is a daily ritual regardless.[35]

Other behavioral practices relate less clearly to humoral medical theory. Asmah, from Kedah, ground cinnamon bark with water to apply to her forehead, to keep away wind and to avoid headaches from wind entering the temples. Adibah, from Singapore, maintained that eyesight was poor after birth, and that a mixture of lime, *sepang* bark (*Caesalpinia sappan*) and rose water should be applied on the forehead over the eyes continually to keep the head cool and help restore the eyesight: according to her, then, the body should be kept warm but the head cool. Mak Enjar, a Singapore midwife, explained that the paste on the forehead prevented "white blood" going to the eyes: she ground together for the paste onions, cummin, *kayu serapat* (*Salacia flavescens*), cloves, tailed pepper, *cekur* (*Phyllanthus frondosus*), and guava or *turi* (*Sesbani grandiflora*) leaves.

Further prescriptions protect the newly delivered mother from supernatural risks. Aswah explained that evil spirits were attracted to the mother because she was polluted. Women postpartum tie their hair in a tight bun with a nail through it to ward off evil spirits, and place *daun geroda* over the door for the same purpose.[36] Women should not knit, sew, or cut throughout the confinement, since blood would spurt out of any wound, causing lockjaw and death. Women are considered most vulnerable magically from the 41st to 44th day of their confinement and should be especially careful to observe the behavioral restrictions, avoiding cutting themselves or stubbing a toe at that time.

The above puerperal practices, or variations thereof, are not observed uniformly amongst peninsular Malays. Haslinda from Kuala Pilah, Negri Sembilan, reported that in her village, 3 or 6 days after parturition (but not the 4th or 5th day), the midwife massaged the whole body of the mother to "bring up the womb" as a prelude to binding using pure coconut oil made in the village and prayed over by the midwife. Haslinda was familiar with variations of roasting and smoking but they were not practised in her community: she suggested it was a custom in Johore and Perak and amongst Javanese residing in Negri Sembilan.

As noted above, roasting and smoking are part of a broader set of puerperal behavioral prescriptions aimed at protecting the newly delivered mother from cold and wind, which include her confinement in a room well-sealed against draughts, the use of herbs, and warm water for bathing and wearing heavy clothing. These precautions are reinforced by extensive dietary restrictions.

Like the behavioral precautions, dietary precautions vary throughout the peninsula. Immediately after delivery, a cup of tamarind pulp, sugar and warm water may be drunk by the woman to expel lochia from the uterus.[37] Asmah, a Kedah informant, did not refer to this drink, but recounted that for the first three days postpartum, first thing in the morning she drank a juice from turmeric root (*kunyit*) and rock salt to "tighten her inside." For the next three days, she drank juice from fresh ginger root and rock salt; thereafter she took a concoction of boiled coconut water, lemon grass and herbs. At other times, she drank water boiled with ginger and a little sugar, to warm her and get rid of the "air" inside her. Haslinda from Negri Sembilan took the turmeric and salt juice for the full 44 days postpartum, using about half a kati (c. 300 g) of turmeric root each time; she maintained that this juice helped flatten the stomach, improved the blood and kept the woman looking youthful. Haslinda also drank daily *ubat periuk* from a root boiled in water, believed to be "good for the womb." Adibah from Singapore prepared the juice of turmeric with honey and egg yolk as a morning tonic for the full 44 days, but noted that some women found this mixture unpalatable and ceased after the seventh day. Mak Enjar, the midwife from Adibah's village, prescribed to her patients a daily dose of *ubat periuk* which included in its preparation turmeric and ginger, *seperantu* (*Sindora sumatrana*) and pepper and introduced other herbs or jamu, such as *semangkok* seeds (*Scaphium affine*) after the fifteenth day of confinement. Safiah, another Kedah informant, ground fresh turmeric with seven different flowers and warm water to take for the three mornings from the 39th day of her confinement: she took Dom Perignon champagne for the 44-day period, then *rempah ratus* (100 spices) twice a day for a further month.[38] Others took *makyun*, a mixture of spices and lemon grass fried in coconut oil, to shrink the uterus and to strengthen abdominal muscles. All informants, and the women of the larger survey I undertook, at other times during their confinement drank warm ginger water and occasionally coffee, and strictly avoided plain water, other "cooling" beverages, and usually tea.

Similarly, solid foods are restricted. In general cold foods, including most fruit and vegetables, are proscribed; hot foods are prescribed. Wilson reports an ideal diet of rice, roasted fish, black pepper and coffee, and although the observed diets of young mothers in her study village included some other foods, general proscriptions were observed and had serious implications for the mother's health.[39]

A variety of reasons exist to explain the extensive food proscriptions. Respondents to the survey maintained that cold foods could cause swelling, increase the lochia discharge and make the uterine and vaginal muscles "watery"; failure to observe the proscriptions could cause "aching veins" in later life. Oily foods could also make the uterus "watery." Sharp foods, such as pineapple, vinegar and sour mango, caused rashes and caused veins to swell although certain sharp foods, such as *pangaga* and *maman* shoots, were believed by some women to help the womb shrink. Eggs, "itchy" fish (including a large number of salt water fish and seafood such as crab and prawns), and sometimes also chicken and beef were avoided since they might inhibit the woman's general recovery and prevented healing where the perineum had torn or where the woman had had an episiotomy. Food described as "windy," including cucurbits and tubers, were also generally avoided, although some women argued that the consumption of windy food forced the body to expel other wind or air within the body. Other foods classified in a personalized and arbitrary fashion as "poison" (*bisa*) were again avoided, since they would weaken the woman, inhibit her recovery and could cause convulsions, coma and death.

From key informants and the surveyed women, some 120 foods and groups of foods were listed as proscribed. Over half the women included all cold foods, cold vegetables, or fruit and vegetables; others distinguished particular cold foods only, including certain bananas, coconut, water, cabbage, *kankung* (ipomea leaves), mustard greens, spinach, beans, gourds and cucumbers. Papaya was proscribed, by one informant for three months postpartum, or the woman's stomach would not go down; watermelon would make the uterus weak and "watery." High water content foods in general, including soups (e.g. *laksa*) and watery curries (*kuah*) were to be avoided. Windy foods including yam, taro, sweet potato, cassava, and jackfruit were occasionally considered taboo; sharp foods including mangos, citrus fruit and bamboo shoots were more frequently proscribed. A wide variety of fresh water fish and seafood was also proscribed, although baked or dried fish including *ikan bilis* (anchovy), *ikan kembang* (mackerel) and *ikan parang* (wolf herring) were considered safe and in fact constituted a major part of the confinement diet of Malay women.

Observance of these dietary taboos was variable. Most women followed a traditional confinement and its dietary demands for at least part and usually the full term. However, some 10% of survey respondents ignored traditional procedure and did not modify their diet in any significant manner either because they were under medical supervision, because they were taking (Western) medicine which they believed rendered the traditional precautions unnecessary or because they felt that such practices were too much trouble and had no real effect.

Heat in Confinement in Cross-Cultural Perspective

The extensive behavioral and dietary restrictions described above are by no means peculiar to Malay society. Both Indian and Chinese women in Malaysia similarly believe that a woman loses heat in childbirth. During confinement, observed by both ethnic groups for 30 days, the woman must restore her body to a state of equilibrium and protect herself from catching cold or "wind." Most dietary and other practices relate to these beliefs.

Indian women take hot drinks such as coffee and hot foods such as garlic and onions for the first three days after delivery. On the third day, the newly delivered mother bathes with margosa and tamarind leaves to relieve aches and pains and to encourage lactation. She takes special spicy food, such as a curry of coriander, chili and salt fish and avoids all cold foods including most fruit and vegetables. For the first 15 days of confinement, she takes a tonic which includes garlic, ginger, pepper, rice, nutmeg and cummin and which is said to relieve backache and aid lactation; she also eats daily a cummin seed, asapheotida tide and palm sugar mixture.[40]

Similarly Chinese women should only eat hot foods. Only ginger water, a broth made from fried rice and ginger, may be drunk. Chicken should be dry-baked in hot salt, steamed with wine, or stewed with sesame oil and rice wine. Pork liver may be eaten, fried with ginger and linseed oil, to "renew the blood." Turmeric may be taken to expel wind and to tighten the uterine muscles: ginger steamed with Chinese medicine (*leng seng yuen*) is also taken to expel wind; a drink (*char lat*) made from cockroach droppings and dried eggshell serves the same purpose. Cold foods, including food cooked the previous day, plain water, fruit and vegetables, are proscribed for fear of asthma, rheumatism, arthritis and other aches and pains.[41] Bathing is proscribed until the twelfth day of confinement, and then only in warm water; after bathing the woman should drink warm rice wine with pork and ginger to protect herself against wind. Hair may not be washed for the first 21 days to avoid headaches and wind.[42]

Variations of these practices are common in other Indian and Chinese societies. Pillsbury reports extensive taboos applied for a full month of convalescence in Taiwan. When women "sit out the month" to restore the body's imbalance and to prevent ailments in later life, restrictions include refraining from bathing and hair-washing; confinement to the home; the proscription of cold and prescription of hot foods; and avoiding exposure to wind, including from a fan or air conditioning. Other restrictions involved are based on belief in the polluting powers of placental blood.[43] Studies of women in India provide similar evidence of therapeutic measures to restore lost heat. Katona-Apte reports that in South India, confinement may last from 10 to 40 days. The woman is considered dirty and defiling, and often stays within a small poorly lit and ill-ventilated area of the house. For the first 3 days postpartum, she takes only coffee; for as long as 6 weeks, her diet is severely restricted.[44] Shosh reports a similar restricted diet for 9 days postpartum; Eichinger Ferro-Luzzi provides extensive details of food taboos, particularly of foods classified as cold or windy (*vayu*), which are observed for the first month after delivery.[45] Many of the food proscriptions relate to the ascribed effect of the food on the infant, transmitted through breast milk, as well as the effect of the food on the mother in terms of hot and cold.

Whilst dietary restrictions, physical confinement and restrictions on drinking, bathing and washing hair in ordinary water are common, the particular practices of the external application of heat, including "mother roasting," appear to be confined in Asia to the Southeast Asia region.

Several descriptions exist of mother roasting and related puerperal prescriptions in Thailand.[46] In its traditional form, women lie by a ritually lit and extinguished fire (*yu fai*), covered with turmeric to prevent burning, for much of the confinement period.[47] Hanks argues in her description of the ritual that whilst drying out the womb is a manifest function, lying by the fire serves several purposes: the fire magically perfects the mother as a compassionate and moral being; strengthens and restores her health by ridding her of bad blood and dangerous fluids; transforms her to a better nourisher, granting her lasting and beneficial nursing habits; and strengthens her *khwan* or soul to withstand spirits. Lying by the fire, then, treats the physical effects of child-birth but serves also to bring the woman to full maturity as a mother: "Maturity did not come just by bearing a child. The fire brought about the transformation."[48] Hanks notes that the "fire-rest" was optional rather than mandatory, but most women in Bang Chan underwent the ritual al least once.

Mougne reports three alternative methods to lying by the fire in northern Thailand. In one, *khao sao* ("entering the tent"), a well-heated stone or brick is placed in a freshly dug pit in the floor of the house, over which the woman con-structs a tent from a woven mat and towelling or cloth. She then places leaves and/or bark on the stone, squats over it and pours boiling water onto it, thereby creating steam causing her to sweat heavily. In a second method, *rom ya* ("to inhale medicine"), the woman squats over a pot of boiling herbs and bark, again under a tent or a blanket to concentrate the steam. Lying by the fire continues for a 15-day period, whilst the two smoking/steaming methods are undertaken for 2–3 days, for half an hour at a time, towards the end of the confinement. A third alternative to lying by the fire, undertaken nightly from the fourth or fifth day postpartum and for as long as the woman wishes, involves the application to the woman's ab-domen of a heated brick with pounded herbs and bark, wrapped in a cloth.[49] Women believe that drying out the womb is an effective means of birth control as well as relaxing the mother and protecting her from ailments.

Amongst Thai women as amongst Malays, lying by the fire and variants of smoking/steaming are only part of the confinement, which includes physical con-finement, restrictions on bathing, heavy clothing, stomach binding, avoidance of smells, the proscription of a wide range of foods and the prescription of a wide range of foods and the prescription of especially hot foods. Hanks, for example, re-ports a strict diet of rice with salt, dried fish, baked banana and boiled water.[50] Mougne notes also the proscription of unboiled water which is believed to congeal blood in the womb; her informants drank throughout confinement a special drink from water boiled with a root (*Zingiber cassumunar*) and ate a limited amount of rice cake and salt, roast pork and certain vegetables.[51]

Variations of these confinement practices occur elsewhere in Southeast Asia also. In Burma, women observe a 7-day confinement to the delivery room, with steam bathing, sitting on hot rocks or bricks, smearing the body with turmeric, regularly drinking turmeric powder in water to encourage sweating, following a special diet of salt fish and avoiding cold foods (including in this instance meat, eggs and mill, as well as fruit and vegetables), all to purify the mother and restore bodily balance.[52] Lao women similarly roast and inhale hot water for a 25-day confinement.[53] Vietnamese women remain in a well-sealed and darkened room for 30 days; like Malay women, they lie on a bed over a charcoal burner for the full month, take a herbal steam bath thrice daily, are massaged with ginger and saffron, place warm bricks or warm salt on their abdomen, strictly avoid cold and toxic food and ideally eat only rice gruel with salt and pepper.[54] Filipino women may be roasted by lying beside a stove for up to 30 days after delivery to stop the lochia, restore the uterus to pre-delivery position, and to alleviate soreness; alternatively they may squat over a clay stove with live coals under an improvised tent or sit on a chair over hot water, stones, and burning twigs. In some areas, women are "bathed" in smoke from smouldering leaves; they are massaged with coconut oil; and are forbidden cold food, including water and other foods which might cause the uterus to "slip" or cause hemorrhaging.[55] Similarly, Iban women, nominally Christians, apply a poultice of ginger to their abdomen and sit with their back to the fire to "dry out"; ginger water only may be drunk for the first 3 days postpartum and their intake of ordinary water is limited for the first 7 days. Here, however, postpartum food taboos in general appear to relate to nonhumoral beliefs about the effects of foods.[56] Acehnese women in North Sumatra again lie on a platform over hot bricks for from 20 to the full 44 days of confinement, bathe minimally and are massaged with coconut oil. Food taboos are introduced only after the seventh day but may continue for 5 or more months: these taboos appear also to be peculiar to the region.[57] By contrast, there is no evidence of the treatment of puerperal women with heat in Java and Geertz reports a prescribed potion designed to cool, not heat, the mother.[58]

But mother roasting and like practices are not isolated to a Southeast Asian stage. Ethnographic data from societies with a history of humoral medicine provide evidence of the extensiveness of the taboo on cold foods during confinement as a therapeutic and protective measure for both the mother and child. In a number of cases (but not all), these dietary measures are reinforced by behavioral precautions which stress the avoidance of cold (e.g. proscriptions on bathing, confinement to a well-sealed room) and the application of heat (warm clothing, lying by a fire). Kelly and Manzanedo, for example, report for Mexican women an ideal diet as restrictive as that prescribed Malay women, to be observed for a 40-day confinement; additionally women avoided bathing, took herbal potions and douched with or bathed in the smoke of local plants.[59] Elsewhere, Kelly reports that the postparturient "cannot leave the house; she remains in her room; going out, she would be exposed to 'air.' This would give her sharp pains in the temples and eyes and would weaken her vision."[60] Kelly also reports a postpartum herbal bath in a makeshift sweathouse, believed to be vital to restore the health of the new mother.[61] Wiese reports that Haitian women customarily take a hot leaf bath and avoid cold foods during confinement.[62] Saunders refers to women standing in the smoke of dried petals over hot coals to prevent postpartum haemorrhage.[63] Griffin observes that amongst the Seri Indians of Mexico, the confined parents (both mother and father) lie beside a ritual fire for 4 days postpartum.[64] Métraux refers to the application of hot flat stones to the stomach of newly delivered mother on Easter Island where humoral medicine had been borrowed from Chileans.[65] Morgenstern provides instances of a 40-day confinement with mother roasting amongst Muslim Albanians, and a 40-day confinement with a taboo on bathing amongst the Bedouin of the Arabia desert.[66] The Hausa-Fulani of Nigeria again confine the newly delivered mother to a small room for a 40-day period, during which time she lies on a bed over a fire in order to "keep away the cold"; daily or twice daily she is bathed in near scalding water also.[67] And Bagnall reports that North African women squat over hot herbal water; Pondo women also lie by a fire.[68]

Further, puerperal practices relating to heat are not confined to areas where humoral medical theory was observed historically or where it is a living tradition.

In Anglo-Australian society, there is evidence of the treatment of confinement with heat that perhaps derived from medieval humoral medical practices. An Irish-born witch/herbalist/midwife who lived and practiced throughout her life (1888–1963) in a large Australian country town regarded the immediate postpartum period as a time in which the mother was vulnerable both physically and mentally. A woman over whose delivery she had presided was given a hot herbal bath in a large wooden tub 3–4 hours after delivery; she was then kept in a bed warmed with hot stones, water bottles, or earthenware carney jugs for the next 48 hours on a restricted diet, during which time the infant was not separated from its mother.[69]

In contrast, Janice Reid[70] has provided details of steaming/smoking ceremonies amongst a northern Australia Aboriginal community (the Yolngu) where there is no evidence of classical humoral theory; here, the ceremonies serve to purify individuals from a ritually or physiologically polluted state, including men following rites of revelation (initiation ceremonies), girls following their first menstrual period, and women postpartum. According to a male informant:

> And the baby—when it was born we didn't have a big hospital. We had a different law. When the baby was carried in the stomach and baby would be born in some place, the relatives would hold the woman round the chest and massage downwards so the baby was born himself. The mother (the mother's mother) made a fire with a stone in it and got the skin (inner bark) of the stringy bark tree (*Eucalyptus tetrodonta*) and put it in water and stringy-bark and leaves (put on top of the fire) and the woman sits (squats over) the fire which is a little bit hot. This makes them feel good so that the baby won't die. And they put their breasts in the fireplace to make plenty of milk for the baby to drink.

Traditionally, two ceremonies were held: the one described above immediately following delivery to promote the health of the infant, to encourage lactation, to provide protection against early re-conception, and to heal any perineal tearing; the second following the cessation of the lochia flow to free the mother of food taboos. Today, the two appear to have been collapsed into a single ceremony conducted, where the mother has delivered in a Western hospital, after her discharge.

Further instances of roasting, smoking, and dieting, presumably independent of the humoral classification of the puerperium as cold, follow a common theme. Cherokee Indians, for instance, massage the parturient with a fire-warmed hand to expel the placenta; the new mother should not eat any fish for the first few days postpartum "because fish have cold blood, and they would therefore chill the blood that has still to come out of her and would cause it to clot."[71] Among the Jivaro and the Kurtatchi, heat is applied directly to the vulva to stop the lochia flow; amongst the Tanala, women lie beside a smouldering fire for 8 days: amongst the Tabatulabal, women lie on a mat in a hot trench for 6 days.[72] Trobriand Island women traditionally lie for much of a month on a bed over a fire; according to Malinowski, "this is a matter of hygiene, as the natives consider such baking and smoking to be very beneficial for the health and a sort of prophylactic against black magic."[73] Thompson and Sahlins both note that in the past in Fiji the newborn infant was ritually steamed over a wooden bowl of cut leaves, water, and hot stone on the fourth day after birth: Sahlins notes too that the mother of a royal child was symbolically "cooked" (in fact steamed) following the birth of her first child.[74] Sahlins also reports that "a smouldering fire is kept burning near the mother and infant for ten days in the rear, sacred section of the house of confinement, and the doors of the house are tightly shut."[75] According to Teckle, in contemporary Fijian society heat is rarely applied directly either by steaming or by fire. However the notion of heat remains extremely important both for women during pregnancy and lactation and for the neonate. Women wear several layers of clothing and are massaged throughout pregnancy and during labor to keep their breasts and abdomen warm. A fire is lit as soon as possible after the onset of labor to prepare food for the mother: this food is eaten whilst it is still hot. The infant is dressed warmly to "keep out wind": the woman also continues to dress heavily to keep her breasts warm through lactation to ensure the production of milk.[76]

Rationales of Confinement Practices

Cross-cultural borrowing may explain the incidence of practices such as mother roasting in parts of Southeast Asia where there is no evidence of humoral pathology historically as amongst the Iban, but this is by no means the sole nor the obvious explanation of the coincidence of this phenomenon and fails to account either for the apparent autonomous existence of like practices in areas beyond the sphere of humoral influence or for the absence of many heat-related practices in areas with a tradition of humoral pathology. The preexistence and the indigenous origin of the treatment of birth with heat is therefore equally credible: accordingly, mother roasting and other treatments with heat of the new mother and infant were common in Southeast Asia and elsewhere; the introduction of humoral medical theory, with its diagnosis of pregnancy and confinement in terms of hot and cold, provided a new rationalization of these practices and reinforced their observation.

Western medical practitioners (and scholars) remain in disagreement about the value of the application of heat in response to birth; the proscription of fruit and vegetables has been attacked especially. But certain aspects of traditional confinement are accredited with some scientific basis: the confinement of the postpartum woman to the home ensures that she rests and avoids contact with carriers of infection; the emphasis on keeping the mother warm and out of draughts provides further protection in colder climates (e.g. China); the prescription of protein-rich foods provides her with nourishment which she may not ordinarily enjoy.[77] Thus certain puerperal practices may simply formalize through a set of rules the commonsense care of the woman and the neonate.

However, emic rationales provide the more substantial explanation for the endurance of the use of heat after birth. According to respondents, the taboo on cold foods, the consumption of hot foods and the direct application of heat relate to the need to expel the blood and to dry out the womb. Coldness, either from "cold" foods or the weather, may congeal the blood and inhibit its discharge. Harwood reports that Puerto Ricans believe that if the lochia is not expelled, it will flow to the head and cause "nervousness" or even insanity.[78] Many cultures force the post-parturient to remain upright for the first few days after birth to ensure that the lochia is discharged; others avoid cold environmentally and through ingestion to this end. Heat serves positively to "dry out" the womb, although it is not the only means by which the drying is achieved: other practices include the consumption of large quantities of salt or salty food (for example, among the Hausa-Fulani and Thai and Malay women), bathing in a strong saline solution, or, as in the case for women of Oman, South Arabia, salt-packing the vagina).[79]

The importance of measures to dry out the womb leads to a second rationale, whereby lochia like menstrual blood is considered to be defiling, and the woman polluted ritually and physically whilst the flow continues. In most societies where the confinement of women postpartum is strictly prescribed, women in fact are considered to be in a state of ritual pollution, and their participation in devotional, social and sexual activities may be prohibited or strictly limited. The use of heat in an institutionalized and circumscribed manner provides for the ritual cleansing of the newly delivered mother and establishes the means by which she may re-enter society.

But the use of heat, whilst significant, is only a constituent of the confinement practices which as a whole function to mark the final stage of the *rite de passage* of mother-becoming. Levi-Strauss extends the application of direct heat in various *rites de passage* to argue for the symbolic connotation of the use of heat whereby individuals who are "cooked" are always those deeply involved in a physiological process.[80] Accordingly the puerperal woman, by contact with heat, is "mediatized" and socialized.[81] Hanks pre-empted this argument when she argued, as outlined above, that no parturition, but the fire itself, made the woman a mother and brought her to maturity. Even it we reject this critical symbolic role of heat during confinement, the use of fire, hot water, hot food and so on provide the grammar to mark out birth. The use of heat-related practices marks as culturally and psychologically significant a biological-medical event; this in itself explains the persistence of particular confinement precautions regardless of the extent to which childbirth has been medicalized and subsumed within a Western health care system. For some women traditional postpartum practices are considered redundant: institutionalized care and Western medicine are believed to provide sufficient protection for both the new mother and child. However, in other cases Western medicine, treatment, and materials are incorporated into a traditional schema and the essential rationale for confinement behavior remains unchanged. Thus the perineal heat lamp, used to heal episiotomy wounds in Western-style hospitals in north Thailand, is rationalized as a Western development for "drying out the womb."[82] Northern Thai women place hot water bottles and metal containers filled with charcoal on their abdomens instead of lying by the fire;[83] Vietnamese women similarly replace charcoal braziers with hot water bottles, electric blankets, and radiators.[84] And, as noted above, Malay women replace the lime poultice and traditional *bengkung* binder with alcoholic spirits and a Western corset.

Ultimately, it is as a medium by which women are able to become mothers (and come to terms with becoming mothers) that the behavioral and dietary precautions of the puerperium are important. Medical personnel may indeed believe, like the doctor in Alma de Groen's play *The Joss Adams Show*, that giving birth is easy, "like having a shit after breakfast."[85] But for the expectant mother pregnancy, parturition and confinement remain events essentially unknown and understood until directly experienced. Prescriptions governing the diet and behavior of women which derive from traditional medical theories, including those from humoral pathology and those which draw independently on the virtue of heat, offer scripting for both the pre- and postpartum periods, thereby providing the mother and those around her with a specific cultural framework within which to manage birth.

References

1. In modern industrialized societies, ante-natal and postnatal classes provide critical support both institutionally and from non-kin peers, replacing in part support provided elsewhere by the mother, grandmother, aunts, and older sisters of the expectant mother and by other older non-related women. Ante-natal classes ensure that the expectant mother understands the physiology of pregnancy: hospital tours familiarize her with the birthplace. Even so, women attending ante-natal classes (at least in Australia) are usually shown all but the labor ward, and the experience of labor retains its mystery. Class members tend to reinforce each other's fears by recounting stories of difficult and prolonged labors, painful parturition and unhappy and problem-fraught early mothering experiences.

2. Raphael, D. Matrescence, becoming a mother, a 'new/old' *rite de passage*. In *Being Female. Reproduction, Power and Change* (Edited by Raphael D.), p. 66. Mouton, The Hague, 1975.

3. Raphael, *op. cit.*, pp. 66–67. Kitzinger notes that women may not even be considered wives until they have given birth to, and sometimes even weaned, the first child. See Kitzinger, S. *Women as Mothers*, p. 74. Fontana Books. Glasgow, 1978.

4. Anne Banning has recounted this social assumption of motherhood in an Australian setting. "Recently I visited a new mother and father who were leaving a maternity hospital with their five-day old baby girl: I saw re-enacted the age-old hospital custom symbolizing the hospital's ownership of the child unto mother and baby are discharged: the hospital sister carried the baby outside the hospital and was not allowed to hand over the baby until the father had brought the car to the hospital entrance.

"Then there was the ceremonial handing-over of the baby, with the hospital having discharged its responsibility. The excuse given was that the hospital maintains liability (and may be sued) while the baby is on the premises. The mother has very little responsibility (and therefore no ownership) while the baby is in the hospital. The father has no responsibility at all and is only allowed to see his baby by courtesy of the hospital, at times allocated to visiting." Banning A. Who owns the child. *The Australian*, p. 7. 1411 May, 1980. See also Raphael, *op. cit.*, p. 67.

5. This research was funded by grants from The Australian Research Grants Committee and The University of Sydney, and was undertaken by the author as a post-doctoral research fellow with the Department of Indonesian and Malayan Studies, the University of Sydney. Fieldwork in Malaysia was conducted in association with the Department of Malay Studies, The University of Malaya, and with the generous co-operation of the Medical and Health Departments in Kuala Lumpur and the five study slates. An earlier version of this paper was presented to the Department of Anthropology, The University of Adelaide. I am grateful to Janice Reid and Clive S. Kessler for their comments.

6. For a guide to the literature, see Logan, M. H. Selected references on the hot-cold theory of disease. *Med. Anthrop. Newslett.* 6, 8, 1975.

7. Lloyd, G. E. R. The hot and the cold, the dry and the wet in Greek philosophy. *J. Hellen. Stud.* 84, 92. 1964.

8. Basham, A. L. The practice of medicine in ancient and medieval India. In *Asian Medical Systems. A Comparative Study* (Edited by Leslie, C. S.), pp. 18–43. University: of California Press, Berkeley. 1976.

9. Anderson notes the temporally coincidental maturation of Greek, Ayurvedic, and Chinese medical traditions and suggests that the hot-cold classification was introduced from West Asia to China around the time of the Wan dynasty, where it integrated with the older Chinese concepts of *yin* and *yang.* See Anderson, E. N. "Heating" and "cooling" foods in Hong Kong and Taiwan. *Soc. Sci. Inform.* 19, 242, 1980. For an extensive discussion of hot and cold, yin and yang in Chinese society, see Ahern E. M. Sacred and secular medicine in a Taiwan village: a study of cosmological disorders. In *Medicine in Chinese Cultures: Comparative Studies of Health Care in Chinese and Other Societies* (Edited by Kleinman, A., et al.), pp. 91–113. Fogarty International Center, Bethesda, 1975. See also Gould-Martin, K. Hot cold clean poison and dirt: Chinese folk medical categories. *Soc. Sci. Med.* 12B, 39, 1978.

10. Hart, D. V. *Bisayan Filipino and Malayan Humoral Pathologies: Folk Medicine and Ethnohistory in Southeast Asia.* Data Paper No. 76, Department of Asian Studies Southeast Asia Program, Cornell University. Ithaca, NY, 1964.

11. Manderson, L. Traditional food classification and humoral medical theory in Peninsular Malaysia. *Ecol. Food Nutr.*, 11:1-8, 1981.

12. However, Anderson, *op. cit.*, p. 244, and Manderson, *op. cit.* report for Chinese and Malays respectively a loose system of ranking whilst the Burmese observe a sophisticated ranking system which distinguishes three types of hot, three of cold, one bland and two neutral categories of food, with other foods unclassified and excluded from the system. See Nash, M. *The Golden Road to Modernity: Village Life in Contemporary Burma*, p. 196. Wiley, New York. 1965. The wet/dry dichotomy continues notably in Chinese culture but covers few foods and is not very important, see Anderson, *op. cit.*, p. 245.

13. Whilst the ascribed physical effect emerges as the major criterion by which foods are classified as hot or cold, other factors may be used also. Logan reports that in Guatemala, the

origin of food, its colour, sex, nutritive value, physical effect and medicinal use all serve as criteria for identification; Anderson and Anderson argue that food which takes a long time to cook and is exciting to eat is hot whilst fresh and bland food is cold. See Logan M. M. Humoral medicine in Guatemala and peasant acceptance of modern medicine. *Hum. Org.* 32, 1973; Anderson, E. N. and Anderson, M. L. Cantonese ethnohoptology. *Ethnos* 34, 113, 1969; see also Anderson, *op. cit.*

14. My analysis of foods classified as hot and cold by Malaysian respondents (predominantly Malays and Chinese) indicated that cold foods have a higher water content, less protein, less fat, lower carbohydrate content, and fewer calories than hot foods but the range was broad. Frequently, too, there were contradictions: mutton and certain fruit such as rambutan (*Nephelium lappaceum*) and watermelon were classified by some respondents as hot, others as cold. See Manderson, *op. cit.* The generality is maintained but the contradictions more marked cross-culturally: Lewis, for example, reports that his Mexican respondents considered meat to be cold, see Lewis, O. *Tepoztlan: Village in Mexico*, p. 12. Holt, Rinehart & Winston, New York, 1960.

15. Manderson, L. Traditional food beliefs and critical life events in Peninsular Malaysia. *Soc. Sci. Inform.* 20:947-975, 1981.

16. Topley, M. Cosmic antagonisms: a mother-child syndrome. In *Religion and Ritual in Chinese Society* (Edited by Wolf, A. P.), p. 237. Stanford Univ. Press, Stanford, 1974.

17. Manderson, L. and Mathews, M. Vietnamese attitudes towards maternal and infant health. *Med J. Aust.* 1, 70, 1981. Both physical states and foodstuffs may be classified as tonic or anti-tonic, tonicity being applied to indicate items which increase the volume of blood and promote health and energy.

18. Mougne, C. An ethnography of reproduction. Changing patterns of senility in a Northern Thai village. In *Nature and Man in South East Asia* (Edited by Stott, P. A.), p. 73. School of Oriental and African Studies, London, 1978.

19. Both Harwood and Lieberman report that Puerto Ricans traditionally classify pregnancy as a hot state and thus avoid hot-classified foods. See Harwood, A. The hot-cold theory of disease. Implications for treatment of Puerto Rican patients. *J. Am. mod. Ass.* 216, 1157,1971; Lieberman, L. S. Medico-nutritional practices among Puerto Ricans in a small urban northeastern community in the United States. *Soc. Sci. Med* 13B, 193, 1979. Currier notes that Mexicans too classify pregnancy as hot but states that they avoid cold, not hot, foods. O'Grady reports the restriction of both hot and cold foods amongst Mexican-American women: this is also the case in Peru. See Currier, R. L. The hot-cold syndrome and symbolic balance in Mexican and Spanish-American folk medicine. *Ethnology* 5, 257, 1966; O'Grady, I. P. Childbearing practices of Mexican-American women in Tucson. Arizona. Master's diss. University of Arizona. Tucson, 1973, cited in Snow, L. F. and Johnson, S. M. Folklore, food, female reproductive cycle. *Ecol. Food Nutr.* 7, 44, 1978; Wellin, E. Pregnancy, childbirth and midwifery in the Valley of Ica, Peru. *Hlth Inform. Dig. Hot Count.* 3, 15, 1956. In contrast, according to the Costa Rica system, the pregnant woman is said to be excessively hot whilst the womb gradually becomes excessively cold, reaching a peak in the last month of pregnancy and continuing for 40 days postpartum, see Orso, E. Hot and cold in the folk medicine of the Island of China, Costa Rica, pp. 38–9. Monograph and Dissertation Series No. 1, Latin American Studies Institute, Louisiana State University, Baton Rouge, 1970.

20. For example, amongst Tamils, Thais, Puerto Ricans and Malays, see Eichinger Ferro-Luzzi, G. Food avoidances of pregnant women in Tamilnad, *Ecol. Food Nutr.* 2, 00, 1973; Mougne, *op. cit.*,

Harwood, *op. cit.* and Manderson, Traditional food beliefs . . . *op. cit.* Kelly and Manzanedo report that Mexican women take hot drinks to accelerate delivery, see Kelly, I. and Manzanedo, M. G. *Santiago Tuztla, Veracruz. Culture and Health.* p. 106. Institute for Inter-American Affairs, Mexico, 1956. Metraux refers to the external application of heat, using a large stone heated in an open fire, placed under the woman to induce labor pains. See Metraux, A. *Ethnology of Easter Island,* p. 102. Bulletin 160, Bernice P. Bishop Museum, Honolulu, 1940.

21. Haiti may be an exception to this rule: Wiese maintains that a woman is in the hottest of stages during her first three months postpartum. However, this is perhaps an error in the interpretation of field tests since the foods prescribed to women postpartum are predominantly cold, not hot, foods, in accordance with dietary restrictions observed in other cultures where the puerperium is clearly seen as a cold state. See Wiese, H. J. C. Maternal nutrition and traditional food behaviour in Haiti. *Hum. Org.* 35, 198, 1976.

22. See for example Pillsbury, B. L K. "Doing the Month": Confinement and convalescence of Chinese women after childbirth. *Soc. Sci Med.* 2B, 16, 1978; Manderson in Mathews, *op. cit.,* p. 70.

23. Hart, *op. cit.*

24. Newbold, T. J. *Political and Statistical Account of the British Settlements in the Straits of Malacca, viz. Pinang, Malacca,, and Singapore: With a History of the Malayan States on the Peninsula.* John Murray, London. 1893; Maxwell, W. E. Shamanism in Perak. *J. Straits Br., R. Asiat. Soc.* 12, 222, 1883; Skeat, W. W. *Malay Magic: Being an Introduction to the Folklore and Popular Religion of the Malay Peninsula.* Dover, New York, 1967 (1st publ. 1900); Gimlette, J. D. *Malay Poisons and Charm Cures.* Oxford Univ. Press. Kuala Lumpur 1971 (1st. publ. 1913).

25. McArthur, A. M. Malaya—12. Assignment Report June 1958–November 1959. W.H.O. Regional Office for the Western Pacific, Kuala Lumpur. 1962 (not a publication).

26. Wilson, C. S. Food beliefs and practices of Malay fishermen: an ethnographic study of diet on the east coast of Malaya. Ph.D. diss., Univ. of California. Berkeley, 1970.

27. Laderman, C. Giving birth in a Malay village. In *An Anthropology of Birth* (Edited by Kay M.). Davis, Philadelphia. 1982.

28. Wilson, C. S. Food taboos of childbirth: the Malay example. *Ecol. Food Nutr.* 2, 267, 1973, Siti Hasmah, binti Mohamed Ali. Effect on a basic attitude: *Health. Intisari* I, 30, 1963; Chen, P. C. Y. An analysis of customs related to childbirth in rural Malay culture. *Trop. Geogr. Med.* 25, 197, 1973; Fraser, T. M. *Fishermen of South Thailand: The Malay Villagers,* pp. 60, 70. Holt, Rinehart & Winston, New York, 1961; Millis, J. Modification in food selection observed by Malay women during pregnancy and after confinement. *Med. J. Malaya* 13, 139, 1958.

29. Wilson, *op. cit.* (1973), p. 268

30. Chen, *op. cit.,* p. 201.

31. The terminology is problematic. *Bersalin,* used by Wilson to describe both roasting and the lying-in period, conventionally refers to parturition. *Berdiang,* used by Chen for roasting but by my Kedah informants for smoking, literally translates as "to sit near a fire to warm oneself." *Ganggang* was used by Singapore informants for smoking but literally means either to dry over a fire or to warm oneself by a fire. McArthur (p. 27) reports that her respondents used *bersalai* for roasting: this term may also be used for drying. Similarly Chen uses *tungku,* correctly, for a large cooking stone: my Kedah informants used *tungku* to describe a traditional iron.

32. Dr. Alias. Personal communication.

33. Fraser, *op. cit.* p. 195.

34. Siti Hasmah similarly reports that Kedah Malay women sit on a high stool over a burner after bathing, thereby smoking the birth canal to assist stopping the lochia: she also reports mas-

sage with embrocation, the application of a hot stone brick, or iron on the woman's abdomen for half an hour to an hour each day and the use of lime (*kapur*) with binding. S. Hasmah, *op. cit.*

35. Mak Enjar, the midwife/masseuse (*tukang urut*) practicing in Adibah's village, provided the alternative spices whilst confirming the procedures and their order: guava leaves, turmeric leaves, lemon grass and ginger were boiled in the bath water; only *kemenyan samsu* was used with the charcoal for the *ganggang*. She used coconut oil with lime and lime juice on the woman's abdomen before binding, but also prepared a special massage oil with pound ginger and turmeric root, tailed pepper, cummin, black pepper, *kayu tarek angin, akar kelor* and *cekur*. See also Kuah, K. B. Malay customs in relation to childbirth. *Med. J. Malaysia* 27, 83. 1972; and Wylde, E. M. Some superstitious customs surrounding childbirth noted in Kuala Lumpur. In *Applied Nutrition in Malaya* (Edited by Simpson, I. A.), p. 132. The Caxton Press, Kuala Lumpur, 1957.

36. The nail in the bun protects the confined woman particularly from *pontianak*, vampire ghosts of women who died in childbirth, whose prey are newly-delivered mothers and any unsuspecting men. Women will not become *pontianak* if a nail is driven into their coffin, and will return to the grave if their victim can drive a nail into the characteristic hole in the nape of their neck.

37. S. Hasmah, *op. cit.*, p. 31. Judith Djamour reports that her Singapore Malay women took hot water and turmeric juice immediately after delivery, see Djamour, J. *Malay Kinship and Marriage in Singapore*, p. 90. Monograph on Social Anthropology No. 21, Athlone Press, London, 1959.

38. *Rempah ratus* includes coriander, cummin, fennel, turmeric, garlic, black pepper and cinchona bark. S. Hasmah, *op. cit.*, p. 31, provides a full list of the spices

39. Wilson, *op. cit.* (1973). p. 273. See also Chen, *op. cit.* p. 200.

40. Colley, F. C. Traditional Indian medicine in Malaysia. *J. Malay, Br. R. Asiat. Soc.* 11, 94, 1978. One of my Indian informants placed especial value on garlic as protection against infection and an aid to lactation: daily during her confinement, her mother roasted for her half a kati (c. 300 gm) of garlic until the skin had charred and the cloves part-cooked, she then ate the cloves whilst they were still warm.

41. One Chinese informant stated that watermelon was so cold that it should be avoided for 100 days after delivery.

42. Pillsbury, *op. cit.*, p. 13 reports that Taiwanese women either avoid washing throughout their confinement or wash in specially prepared water such as water in which fresh ginger root peel and pomelo leaves have been boiled.

43. Pillsbury, *op. cit.*, p. 14. See also Ahern, E. M. The power and pollution of Chinese women. In *Women in Chinese Society* (edited by Wolf, M. and Witke, R.). Stanford University Press, Stanford, 1975.

44. Katona-Apte J. The relevance of nourishment to the reproductive cycle of the female in India. In *Being Female. Reproduction. Power, and Change* (Edited by Raphael D.), pp. 46–7. Mouton, The Hague, 1975.

45. Shosh, B. N. An exploratory study on midwifery. *Ind. J Publ. Hlth* 12, 159, 1968; Eichinger Ferro-Luzzi, G. Food avoidances: during the puerperium and lactation in Tamilnad. *Ecol Food Nutr.* 3, 7, 1974. Sundaraj and Pereira also note food taboos believed to prevent both the mother and infant from becoming cold see Sundaraj, R. and Pereira, S. M. Diet of lactating women in South India. *Trop. Geogr. Med.* 27, 189, 1975.

46. Hanks, J. R. *Maternity and Its Rituals in Bang Chan.* Data Paper No. 51. Southeast Asia Program Department of Asian Studies, Cornell University Ithaca, N.Y., 1963. Rajadhon, P. A. Customs connected with the birth and the rearing of children. In *Southeast Asian Birth Customs: Three Studies in Human Reproduction* (By Hart, D. V., Rajadhon, P. A., and Coughlin, R. J.), pp. 115-204. HRAF

Press, New Haven, 1965; Pedersen, L. R. Aspects of woman's life in rural Thailand. *Folk* 10, 111, 1968; Mougne, *op. cit.*

47. The confinement and drying period is variable. Mougne (*op. cit.*, p. 78)) states that the total confinement runs to some 30 days, but lying by the fire is observed only for 15 days. Rajadhon (*op. cit.*, p. 149) records a 3-day period for lying by the fire; Pedersen (*op. cit.*, p. 143) 15 days for a primapara and as few as 7 days for other women; Hanks (*op. cit.* p. 541) observed confinements of from 11 to 13 days.

48. Hanks, *op. cit.*, p. 71.

49. Mougne, *op. cit.*, p. 81.

50. Hank, *op. cit.*, p. 54.

51. Mougne, *op. cit.*, p. 79. Pedersen (*op. cit.*, p. 144) reports that Thai women eat mainly plain rice and are recommended rice spirit as an effective agent for drying out the womb.

52. Nash, *op. cit.*, pp. 257–8; also Brant, C. S. Tagadale, *A Burmese Village in 1950*, p. 18. Data Paper No. 13, Southeast Asia Program, Department of Asian Studies, Cornell University, Ithaca, NY, 1954.

53. Halpern, J. *Laos Health Problems*, p. 4. Laos Project Paper No. 21. University of California, Los Angeles, 1961.

54. Coughlin, R. J. Pregnancy and birth in Vietnam. In *Southeast Asian Birth Customs: Three Studies in Human Reproduction* (By Hart, D. V., Rajadhon, P. A., and Coughlin, R. J.), pp. 243–4. HRAF Press, New Haven, 1965; Hickey, G. C., *Village in Vietnam*, p. 108. Yale Univ. Press, New Haven, 1964. Chung and Manderson and Mathews provide some detail on Vietnamese postpartum taboos in conflict with Western medical systems see Chung, H. Y. Understanding the Oriental maternity patient. *Nurs. Clin. N. Am.* 12, 73, 1977; Manderson and Mathews, *op. cit.*

55. Hart, D. V. From pregnancy through birth in a Bisayan Filipino village. In *Southeast Asian Birth Customs: Three Studies in Human Reproduction* (Edited by Hart, D. V., Rajadhon, P. A., and Coughlin, R. J.), pp. 65-71. HRAF Press, New Haven, 1965. See also Crispino, J. B., and Bailon, S. A survey of beliefs and practices during pregnancy and childbirth in Bay, Laguna. *ANPHI Papers* 5,5 1970.

56. Jensen, E. Iban birth. *Folk* 8, 165, 1966.

57. Siegel, J. T. *The Rope of God.* pp. 159–60. University of California Press. Berkeley. 1969.

58. Geertz, H. *The Japanese Family*, p. 90. The Free Press of Glencoe. New York 1961.

59. Kelly and Manzanedo, *op. cit.*, p. 111.

60. Kelly, I. *Folk Practices in North Mexico: Birth Customs, Folk Medicine, and Spiritualism in the Laguna Zone*, p. 16. Latin American Monographs No. 2. Published for The Institute of Latin American Studies, The University or Texas. The University of Texas Press, Austin, 1965.

61. Kelly I. The anthropological approach to midwifery training in Mexico. *J. Trop. Pediatr.* 1, 203. 1956.

62. Wiese, *op. cit.*, p. 194.

63. Saunders, L. *Cultural Difference and Medical Care: the Cure of the Spanish-speaking people of the Southwest.* p. 157. Russell Sage Foundation, New York, 1954.

64. Griffin, W. B. *Notes on Seri Indian Culture. Sonora, Mexico.* Latin American Monograph Series No. 10. University of Florida Press, Gainesville, 1959.

65. Metraux, *op. cit.*, p. 103.

66. Morgenstern, J. *Rites of Birth. Marriage, Death and Kindred Occasions among the Semites*, pp. 13, 27. Ktau, New York. 1973.

67. Fillmore, S. J., and Parry, E. H. O. The evolution of peripartal heart failure in Zaria, Nigeria: Some etiologic factors. *Circulation* 56, 1060, 1977.

68. Bagnall, D. Obstetric rituals and taboos. *Nurs. Times* 70, 1132, 1974.

69. McMann, M. Personal communication. This midwife assisted only a select number of women reluctant to place their pregnancy under medical/hospital care. She delivered some 12 infants per annum, with payment to her either in cash or kind, and according to the woman's ability to pay. Expectant mothers visited her from relatively early in the pregnancy and were massaged every 4–6 weeks from the fourth month with additional irregular visits in the event of any unusual indication. The sex of the infant was determined at 5 months. Delivery and lying-in were at the midwife's home. Massages were given to the newly delivered mother every 2 or 3 days for 6 to 8 weeks after delivery to expel impurities and to restore the woman's muscles. Whilst the bathing and warm bed are in line with conventional humoral practices, the diet during the lying-in period was comprised of "cold" foods: meat was proscribed and the mother was fed on fresh vegetables, salads, and fruit juices. Milk was restricted particularly if the mother was lactating heavily, but used to encourage lactation where a mother was having difficulty establishing a milk supply.

70. Reid, J. Personal communication.

71. Olbrechts, F. M. Cherokee belief and practice with regard to childbirth. *Anthropos* 26, 29, 1931.

72. Ford, C. S. *A Comparative Study of Human Reproduction*, pp. 66–7. Yale University Publications in Anthropology No. 32, HRAF Press, New Haven, 1964 (1st pub. 1945).

73. Quoted in Ford, *op. cit.*, p. 67.

74. Thompson, L. *Southern Lau, Fiji: An Ethnography*, pp. 84–5. Bulletin 162. Bernice P. Bishop Museum, Honolulu, 1940. Sahlins, M. The Stranger-King, or Dumezil among the Fijians, p. 30. Presidential address, Anthropology section, ANZAAS Jubilee Congress, Adelaide, May 12, 1980.

75. Sahlins, *op. cit.*, p. 40.

76. Teckle, N. Personal communication.

77. Pillsbury, *op. cit.*, pp. 16–17.

78. Harwood, *op. cit.*, p. 1157.

79. Doorenbos, H. Post-partum salt packing and other medical practices: Oman, South Arabia. In *Medical Anthropology* (Edited by Grolling, F. X., and Haley, H. B.), pp. 109–11. Mouton, The Hague, 1976.

80. Levi-Strauss, C. The Raw and the Cooked. Introduction to *The Science of Mythology* (Trans. by Weightman, J., and Weightman, D.), pp. 335–6. Jonathan Cape, London, 1970 (1st pub. 1964).

81. Ibid.

82. Muecke, M. A. Health care systems as socializing agents: childbearing the North Thai and Western ways. *Soc. Sci. Med.* 10, 381, 1976.

83. Mougne, *op. cit.*, p. 80.

84. Manderson and Mathews, *op. cit.*

85. De Groen, A. The Joss Adams Show. In *Going Home and Other Plays* (By de Groen, A.), p. 125. Currency Press, Sydney, 1977).

Editor's Introduction   9
Sudden Infant Death Syndrome in Cross-Cultural Perspective: Is Infant-Parent Cosleeping Protective?

JAMES J. MCKENNA

JAMES MCKENNA IS A PROFESSOR at the University of Notre Dame where he runs the Mother-Baby Behavioral Sleep Laboratory and is an expert on the impact of co-sleeping on Sudden Infant Death Syndrome (SIDS). SIDS or crib death is the greatest cause of mortality among infants aged one to twelve months in the United States, and is believed to be responsible for approximately 7,000 infant deaths per annum. The peak time of danger seems to be between two to four months and the majority of deaths in the northern hemisphere occur in the winter. There are competing theories as to the cause of SIDS, but one theory relates its onset to sleep apnea, or lapses in breathing.

In chapter 9 (taken from *Annual Review of Anthropology* 25 [1996]: 201–216), McKenna investigates the possible effects of co-sleeping or bed-sharing on the occurrence of SIDS. He explores this topic in depth in a number of other papers, as well, for example, M. T. Stein, C. A. Colarusso, J. J. McKenna, and N. G. Powers, "Cosleeping (bedsharing) among Infants and Toddlers," *J Dev Behav Pediatr* 22, no. 2 Suppl. (2001): S67–71; and J. J. McKenna and L. M. Gartner, "Sleep Location and Suffocation: How Good Is the Evidence?" *Pediatrics* 105, no. 4 Part I (2000): 917–919. In other essays, McKenna focuses on breastfeeding as well as co-sleeping and their impact in reducing SIDS. See J. J. McKenna and N. J. Bernshaw, "Breastfeeding and Infant-Parent Co-Sleeping as Adaptive Strategies: Are They Protective against SIDS?" in *Breastfeeding: Bicultural Perspectives*, edited by P. Stuart-Macadam and K. A. Dettwyler (New York: Aldine de Gruyter, 1995), 265–303.

SIDS is not new as it appears to be mentioned in the Old Testament. In the celebrated story of King Solomon's judgment, awarding a newborn baby to one of two claimants, the false woman's "child died in the night; because she overlaid it" (I Kings 3:19). Inasmuch as SIDS has been reported in many industrialized countries, it is to be expected that research has been carried out in numerous sites. SIDS International conferences bring together scholars from a variety of disciplines. See, for example, T. O. Rognum, ed., *Sudden Infant Death Syndrome: New Trends in the Nineties* (Oslo: Scandinavian University Press, 1995).

In 1990, some mothers were told to place their newborn infants on their stomachs to sleep to prevent these infants from possibly choking on their vomit. By 1994, however, conventional wisdom had changed. Then women were instructed to do the reverse, that is, place their sleeping infants on their backs so that they would not be suffocated by their bedding. Supine positioning of infants continues to be strongly recommended. See, for example, A. K. Knight, "Positioning to Reduce the Risk of Sudden Infant Death Syndrome (SIDS): Current Trends and Research," *Physical Occupational Therapy in Pediatrics* 18 (1998): 137–148.

McKenna's essay raises serious questions about American parents taking for granted the wisdom of placing a newborn infant's sleeping quarters in a separate room. In the light of cross-cultural evidence, parents may want to reconsider where a baby should be placed to sleep (with the nursing mother or apart).

Sudden Infant Death Syndrome in Cross-Cultural Perspective: Is Infant-Parent Cosleeping Protective?

9

JAMES J. MCKENNA

Introduction

NOWHERE ARE THE CULTURAL VALUES, expectations, and preferences of the Western industrial world more strongly reflected than in its clinical models of "normal" infant sleep and "normal" infant sleeping arrangements in the first year of life. From popular parenting books[18,77] to the most widely respected scientific literature[2–4,82] in the field of pediatric sleep medicine, cultural rather than biological understandings predominate, often without scientists' awareness.[91] The nearly universal, species-wide pattern of infant sleep, which involves infants and parents sleeping within sensory proximity of one another,[10,36,41,44,52,89] is either ignored altogether or regarded as inherently unhealthful, psychologically damaging to the infant or child, and potentially threatening to the husband-wife relationship.[14,33,69] Suffocation by overlying is considered an inevitable outcome of cosleeping, especially when bedsharing, and the ability to condition infants and children to sleep alone throughout the night, as early in life as possible, is a developmental goal around which both infant-child maturation and parenting skills are evaluated and rated.[4,12,18,63,77,88]

As Abbot[1] discussed, Western industrial values thus seem to favor early autonomy and individualism over familial interdependence.[31] While this preference is not especially startling, given the apparent economic and professional needs of people whose lifestyles demand more and more time away from their infants and children, it has led scientists to define the best biological interests of infants and children according to the social interests of their parents. In so doing—and this is based on anthropological evidence—scientists push too far the notion of the infant's physiological independence from its caregivers, confusing the infant's preparedness to adapt with actual adaptation,[50,51] and confusing widespread underlying cultural assumptions with established scientific facts.

This review examines the sudden infant death syndrome (SIDS, cot or crib death), the leading cause of non-accidental death in industrialized countries for infants younger than one year of age. SIDS is reviewed in the context of how Western cultural conceptualizations of infant sleep, rather than species-typical patterns, have influenced and constrained SIDS research. For example, measurements of so-called normal infant sleep physiology have been derived exclusively from studies of non-breastfeeding, solitary-sleeping infants, a context that, for the species, is neither biologically nor socially normal at all. In addition, I explore SIDS rates cross-culturally to highlight how much childcare practices generally, and sleeping arrangements in particular, may potentially be linked to the ease by which certain types of infantile defects suspected to be involved in SIDS find expression. A laboratory-based study comparing physiological and behavioral differences between social- and solitary-sleeping mother-infant pairs is presented to illustrate the effect that "choice" of childcare practice has on factors that could potentially mitigate the suspected deficiencies of some SIDS victims.

One purpose of this review is to demonstrate just how powerful anthropological concepts can be in helping to reconceptualize fields of research, such as sleep, not traditionally within the discipline's purview. Unfortunately, few anthropologists are involved in SIDS or pediatric sleep research, and even fewer have considered, for example, the paleoecology of hominid sleep and its implications for the evolution of human sleep in general.[19,55] Perhaps this review will stimulate additional interest by anthropologists whose research knowledge and expertise are precisely relevant to these areas and demonstrate to nonanthropologists that their own research in sleep can benefit from evolutionary and cross-cultural perspectives.

What Is SIDS or Cot or Crib Death?

Responding to the increasing need for more in-depth, on-the-scene environmental data and family history as part of the pathologist's criteria for a SIDS diagnosis, the National Institutes of Child Health and Human Development (NICHD) recently modified the definition of SIDS to read as follows: "The sudden death of an infant under one year of age which remains unexplained after a thorough case investigation, including performance of a complete autopsy, examination of the death scene, and a review of the clinical history."[90] The most intriguing clue to understanding SIDS is the unique age distribution of its victims. No other human malady except infant botulism is so heavily concentrated around such a narrow developmental period. Ninety percent of SIDS deaths occur before six months of age, mostly between two and four months; rarely do such deaths occur beyond 12 months of age. In all societies studied to date, boys die more frequently from SIDS than girls.[6]

What Are the Possible Causes of SIDS?

The primary causes of SIDS are still unknown, but the most compelling general hypothesis is that the fatal event is related to the control of breathing and/or arousal during sleep. As a result, the architecture of infant sleep, breathing patterns, and arousal have been intensely studied by SIDS researchers, as have the neurostructural, neurochemical, and physiological systems that underlie, influence, or control these activities. Researchers note that SIDS tends to occur after abnormalities of the cardiorespiratory control system have failed to monitor some combination of oxygen levels, breathing, heart-rate rhythmicity, body temperature, or the arousal responses needed to reinitiate breathing after a normal breathing pause or apnea. Essentially, the cardiorespiratory system is thought to collapse.[26,28,32,35,49,70,72,75]

The unfolding pattern of sleep itself, including how and when human infants arouse or awaken from sleep, is believed to be controlled by the primitive brain stem, located at the central base of the brain. This area is composed of clusters of differentiated cells that receive and send messages to and from the heart, hormonal centers, lungs, muscles surrounding the ribs, diaphragm, and airway passages, as well as structures that specifically help to balance the proper amounts of oxygen and carbon dioxide in the blood. Also controlled by the brain stem is the amount of time spent in various stages of sleep during any given sleep period—e.g. during light sleep (stages 1 or 2), deep sleep (stages 3 or 4), or rapid eye movement (REM), i.e. active sleep.[26,28] In addition, sleep architecture, including the form and timing of arousals, is also influenced by external stimuli such as feeding method and the presence of a cosleeping partner and must, therefore, be considered alongside internally based sleeping mechanisms.[57]

Most recently, Kinney et al.[35] studied an area of the brain, the arcuate nucleus, located on the ventral surface of the brain stem, an important area that monitors the proper balance of CO_2 and O_2. Recall that when CO_2 builds up in the blood, the respiratory neurons are activated to expel it, thereby causing fresh O_2 to be inhaled, reducing the acidity of the blood. A significant number of SIDS victims compared with control infants had fewer acethecoline-binding sites in this area of the brain. This suggests that in a variety of different circumstances, prone sleeping included, infants may not have the optimal or even minimal ability to arouse to reinitiate breathing following some type of apnea or exposure to their own exhaled CO_2 if it is trapped, for example, in a mattress as the baby lies face down, or if the infant is under thick blankets. Or it might mean that infants simply cannot arouse to breathe after particularly long breathing pauses or apneas. It is a promising clue.

Some SIDS victims may differ from surviving healthy babies not so much in kind as in degree.[71] These SIDS infants appear to suffer from subtle deficits that develop during intrauterine life and are not apparent in the neonate.[85,86] Researchers believe that the actual expression of the fatal deficit is likely to be influenced by, if not dependent on, a number of cofactors that converge at a vulnerable moment in the infant's life.[9,70] Nobody can yet delimit all the appropriate SIDS cofactors or explain why cofactors seem to have differential effects on infants. However, it is extremely likely that certain factors are more relevant to some SIDS victims than to others. For example, for some infants a contributing SIDS risk factor might be the lack of breastfeeding,[27] while for others it might be sleeping face down (prone) in the presence of an upper-respiratory infection that diminishes the potency (muscle tone) of airway passages.[11] In certain predisposed infants, efficient respiratory control might also be jeopardized by infantile hyperthermia, induced by atmospheric temperature, humidity, or too much bundling up (overheating) in cold weather.[6,7] One group of researchers suggests that between 28 and 52% of SIDS victims found "faces straight down" may have actually suffocated, especially those who were sleeping on beanbag cushions. Unable to dislodge themselves from the pockets formed by such cushions, the infants may have been forced to re-breathe lethal doses of their own expelled CO_2.[34]

Epidemiological Overview

Although this may be changing with recommendations to position infants in a supine position—on the back—for sleep, SIDS occurs most frequently in winter, and usu-ally in the early morning or evening hours, when the infant is out of sight of the care-giver and presumably asleep. However, SIDS also occurs while babies are riding around in strollers, sitting in car seats, dozing in baby carriers, and even sleeping on their mother's chests following a breastfeeding episode.[24,50]

The SIDS population remains exceedingly heterogeneous. No single consistent criterion or pathological marker can be used to either predict potential SIDS victims or identify them upon postmortem autopsy. Nor is there an animal model of SIDS; it is not known to occur in any species other than human beings.[70]

In the United States, SIDS rates are highest among both Native Americans and poor African Americans whose mothers are less than 20 years of age, smoke during their pregnancies, are unmarried, and lack access to prenatal care.[27] SIDS rates are lowest in most Asian cultures, as well as Swedish, Finnish, Norwegian, English, and Israeli populations, where mothers tend to be a bit older, do not smoke during preg-nancy, and place their infants in the supine or side position for sleep, and where par-ents, Asians especially, sleep either near or in contact with their infants during the first year of life and/or breastfeed intensively for the first six months of life.[21,87] SIDS is virtually unknown in China, although there could be serious reporting problems there, but it is as high as 9–15 per 1000 live births among impoverished Canadian Indians.

About 18% of all SIDS deaths involve premature infants. Low birth weight is a risk factor, as is the experience of one or more of an apparent life-threatening event (ALTE), which is characterized by a loss of muscle tone accompanied by gasping or choking, listlessness, color changes, or a cessation of breathing. Approximately 6% of infants who experience an ALTE die from SIDS.[6]

Various studies report that before their deaths, some SIDS infants slept for longer periods, awoke less often, and had more difficulty awakening or arousing than healthy infants with whom they were compared.[15,26] At birth some SIDS infants received lower Apgar scores and gained weight more slowly. Some exhibited less frequent but more sustained heart-rate variability and fewer but longer breathing pauses (apneas).[6]

In a major study funded by the National Institutes of Child and Maternal Health, 756 SIDS victims were compared with 1600 control infants. The research team found that many SIDS victims had had colds and bouts of diarrhea or vomiting within two weeks of death. A significant number had also exhibited droopiness, irritability, or some form of breathing distress involving a rapid heartbeat 24 hours before they died. However, researchers believe that all these symptoms were acting in a secondary fashion rather than as primary causes of SIDS.[27] As few as 10% of all SIDS victims have had any symptoms associated with a potential SIDS event before their deaths. This figure includes full-term infants with clinical histories of apneas as well as preteen underweight babies who experienced "apneas of prematurity."[6]

Only a relatively low number of symptomatic infants actually die of SIDS. As a result, the medical community is engaged in a volatile debate about whether infants with a history of repeated apneas should be sent home from the hospital with breathing monitors. At any given time, between 40,000 and 45,000 monitors are in use in the United States; yet no data indicate that monitors prevent SIDS deaths, and no data suggest how or under what circumstances infants die from SIDS when monitors are in use. At present, the effectiveness of home monitors in preventing SIDS deaths is highly questionable.[6]

The Importance of Child-Care Practices:
The Surprise of the Decade

In the past decade child-care practices have proven to be the single most important set of factors for reducing the chances of an infant dying of SIDS.[25] The discovery that just by placing infants in the supine (back) rather than in the prone (belly) sleep position could cause a decline in SIDS rates by as much as 90% in some countries (table 9.1) continues to astonish many SIDS researchers around the world. Many renowned investigators, including Johnson,[29] now accept an idea suggested by some researchers

Table 9.1.   Reduction in SIDS Rates per 1000 Live Births Following Public Campaigns Recommending the Supine Rather than Prone Infant Sleep Position.* Before Campaign: Prone Position; After Campaign: Supine Position

Country	Year: SIDS rate	Year: SIDS rate	Decline
Ireland	1986: 2.5	1993: 0.6	76%
Denmark	1991: 1.8	1993: 0.5	72%
Sweden	1991: 1.1	1993: 0.75	31%
New Zealand	1989: 4.0	1992: 2.2	45%
West Germany	1988: 1.8	1992: 1.2	33%
Great Britain	1989: 3.5	1992: 0.03	91%
Austria (Graz)	1990: 1.9	1994: 0.8	57%
Holland	1985: 1.07	1991: 0.44	58%

*Statistics reported at the Third International SIDS Conference, Stavanger, Norway, 1994.

nine years ago that the overall environment in which SIDS deficits find expression may be as important (to understanding SIDS) as the primary deficits themselves. Had researchers been asked just five years ago to prioritize SIDS research areas according to their likelihood in yielding clues about reducing SIDS risks quickly and significantly, child-care practices over which both parents and professionals assert control would not have been ranked very high. However, epidemiological findings across cultures now show consistently that, in the absence of maternal smoking, and where child-care patterns integrate the supine infant sleep position, breastfeeding, increased infant holding, maternal responsiveness, and cosleeping, SIDS rates are low compared with the rates in societies where mothers smoke, fail to breastfeed, infants sleep prone, and early parent-infant separation, including solitary infant sleep, is encouraged.[8,13,17,21,40,80,81]

From an anthropological perspective, it is not surprising that child-care practices in relationship to SIDS prevention should prove so important. Several different lines of evidence indicate that the social care of infants is practically synonymous with physiological regulation, since the infant's brain is only 25% of its adult brain weight, making the human infant the least neurologically mature primate of all primates and subject to the most extensive external regulation and support for the longest period. Hence for infants to survive, and for human (parental) reproductive success to be maximized, natural selection likely favored the coevolution of highly motivated caregivers on one hand and highly responsive infants on the other—infants designed to respond to and depend on external parental sensory signals and/or regulatory stimuli available in a microenvironment within which mothers and infants are almost always in contact. From both an evolutionary and developmental perspective, then, parental contact and proximity with infants (while awake and asleep) can be seen to represent a developmental bridge for the infant, extending into postnatal environments the role that the mother played prenatally in regulating important aspects of her infant's continuing development.[53]

Recent laboratory studies corroborate the importance of maternal contact.[42,60,65–68] Many studies show beneficial physiological effects of mothers holding their preterm and newborn infants using, for example, the kangaroo method of baby care, or skin-to-skin contact, which has the effects of increasing the infant's skin temperature, stabilizing heart rates, and reducing apneas and crying, all of which are consistent with an evolutionary perspective on how human infants develop optimally.[5,46–48] Years ago, Korner and Thoman[39] and Korner et al.[38] demonstrated that vestibular (rocking) stimulation of neonates and infants could reduce infant crying and the number of apneas experienced during sleep. Laboratory studies also confirm that for slow-developing monkey and ape infants, even short-term separation from their mothers induces deleterious physiological consequences such as loss of skin temperature, cardiac arrhythmias, depressed immune responses, and increased stress involving adrenocorticotrophic hormone release and, in some cases, a reduction in the number of antibodies in the infants' blood.[64,66]

SIDS Rates in Cross-Cultural Perspective

If we assume, for the moment, that the most predominant known SIDS risk factors (maternal smoking, prone sleeping, not breastfeeding) can be held constant, and that no genetic factors predispose some populations more than others to SIDS, we should find lower SIDS rates in societies—or in segments within a society—in which maximum body contact between the mother and infant occurs. An evolutionary perspective on infants would suggest that intense and prolonged mother-infant contact evolved specifically to buffer infants from various kinds of environmental assaults, infantile vulnerabilities, or physiological deficiencies, including SIDS.[43,50,78,79]

Cross-cultural data from urban industrial Asian countries generally support aspects of this prediction, but such comparisons are, admittedly, difficult to make. In Japan, for example, where infant-mother cosleeping on futons remains the norm,[74,80] current published rates for SIDS are among of the lowest in the world: 0.15/1000 births in Tokyo in 1978; 0.053/1000 in Fukuoka in 1986; and 0.22/1000 births in Saga.[81] The most recent estimate for the national SIDS rate in Japan is 0.3/1000 live births. These data do not, of course, prove that cosleeping is protective against SIDS. It may well be that SIDS is underreported in Japan, or that it is misdiagnosed as infantile suffocation. Japanese medical scientists have not participated in international SIDS research studies to the extent of American and European scientists, so the postmortem procedures they employ to identify SIDS may not be appropriate. Nevertheless, these low SIDS rates deserve explanation and further research.

In 1985, Davies[13] reported on the rarity of SIDS in Hong Kong. He used postmortem diagnostic protocols that, on review for a follow-up study by Lee et al.,[40] were judged comparative to Western diagnostic standards by John Emery,[16] a renowned SIDS researcher from Great Britain. Davies found that even in a context of poverty and overcrowded conditions, where the incidence of SIDS should be high, the rates were 0.036/1000 live births, or approximately 50 to 70 times less common than in Western societies. This finding is even more surprising because breastfeeding is not common (of 175 infants at two, four, and six months of age, the percentage of infants nursing was 9, 4, and 2, respectively), although cosleeping and the supine sleep position for infants represent the cultural norm.[13]

Davies proposed that proximity to the parent while the infant is asleep may be one reason why the rates are so low, as well as the typical (supine) sleeping position of Chinese infants. The author asked whether the possible influences of lifestyle and caretaking practices in cot death are being underestimated in preference for more exotic and esoteric explanations[13]—a viewpoint not unlike that of Emery,[16] who also implicated, for some English infants, the importance of caregiving environments and other behavioral and socioeconomic factors. A follow-up on Davies's work by Lee et al.[40] confirmed the relative rarity of cot deaths in Hong Kong, finding a slightly higher rate of deaths per 1000 live births (0.3, compared with 0.04/1000 reported by Davies).

A third study confirmed the rarity of SIDS in infants of Asian origin living in England and Wales, particularly infants of mothers born in India and Bangladesh but also infants of mothers with African origins. As the authors pointed out, Asian women have few illegitimate births and few births at younger ages, and few of them smoke,[8] all of which seems to reduce the risks of infants dying of SIDS. No mention was made of any possible differences in sleeping patterns that could explain the lower SIDS rate among the Asian subgroup, although it is likely that these infants were sleeping near their parents.

These low SIDS rates continue in Asian ethnic groups even after they immigrate to Western (non-cosleeping) cultures, where most continue their traditional care-giving practices, which include cosleeping.[21] One study reports that among five Asian American subgroups living in California, the incidence of SIDS ranged from a low of 0.9/1000 live births to a high of 1.5/1000. The variability was related directly to the duration of residence in the United States: The longer the group lived in the United States, the higher the SIDS rates,[23] which leads us to ask whether the trend toward higher SIDS rates reflects the adoption of more "American" patterns of infant sleep management, i.e. solitary infant sleep, among other things.

Within Western societies it can be particularly difficult to show a correlation between cosleeping and reduced SIDS because usually the groups of people that practice bedsharing (or at least admit to practicing bedsharing) exhibit multiple risk factors for SIDS, much more so than do lower-risk groups. Consider, for example, the results of one of the very few studies of sleeping arrangements in the United States. In their study of parent-infant cosleeping among urban Americans in New York City, Lozoff et al.[45] found that 35% of poor urban whites and 79% of poor urban blacks routinely slept with their children, who ranged in age from six months to four years (beyond the peak age for SIDS). If these data are representative of younger infants, why are the SIDS rates for black Americans in New York City higher rather than lower, since they bedshare? One reason could be that lower-risk groups underreport bedsharing because it violates the cultural norms. However, another more important factor has to do with the overall characteristics of the social and physical environment within which bedsharing is occurring. For African Americans the potential benefits of cosleeping may be overridden by the fact that black mothers ordinarily have their infants at a younger age (< 20 years), smoke during their pregnancies, live in impoverished conditions, are less likely to be married, lack access to education on both parenting and prenatal care, and do not breastfeed.[84] All these factors are known to increase the chances of an infant dying from SIDS.[27,59]

Physiological and Behavioral Studies of Infant-Parent Cosleeping: The Physiological Effects on Mother and Infant

My colleagues and I have attempted to understand infant-parent cosleeping by studying this behavior in a sleep laboratory, where differences between the solitary and bedsharing environments can be quantified and where both the behavioral and physiological findings can be interpreted in the context of known SIDS risk factors. We have hypothesized that under safe sleeping conditions, including those where mothers do not smoke, and for the vast majority of infants, infant-parent cosleeping should be inherently beneficial. More specifically, we suggest that the sensory-rich cosleeping microenvironment may change the sleep physiology and architecture of the human infant in ways helpful in resisting some types of SIDS.[50,53,57,58,61,62]

Two preliminary studies[56,58,61] and one more extensive NICHD funded study have been completed to date. The most recent study included 35 healthy Latino mother-infant pairs (20 routine bedsharers and 15 routine solitary sleepers). All mothers and infants chosen for the study breastfed nearly exclusively, as determined by an analysis of logs kept by mothers at home and used to categorize them according to whether they routinely slept with their infants or routinely slept apart. Strict criteria were used to distinguish these two groups.[57,62] At the time of the study, the infants were approximately three months old (the peak age for SIDS vulnerability) and healthy. Once in the laboratory, and after retiring for bed, polysomnographic machines monitored all the relevant physiological variables of mother-infant pairs simultaneously, including EEG, eye movements, and breathing and heart rates. Among the infants, body temperatures, O_2 saturation levels, and nasal airflow rates were also monitored. The first night (the adaptation night) mothers and infants slept in their routine home condition (either in the same bed or in adjacent rooms). On the second and third nights (the order being randomly chosen), mother-infant pairs alternated between repeating their home (routine) condition and completing an experimental night wherein routine cosleepers slept in adjacent rooms, while routine solitary sleepers slept in the same beds. In addition to polysomnography, all behavioral interactions, including breastfeeding, were recorded throughout the nights for later analysis using infrared-sensitive audio/video camcorders.

Among other things discussed elsewhere, the data revealed that: (a) bedsharing mothers and infants exhibit high levels of arousal overlap, both longer epochal and smaller physiologically defined transient arousals; (b) infants exhibit more frequent stage shifts, i.e. they move from one stage of sleep to another, or awaken more frequently, while bedsharing and spend more time, at the same time, in the same sleep stage (stages 1–2, 3–4, or REM) or awake condition as their mother, compared with when they sleep apart from their mothers; and (c) compared with when they sleep alone, bedsharing infants spend less time in deep stages of sleep (stage 3 or 4).[50,56–58,61,62]

Behavioral analysis of the videotapes revealed that during the bedsharing night, infants faced toward their mothers for the vast majority of the night (between 72 and 100% of the time), and they almost doubled their number of breastfeeding episodes compared with what occurred on the solitary night. Also of importance is that on the bedsharing night, the average breastfeeding interval was reduced by approximately one half, and the average total nightly duration of breastfeeding practically tripled compared with the solitary nights.

One additional observation is that when infants shared their mother's bed, almost always their mothers placed them in the safer supine position rather than in the prone or more risky infant sleep position. Watching our videos made it clear that if infants are breastfeeding they cannot get to or away from their mothers' breasts and nipples or, indeed suck milk if lying prone. Supine sleeping infants arouse more frequently, too, and in general they have far more control over their environment (throwing blankets off or awakening their mothers by arm movements to breastfeed) than prone sleeping infants. This is important because supine sleeping infants are at a significantly reduced risk of dying from SIDS,[25] compared with prone sleeping infants. Prone sleeping is associated with infants being placed in a crib to sleep alone and not with bedsharing, according to our data.

Relevance of the Data to SIDS Prevention

At present, our laboratory is the only one in the world to have quantified both physiological and behavioral differences between bedsharing and solitary-sleeping mother-infant pairs. While this laboratory work does not prove that bedsharing protects infants from SIDS, several of our findings suggest that bedsharing, under safe environmental circumstances, could potentially reduce SIDS rates. For example, the finding that bedsharing mothers and infants exhibit synchronous, partner-induced physiological arousals, although not very surprising, is potentially important because of the suspected relationship between infantile arousal deficiencies and some cases of SIDS. As described earlier, Kinney et al.[35] found that some SIDS victims had fewer neurotransmitter receptor sites in the brain stem, which suggests that arousals may be impaired in this group of SIDS infants. With increases in the type and number of arousals, bedsharing could potentially compensate for such a deficiency,[62] possibly by providing the infant with more opportunities to practice arousing, thereby enabling it to become more proficient at it, or through its being closer to the mother, permitting her to intervene should she see or hear a distress signal from her infant.

Our finding that bedsharing infants spend less time in deep sleep—stages 3 and 4—and more time in light sleep—stages 1 and 2—is also potentially important. It is more difficult for infants to arouse to terminate apneas to reinitiate breathing from deep stages of sleep than it is for them to arouse from lighter stages. Arousals are protective responses required of the infant to terminate life-threatening, prolonged apneas. Solitary infant sleeping environments may accelerate, then, the maturation of deep sleep in infants prematurely, before the infant's arousal mechanisms are able to effectively handle it. This problem could be exacerbated in infants born with arousal deficiencies.

Finally, that infants exhibit significantly more breastfeeding activities while bedsharing is potentially very important with respect to protection from SIDS. Two recent epidemiological studies suggested that breastfeeding lowers the risk of SIDS,[27,59] while two others suggested that the extent of protection may be dose specific, i.e. the more breastfeeding, the greater the protection.[20,30] While a protective effect has not been found in every study,[22] many international SIDS prevention campaigns, including those in the United States, encourage or recommend breastfeeding as a way to help reduce SIDS.

Note that in New Zealand, and among the Maori, a positive association has been found between bedsharing, maternal smoking, and increased risks of SIDS.[73] This association is important and justifies a recommendation against Maori bedsharing in cases where mothers smoke. However, the special characteristics of the populations on which these findings are based do not justify the investigators' sweeping conclusion, namely, that under all circumstances and in all families and cultures, bedsharing in whatever form causes or necessarily increases the risk of SIDS and should therefore always be advised against. It is imperative that we reconceptualize, from a biological and not strictly a cultural point of view, the appropriateness of parents and infants sleeping alongside one another. The existence of dangerous cosleeping conditions is no more an argument against the potential benefits to infants and parents of sleeping together than the existence of dangerous solitary infant sleep environments constitutes a valid argument against the safety of all solitary infant sleep. No environment is risk free.[53]

While recent cultural changes in Western societies stressing individualism over interdependence may help to support Mitchell and Scragg's recent suggestion that "cosleeping has outlived its historical usefulness,"[59] the kinds of data being collected in our laboratory force us to ask whether cosleeping outlived its biological usefulness to the infant. We must conclude that it has not. In fact, there is far more evidence suggesting negative socioemotional and physiological consequences to infants sleeping socially distant from their parents than evidence suggesting inherent negative effects of increased contact or proximity.[50] Moreover, not one scientific study documents the presumed socioemotional, psychological, or physiological benefits of solitary infant sleep, except where "benefits" are defined according to parental interests, other cultural values, or expectations, or where forms of social sleeping occur under unsafe conditions.[53,83]

If a valid understanding of the potential benefits or risks of cosleeping/ bedsharing is ever to be achieved, anthropologists, forensic pathologists, and epidemiologists must work together. New ethnographically sensitive and appropriate epidemiological variables and categories must be defined that more precisely capture, describe, and classify the diverse social and physical environmental factors that characterize and differentiate cosleeping environments, as well as the social and physical characteristics of the participants.

Conclusion

The species-wide, "normal" context of maternal-infant sleep is social. In fact, so entwined is the biology of mother-infant cosleeping with nocturnal breastfeeding that any study that purports to understand biologically normal infant sleep without understanding how these two activities interrelate socially and biologically must be considered incomplete, inaccurate, or both.[37,54] That infant-parent cosleeping represents the evolutionarily stable and most adaptive context for the development of healthy infants is not to say that modern sleeping structures or conditions are always safe. However, it is important to differentiate between the act of mothers and infants sleeping in proximity and contact, which is adaptive, from the conditions within which they do so, which may not be. Much research is still needed to test the hypothesis that increased parental contact during the night reduces the chances of an infant dying of SIDS. Nevertheless, we must now recognize the legitimacy of diverse sleeping arrangements for infants, including diverse forms of cosleeping, in order to reach a complete understanding of SIDS and normal infant sleep.

References

1. Abbott, S. 1992. How can you expect to hold on to them in life if you push them away? *Ethos* 20(1): 33–65.

2. Adair, R., Zuckennan, B., Bauchner, H., Philipp, B., Levenson S. 1992. Reducing night waking in infancy: a primary care intervention. *Pediatrics,* 89:585–88.

3. Anders, T. F. 1919. Night-waking in infants during the first year of life. *Pediatrics* 63: 860.

4. Anders, T. F. 1989. Clinical syndromes, relationship disturbances and their assessments. In *Relationship Disturbances in Early Childhood: A Developmental Approach,* ed. A. Sameroff, R. Emde, pp. 145–65. New York: Basic Books.

5. Anderson, G. C. 1991. Current knowledge about skin-to-skin (kangaroo) care for preterm infants. *J. Perinatol.* 11:216–26.

6. Ariagno, R. L., Glotzbach, S. E. 1991. Sudden infant death syndrome. In *Pediatrics,* ed. A. M. Rudolph, pp. 850–58. Norwalk, Conn.: Appleton & Lange. 19th edition.

7. Azaz, Y., Fleming, P. J., Levine, M., McCabe, R., Stewart, A., Johanson, P. 1992. The relationship between environmental temperature, metabolic rate, sleep state and evaporative water loss in infants from birth to three months. *Pediatr. Res.* 32(4): 417–23.

8. Balarajan, R., Raleigh, V. S., Botting, B. 1989. Sudden infant death syndrome and postneonatal mortality in immigrants in England and Wales. *Br Med J.* 298: 716–20.

9. Barnett, H. 1980. Sudden Infant Death Syndrome. Child Health Hum. Dev., US Dept Health Hum. Serv. Bull.

10. Barry, H. III., Paxson, L. M. 1971. Infancy and early childhood: cross-cultural codes. *Ethology* 10: 466–508.

11. Blackwell, C. C., Saadi, A. T., Raza, M. W., Weir, D. M., Busuttil, A. 1993. The potential of bacterial toxins in sudden infant death syndrome (SIDS). *Int. J. Legal Med* 105: 333–38.

12. Cuthbertson, I., Schevill, S. 1985. *Helping Your Child Sleep through the Night.* New York: Doubleday.

13. Davies, D. P. 1985. Cot death in Hong Kong: A rare problem? *Lancet* 2: 1346–48.

14. Douglas, J. 1989. *Behaviour Problems in Young Children.* London: Tavistock/Routledge.

15. Einspieler, C., Widder, J., Holzer, A., Kenner, T. 1988. The predictive value of behavioral risk factors for sudden infant death. *Early Hum. Dev.* 18:101–9.

16. Emery, I. 1983. A way of looking at the causes of crib death. In *Sudden Infant Death Syndrome.* ed. J. T. Tildon, L. M. Roeder, A. Steinschneider, pp. 123–32. New York: Academic.

17. Farooqi, S., Perry, I. J., Beevers, D. G. 1991. Ethnic differences in sleeping position and in risk of cot death. *Lancet* 338:1455.

18. Ferber, R. 1985. *Solve Your Child's Sleep Problem.* New York: Simon & Schuster.

19. Foley, R. 1992. *Another Unique Species: Patterns in Human Evolution: Ecology.* Harlow: Essex.

20. Fredrickson, D. D., Sorenson, I. F., Biddle, A. K. 1993. Relationship of sudden infant death syndrome to breast-feeding duration and intensity. *Am. J. Dis. Child* 147: 460.

21. Gantley, M., Davies, D. P., Murcott, A. 1993. Sudden infant death syndrome: links with infant care practices. *Br. Med J.* 306.

22. Gilbert, R. E., Wigfelt, R. E., Fleming, P. J. 1995. Bottle feeling and the sudden infant death syndrome. *Be Med J.* 310: 88–90.

23. Grether, I. K., Schulman, J., Croen, L. A. 1990. Sudden infant death syndrome among Asians in California. *J. Pediatr.* 116(4): 525–28.

24. Guntheroth, W. G. 1989. *Crib Death: The Sudden Infant Death Syndrome.* New York: Futura.

25. Guntheroth, W. G., Spiers, P. S. 1992. Sleeping prone and the risk of sudden infant death syndrome. *JAMA* 267: 2359–63.

26. Harper, R. M., Leake, B., Hoffman, H., Walter, D. O., Hoppenbrouwers, T., et al. 1981. Periodicity of sleep states is altered in infants at risk for the sudden infant death syndrome. *Science* 213:1030–32.

27. Hoffman, H., Damus, K., Hillman, L., Krongrad, E. 1988. Risk factors for SIDS: results of the national institute of child health and human development SIDS cooperative epidemiological study. *Ann. NY Acad. Sci* 533:13–30.

28. Hoppenbrouwers, T., Hodgman, J., Arakawa, K., Stennan, M. B. 1989. Polysomnographic sleep and waking states are similar in subsequent siblings of SIDS and control infants during the first six months of life. *Sleep* 12:265–76.

29. Johnson, P. 1995. Why didn't my baby wake up? See Ref. 70, pp. 218–25.

30. Jura, J., Olejar, V., Dluholucky, S. 1994. Epidemiological risk factors of SIDS in Slovakia. 1993, 1994 (Abstr.). In *Program and Abstr.* 3rd SIDS Int. Conf. Stavenger, Norway, July 31-August 4, p. 98. Oslo: Holstad Grafisk.

31. Kagan, J. 1984. The Nature of the Child. New York: Basic Books.

32. Kahn, A., Picard, E., Blum, D. 1986 Auditory arousal thresholds of normal and near-miss SIDS infants. *Dev Med Child Neurol* 28: 299–302.

33. Kaplan, S. L., Poznanski, E. 1974. Child psychiatric patients who share a bed with a parent. *J. Acad. Child Adolesc.* 13: 344–56.

34. Kemp, J. S., Thach, B. T. 1991. Sudden death in infants sleeping on polystyrene-filled cushions. *N. Engl. J. Med.* 324(26): 1858–64.

35. Kinney, H. C., Filiano, J. J., Sleeper, L. A., Mandell, F., Valdes-Dapena, M., White, W. F. 1995. Decreased muscarinic receptor binding in the arcuate nucleus in sudden infant death syndrome. *Science* 269: 1446–50.

36. Konner, M. J. 1981. Evolution of human behavior development. In *Handbook of Cross Cultural Human Development,* ed. R. H. Munroe, R. L. Munroe, J. M. Whiting, pp. 3–52. New York: Garland STPM Press.

37. Konner, M. J., Worthman, C. 1980. Nursing frequency, gonadal function and birth spacing among Kung hunter-gatherers. *Science* 207: 788–91.

38. Korner, A. F., Guilleminault, C., Van den Hoed, J., Baldwin, R. B. 1978. Reduction of sleep apnea and bradycardia in pre-term infants on oscillating waterbeds: a controlled polygraphic study. *Pediatrics* 61:528–33.

39. Korner, A. F., Thoman, E. B. 1972. The relative efficacy of contact and vestibular-proprioceptive stimulation on soothing neonates. *Child Dev.* 43:443–53.

40. Lee, N. Y., Chan, Y. F., Davies, D. P., Lau, E., Yip, D.C.P. 1989. Sudden infant death syndrome in Hong Kong: confirmation of low incidence. *Br. Med. J.* 298: 721.

41. LeVine, R., Dixon, S., LeVine, S. 1994. *Child Care and Culture: Lessons from Africa* Cambridge: Cambridge University Press.

42. Lipsitt, L. P. 1988. The importance of collaboration and developmental follow-up in the study of perinatal risk. See Ref. 16, pp. 135-50.

43. Lozoff, B. 1982. Birth in non-industrial societies. In *Birth Interaction and Attachment*, ed. M. Klaus, M. O. Robertson, p. 6. Johnson & Johnson Pediatr. Roundtable.

44. Lozoff, B., Brittenham, G. 1979. Infant care: cache or carry. *J. Pediatr* 95(3): 478–83.

45. Lozoff, B., Wolf, A. W., Davis, N. S. 1984. Cosleeping in urban families with young children in the United States. *Pediatrics* 74(2): 171–82.

46. Ludington-Hoe, S. M. 1990. Energy conservation during skin-to-skin contact between premature infants and their mothers. *Heart Lung* 19:445–51.

47. Ludington-Hoe, S. M., Hadeed, A. J., Anderson, G. C. 1991. Physiological responses to skin-to-skin contact in hospitalized premature infants. *J. Perinatol.* 11:19–24.

48. Ludington-Hoe, S. M., Hosseini, R. B., Hashemi, M. S., Argote, L. A., Medellin, G., Rey, H. 1991. Selected physiologic measures and behavior during paternal skin contact with Colombian preterm infants. *J. Dev. Physiol.* 18:223–32.

49. McCulloch, K., Brouillete, R. T., Guzetta, A. J., Hunt, C. E. 1982. Arousal responses in near-miss sudden infant death syndrome and in normal infants. *J. Pediatr.*101:91 1–17.

50. McKenna, J. J. 1986. An anthropological perspective on the sudden infant death syndrome (SIDS): the role of parental breathing cues and speech breathing adaptations. *Med Anthropol.* (special issue): 10(1): 9–53.

51. McKenna, J. J. 1991. *Researching the Sudden Infant Death Syndrome (SIDS): The Role of Ideology in Biomedical Science.* Stony Brook, NY: Res. Found. SUNY, New Liberal Arts Monogr. Ser.

52. McKenna, J. J. 1992. Co-sleeping. In *Encyclopedia of Sleep and Dreaming*, ed. M Carskaden, pp. 143–8. New York: Macmillan.

53. McKenna, J. J. 1995. The potential benefits of infant-parent cosleeping in relation to SIDS prevention: overview and critique of epidemiological bed sharing studies. In *Sudden Infant Death Syndrome: New Trends in the Nineties*, ed. T. O. Rognum, pp. 256–65. Oslo: Scand. Univ. Press.

54. McKenna, J. J., Bernshaw, N. 1995. Breastfeeding and cosleeping as adaptive strategies: Are they protective against SIDS? In *Bicultural Aspects of Breast Feeding*. ed. P. Stuart-Macadem, K. Dettwyler. New York: de Gruyter.

55. McKenna, J. J, Mack, J. 1992. *The paleoecology of hominid sleep.* Presented at Soc. Cross-Cult. Res., Santa Fe. NM, February.

56. McKenna, J. J., Mosko, S., Dungy, C., McAninch, J. 1990. Sleep and arousal patterns of co-sleeping human mother-infant pairs: a preliminary physiological study with implications for the study of sudden infant death syndrome (SIDS). *Am. J. Phys. Anthropol.* 83:331–47.

57. McKenna, J. J., Mosko, S., Richard, C. 1996. Bedsharing promotes breastfeeding among Latino mother-infant pairs. *Pediatr. Pulmonol.* 20:339.

58. McKenna, J. J., Thoman, E., Anders, T., Sadeh, A., Schechtman, V., Glotzbach, S. 1993. Infant-parent co-sleeping in evolutionary perspective: imperatives for using infant sleep development and SIDS. *Sleep* 16: 263–82.

59. Mitchell, E. A., Stewart, A. W., Scragg, R., Ford, R.P.K., Taylor, B. J. et al. 1992. Ethnic differences in mortality from sudden infant death syndrome in New Zealand. *Br. Med. J.* 306: 513–16.

60. Montagu, A. 1978. *Touching.* New York: Harper & Row.

61. Mosko, S., McKenna, J. J., Dickel, M., Hunt, L. 1993. Parent-infant co-sleeping: the appropriate context for the study of infant sleep and implications for SIDS research *J. Behav. Med.* 16: 589–610.

62. Mosko, S., Richard, C., McKenna, J. J., Drummond, S. 1996. Infant sleep and arousals during bedsharing. *Pediatr. Pulmonol* 20: 349.

63. Pinilla, T., Birch, L. L. 1993. Help me make it through the night: behavioral entrainment of breast-fed infants' sleep patterns. *Pediatrics* 91(2): 436–44.

64. Reite, M., Capitanio J. 1985. On the nature of social separation and social attachment. See Ref 65. pp. 223–58.

65. Reite, M., Field, T., eds. 1985. *The Psychobiology of Attachment and Separation.* New York: Academic.

66. Reite, M., Harbeck, R., Hoffman, A. 1981. Altered cellular immune response following peer separation. *Life Sci* 29: 1133–36.

67. Reite, M., Seiler, C., Short, R. 1978. Loss of your mother is more than loss of a mother. *Am. J. Psychiatr.* 135:370–71.

68. Reite, M., Snyder, D. 1982. Physiology of maternal separation in a bonnet macaque infant. *Am. J. Primatol.* 2: 115–20.

69. Robertiello, R. C. 1985. *Hold Them Very Close: Then Let Them Go.* New York: The Dial Press.

70. Rognum, T. O., ed. 1995. *SIDS in the 90's.* Oslo: Scand. Univ. Press.

71. Schwartz, P. J., Sagatini, A. 1988. Cardiac innervation neonatal electrocardiology, and SIDS: a key for a novel preventive strategy. *Ann. NY Acad. Sci.* 533: 21–20.

72. Schwartz, P. J., Southall, D. P., Valdes-Dapena, M. 1988. *The Sudden Infant Death Syndrome: Cardiac and Respiratory Mechanisms and Interventions. Ann NY Acad. Sci.* 533.

73. Scragg, R., Stewart, A. W., Mitchell, E. A., Ford, R.P.K., Thompson, J.M.D. 1995. Public health policy on bed sharing and smoking in the sudden infant death syndrome. *NZ Med. J.* 108: 218–22.

74. Shand, N. 1985. Culture's influence in Japanese and American maternal role perception and confidence. *Psychiatry* 48:52–67.

75. Shannon, D. C., Kelly, D. H., O'Connell, K. 1977. Abnormal regulation of ventilation in infants at risk for sudden-infant death syndrome. *N. Engl. J. Med* 297: 747–50.

76. Smeriglio, F. L., ed. 1981. *Newborns and Parents: Parent-Infant Contact and Newborn Sensory Stimulation.* Hillsdale, NJ: Erlbaum.

77. Spock, B., Rothenberg, M. 1985. *Dr. Spock's Baby and Child Care.* New York: Pocket Books.

78. Stewart, M. W , Stewart, L. A. 1991. Modification of sleep respiratory patterns by auditory stimulation: indications of a technique for preventing sudden infant death syndrome? *Sleep* 14(3):241–48.

79. Super, C., Harkness, S. 1982. The infant's niche in rural Kenya and metropolitan America. In *Cross-Cultural Research at Issue.* ed. L. L. Adler. pp. 47–55. New York: Academic.

80. Takeda, K. A. 1987. A possible mechanism of sudden infant death syndrome (SIDS). *J. Kyoto Prefect. Univ. Med.* 96:965–68.

81. Tasaki, H., Yamashita, M., Miyazaki, S. 1988. The incidence of SIDS in Saga Prefecture (1981-1985). *J. Pediatr. Assoc. J.* 92: 364–68.

82. Thoman, E. B. 1990. Sleeping and waking states in infants: a functional perspective. *Neurosci. Biobehav Rev* 14:93–107.

83. Trevathan, W., McKenna, J. J. 1994. Evolutionary environments of human birth and infancy: insights to apply to contemporary life. *Child. Environ.* 11(2): 88–104.

84. U.S. Government Printing Office. 1984. *Statistical Abstracts of the United States.* Washington, D.C.: USGPO. 104th ed.

85. Valdes-Dapena, M. A. 1980. Sudden infant death syndrome: a review of the medical literature. 1974-1979. *Pediatrics* 66(4): 567–614.

86. Valdes-Dapena, M. A. 1988. A pathologist's perspective on possible mechanisms in SIDS. *Ann. NY Acad. Sci.* 533:31–37.

87. Watanabe, N., Yotsutura, M., Katoi, N., Yashiro, K., Sakanoue, M., Nishida, H. 1994. Epidemiology of sudden infant death syndrome in Japan. *Acta Pediatr. Jpn.* 36: 329–32.

88. Weissbluth, M., Liu, I. C. 1983. Sleep patterns, attention span and infant temperament. *Dev. Behav. Pediat.*: 4: 34–36.

89. Whiting, B. B., Edwards, C. 1988. *Children of Different Worlds. The Formation of Social Behavior.* Cambridge: Harvard University Press.

90. Willinger, M. 1989. SIDS—a challenge. *J. Natl. Inst. Health NIH. Res.* 1: 73–80.

91. Wolfson, A., Lacks, P., Futterman, A. 1992. Effects of parent training on infant sleeping patterns, parents' stress and perceived parental competence. *J. Consult. Clin. Psychol.* 60: 41–48.

Editor's Introduction

10

The Cultural Characteristics of Breastfeeding: A Survey

ARTHUR NIEHOFF AND NATALIE MEISTER

IN CHAPTER 10 (taken from the *Journal of Tropical Pediatrics and Environmental Child Health* 18 [1972]: 16–20), Niehoff (anthropology professor emeritus at California State Los Angeles) and Meister review the variation found in customs and meaning surrounding nursing. As an extension of the nurturing function of pregnancy, breastfeeding allows the mother to continue to furnish sustenance to her growing child. It provides the ideal food for the infant while imparting benefits to the mother such as loss of fat deposits laid down in pregnancy and uterine involution. In addition, it is a free, convenient means of allowing the mother the satisfaction in meeting the nutritional and emotional needs of her infant, and this can be accomplished without the potable water required for the correct use of infant powdered formula.

For a number of reasons, including response to aggressive marketing, mothers in many nonindustrial countries use infant formula, a marked break from a millennia-long commitment to an accumulation of lore regarding nursing. Consider, for example, that grandmothers have been treated with herbs to become wet-nurses in cases of maternal death, a serious commitment in a community with the weaning age of five years (e.g., in Ghana, see L. Goodman, "Obstetrics in a Primitive African Community," *American Journal of Public Health* 41 [1951]: 56–64).

The practice of breastfeeding, like other aspects surrounding birth, is influenced by factors unrelated to health and is subject to trends (see C. M. Obermeyer and S. Castle, "Back to Nature? Historical and Cross-Cultural Perspectives on Barriers to Optimal Breastfeeding," *Medical Anthropology* 17 [1997]: 39–63). In the United States, for example, initial breastfeeding following birth has risen and fallen according to fashion (S. A. Quandt, "Ecology of Breastfeeding in the United States: An Applied Perspective," *American Journal of Human Biology* 10 [1998]: 221–228). In some countries, there are efforts to increase breastfeeding to reverse a trend to forgo nursing infants (cf. J. DaVanzo, J. Sine, C. Peterson, and J. Haaga. "Reversal of the Decline in Breastfeeding in Peninsular Malaysia? Ethnic and Educational Differentials and Data Quality Issues," *Social Biology* 41

[1994]: 61–77). See also D. B. Jelliffe and F. J. Bennett, "Worldwide Care of the Mother and Newborn Child," *Clinical Obst. and Gyn.* 5 (1962): 64–84, which includes discussion of such aspects as breastfeeding position and techniques to increase milk output. For a discussion of the protective effects of breastfeeding (against respiratory illnesses, gastrointestinal illnesses, as well as all illnesses) see M. Beaudry, R. Dufour, and S. Marcoux, "Relation between Infant Feeding and Infections during the First Six Months of Life," *Journal of Pediatrics* 126 (1995): 191–197; and S. P. Srivastava, V. K. Sharma, and S. P. Jha, "Mortality Patterns in Breast versus Artificially Fed Term Babies in Early Infancy: A Longitudinal Study," *Indian Pediatrics* 31 (1994): 1393–1396.

For overviews of issues surrounding nursing, see V. Fildes, *Breast, Bottles and Babies: A History of Infant Feeding* (Edinburgh: Edinburgh University Press, 1986); V. Maher, ed., *The Anthropology of Breastfeeding: Natural Law or Social Construct?* (Providence, R.I.: Berg); V. Hull and M. Simpson, eds., *Breastfeeding, Child Health, and Child Spacing* (London: Croom Helm, 1985); and M. Odent *The Nature of Birth and Breastfeeding* (Westport, Conn.: Bergin and Garvey, 1992).

The Cultural Characteristics of Breastfeeding: 10
A Survey

ARTHUR NIEHOFF AND NATALIE MEISTER

ACROSS-CULTURAL SURVEY OF traditional breastfeeding practices and beliefs, using ethnographic material from the Human Relations Area Files (a social science information retrieval system), was made and is hereby reported with a twofold purpose. Many concerned and knowledgeable persons have felt that information about the cultural characteristics of breastfeeding might be useful to planners of programs aimed at reinstituting breastfeeding. Programs could then be adapted more efficiently to widespread traditional patterns as described in the survey. It was also felt that such information might serve as a basis for suggesting questions to ask and topics to study through field investigations, perhaps administered through UNICEF or another concerned, international organization. The findings of the survey are therefore presented not so much to make definitive cross-cultural generalizations as to suggest characteristics of breastfeeding which might be significant for the purposes mentioned above.

Limitations of the report are due largely to the nature of the HRAF (Human Relations Area Files) material. Information regarding breastfeeding is thorough for some cultural areas but scant for others. Statements about a particular practice may come from a single source in one instance and from several in others. Sources also vary widely in the time period during which the information was gathered. However, despite the unevenness of the material, we believe there was enough to suggest topics to be studied if a thorough survey in the field is to be undertaken and even to suggest tentative guidelines to nutritionists. The particular suggestions will be listed in the "recommendations" section at the end.

Method
Our selection of cultures from HRAF attempted to include large populations only. However, the nature of the material available made it necessary to include some exceptions to

this criterion. In general though, we did not use data from small tribal units even though these are numerous in HRAF.

The distribution and number of cultures surveyed were as follows: Asia–21, Europe–4, Africa–6, Middle East–11, North America–2, Oceania–2, Soviet Union–5, South America–2. A total of fifty-three cultures were covered.

References in the paper may be checked with the assistance of any HRAF curator. Sets of these files are available in the primary social science centers of the United States, usually the major universities. The set used for this study is at the University of Southern California. The first number refers to the particular source. The number-letter combination following it refers to the culture area, and the last number refers to the page.

The data suggested breastfeeding categories of significance as follows: initiation, duration, care of child, supplementary feeding, weaning, and reinforcing attitudes and beliefs.

Initiation of Nursing

A child usually begins to nurse anywhere from immediately after birth to two or three days later, primarily depending on whether the colostrum secreted from the mother's breasts is considered suitable for suckling. Folk beliefs regarding colostrum vary widely; among the Yucatec Maya the newborn was given the breast soon after he was cleaned (2: NV10, 183) while in Tepoztlan, Mexico, it was believed that colostrum was harmful to the infant and to be expressed from the breasts until true milk was secreted (2: NU37, 361).

Substitute nourishments were normally given to infants in cultures where colostrum was regarded unsuitable. Most often this was a mixture of water and sweetening given with a spoon, in a cloth for the infant to suck, or administered from an improvised bottle such as an animal horn with the lip perforated. In Iran (7: MA1, 18) an infant received warm water and dissolved sugar, in Malaya (139: AN5, 90) honey and water, and in Greece (10: EH1, 98) *glykanisso*, anise water and camomile. Less commonly found in the data was the substitution of animal milk such as that of goats among the Tuareg of Africa (1: MS25, 145), cows in Burma (17: AP4, 61) and asses in Greece (10: EH1, 98).

In most cultures it was reported to be quite rare that a woman was unable to nurse her own child. Usually a wet-nurse was obtained only in case of the mother's death or when she was seriously ill. Wet-nurses were most common among the wealthy and privileged of a particular culture. Children of the gentry class in pre-Communist China were regularly nursed by a servant (8. AF1, 115). In Korea women of the middle-class often served as wet-nurses to children of upper-class parents (1: AA1, 357). In some cultures where wet-nursing was practiced, there were strict rules governing the selection of the lactating woman. These will be outlined in a later section of the paper.

The importance of nourishment from human milk, whether that of the natural mother or a wet-nurse, appears to have been common knowledge around the world. In cultures where a wet-nurse could not be procured or where there was no supply of animal milk, as was reported to often be the case among the Serbs, the infant usually died (10: EF6, 106).

In sum, although an infant often received nutritional substitutes the first few days of life, until his mother was able to nurse, in almost all cultures mothers traditionally took responsibility for breastfeeding their own children. Wet-nurses were used only in case of illness or death or among the wealthy and privileged. The importance of breastfeeding seems to have been universally recognized.

Duration of Breastfeeding

How many months or years a child might nurse has varied widely among cultures and also among individuals within a culture. Generally, however, mothers nursed within socially prescribed limits. It was most common for a child to be nursed one to two years, often longer, but very rarely less than one year. Probably the most common limitation on the length of time a child nursed was the birth of a new sibling. Although there were reported instances of mothers suckling two children at a time, the older child was usually weaned before the birth of the new infant.

Weaning during the next pregnancy was sometimes associated with a belief that the milk of a pregnant woman was harmful to her suckling child. This was the case in Senegal (1: MX3, 88) and also among some Arab women (1: M11, 503); yet many continued to nurse as long as their milk lasted. Presumably the advantages of nourishing their children outweighed the believed possible harmful qualities of the milk. In Tepoztlan (Mexico) mothers also continued to nurse despite the widespread belief that their milk was spoiled once they had conceived again.

Nursing might also be terminated when a mother wished to conceive another child. In some cultures termination was associated with the belief that a woman was unable to conceive while she was lactating; this was the case among the fellahin of Egypt (1: MR13, 100). In other cultures, there was a customary taboo to conceiving while an infant was still breastfeeding. A Chagga (Africa) mother was forbidden to cohabit with her husband until the last child was weaned (2: FN4, 105). Kikuyu (Africa) women were also forbidden to conceive while they were still nursing (3: FL10, 19). Islamic law prescribes a two-year nursing period for each child and this has influenced the length of breastfeeding among believers. Exceptions have been made, however. In Jordan the father might give his consent for a child to be weaned after the first year or year and half of nursing (16: MGI, 248).

The sex of a child might also influence how long he or she was suckled. Girl babies among the Wolof of Africa were nursed six months longer than their male siblings because they remained at home and had a closer relationship with their mothers (42: MS30, 219). Among the fellahin, where milk symbolized and was believed to convey "compassion," girls were nursed longer to receive greater measures of this attribute (1: MR13, 100).

Where there were no specific legal, religious or folk guidelines for the duration of nursing, and where a new infant did not replace the nursing child, the length of time a child suckled depended on his need and the mother's convenience. Generally, a child was nursed until he was able to partake of an adult diet and achieved a degree of independence. This turning point was marked among the Gond of India by the child's ability to walk and feed himself (1: AW32, 267) and among the Maori of New Zealand when the child could turn himself over (2: OZ4, 22).

Thus, the specific time length that children were suckled was quite flexible in most places. Often the last child was nursed for many years. It was not uncommon to find evidence of children in many cultures being nursed throughout their early childhood years, particularly while traditional conditions were primarily followed.

Child Care during Nursing

The nursing child in nearly all cultures enjoyed an extremely close relationship with his mother, both physically and emotionally. He was constantly in her company, cradled in her arms, strapped to her back, or lying close by as she went about her daily activities. Among peoples living at the band, tribal, or peasant level, where division of labor usually made it impractical for men to care for their young children, the child was with his mother of necessity.

This close mother-child relationship was reflected in many cultures in the practice of feeding a child "on demand" rather than according to an externally imposed schedule. In Greece where there was a mixture of traditional child-care practices and those based on Western medical knowledge, the rigid schedules recommended in health manuals were little observed in the villages (1: EHI, 139). Scheduled feeding in most instances had replaced "on demand" feeding primarily where Western practices had been influential or where mothers worked and had to follow factory nursing times.

For the most part, however, nursing mothers and their infants followed the Malay pattern where the child took the breast at his leisure and pleasure, either because he was hungry or in need of comfort. He suckled when walking, hiking, and while taking other nourishment (139: AN5, 90). Kha (Laos) babies, where all individuals seem to smoke tobacco, suckle between drags on pipes (Niehoff: personal observation). As among the fellahin, family treatment of the nursling was usually much more protective and attentive than at any other time of his life (1: MR13, 113).

The use of the breast as a pacifier was a fairly widespread custom. Most peoples disliked the sound of a child crying. In Tepoztlan the wails of an infant were usually interpreted as a sign not only of hunger but of neglect (2: NU37. 372). In Jordan the breast was given if the infant showed the slightest sign of restlessness (16: MGl, 93). An Okinawan baby was soothed by the breast when he was ill, in pain, or simply irritable (2: AC7, 463).

The period of life when a child was nursed seemed generally to have been characterized by a close relationship to his mother who kept him near and fulfilled both his nutritive and emotional needs by offering him the breast whenever he cried.

Supplementary Feeding

The survey data indicated an average age of from three to six months when a child received nourishment in addition to his mother's milk. Supplementary food was given both in instances where it was felt that the mother's milk alone was insufficient to nourish the child and where it was part of a gradual process of weaning.

Although three to six months was the usual age to begin giving a child additional food there were instances of earlier and later supplementation. In Malaya breastfeeding was not usually regarded as sufficient and the infant's diet was supplemented from birth (6: AN5, 86). At the other end of the spectrum were the Chukchee who fed infants nothing but mother's milk until after their first year at which time they were given boiled or frozen meat (6: RY2, 23–4).

Usually the first solid foods offered an infant were the staple or staples most available in the culture, mixed with milk or water. The Coorg of India gave six-month-old infants rice mixed with milk and sugar (1: AW5, 93) while the Serbs made a mush of bread and milk (3: EF6, 172).

Giving the infant pre-masticated food was also a fairly common practice. The ptyalin in the saliva of the mother, but absent in the infant, converts insoluble starches into soluble and digestible sugars (3: OZ4, 354). Throughout Southeast Asia it was common for infants to be given pre-masticated rice, sometimes mixed with other foods such as dried fish (17: AP4, 61).

Undoubtedly the economic circumstances of the parents in many cultures influenced the type of supplementary food given. The poorer people in Tepoztlan gave infants a mixture of corn cooked in water and sweetened with brown sugar and cinnamon while wealthier families supplemented the infant's milk diet with more basic foods (2: NU37, 377) In Okinawa, families with rice fields often delayed feeding their children sweet potatoes until the age of three while poor families added sweet potatoes to a child's diet much earlier (1: AC7, 264).

The most important considerations concerning supplementary feeding among any group of people seem to be the age at which it is begun, what types of food are given, and how economic position may affect the kind of food a child receives.

Weaning

Weaning was not regarded as a difficult process in many cultures. It was usually a gradual and relaxed supplementation of the infant's milk diet and the actual termination of breastfeeding happened at the mutual convenience of mother and child.

Where weaning was regarded as difficult, either among a particular group of people or among individuals within a culture, various methods were employed to solve the problem. One of the most common was the application of a bitter substance to the mother's breasts to discourage nursing. Thus, weaning was aided in Greece by the application of quinine (10: EH1, 98), in Korea by putting pepper on the nipples (22: AA1, 95), and among the Maori by using a bitter sap made from a local plant (2: OZ4, 22).

Another weaning method was to frighten the child. An Iranian infant was told that a bogeyman had eaten his mother's breasts which had been smeared with a black substance to show as evidence (7: Ml, 29). In Okinawa black patches, usually used for bruises and aches, were applied to the mother's breasts. The child was then told that his mother was in pain and she would wince if he tried to nurse. Derisive comments were made about the child who persisted. If all else failed, he was separated from his mother for a period of time (2: AC7, 474).

Abrupt weaning by separation, while much less frequent as a general practice, was used in Malaya by sending the child to live with a relative. In China a wet-nurse was sent away for several months at weaning time, then returning to care for the child without nursing (8: AFI, 73). A Kerala (India) mother reported that some women beat their children to stop suckling (12: AW11, 226) but this seemed an extreme exception to the more gradual and gentle practices followed elsewhere in the world.

There were indications in the data that in some cultures weaning was regarded as an emotionally trying, if not traumatic experience for children, particularly younger ones. Among the fellahin, mothers recognized the difficult adjustment required of the weaning child and tried to compensate for his loss by seeking to divert and entertain him: by giving him special foods, and by encouraging him to play with other children (1: MR13, 103). Okinawan children whose suckling period was particularly indulgent and permissive found it difficult to adjust to stricter handling and increased adult expectations (2: AC7, 573).

The weaning child may often have been hungry because he had to adjust to scheduled feeding. He received much less attention from his mother and was often competing with a new baby. Although the psychological difficulties of weaning may have been over-emphasized in these ethnographies due to the bias of Western observers, it may well have been a period of isolation and loneliness for children in many cultures.

That many peoples regarded weaning as an important transition period in a child's life is reflected by the various ceremonies related to weaning or giving the first solid foods in preparation for weaning. The occasion when a child received rice for the first time among the Kerala (south India) was celebrated (6: AW11, 244). Yucatec Mayans marked weaning by bathing the child in a liquid made from a special type of boiled leaf (11: NV10, 212). When a Chamar child in north India received rice for the first time, he was given a feast which included a naming ceremony (22: AWI. 68).

Finally, it has been commonly observed, both by Western ethnographers and the peoples whose cultures they studied, that there seemed to be a correlation between weaning and higher rates of disease and death among children. Many of the health difficulties of weaning children appeared to be due to parasites and bacteria that were ingested with ill-prepared food. Equally important were their increased susceptibility to intestinal ailments and, quite often, simple malnutrition. The increased illnesses and death of weaned children were not always ascribed to causes acceptable in present-day Western medicine. For example, the swollen stomachs of Vietnamese children observed near the turn of the century were attributed to suckling the "unripened" milk of a pregnant woman (136: AMII). This condition, however, would now be regarded as protein deficiency. *Chipilez* was the name given to an important childhood disease in Tepoztlan, Mexico. It was felt to be caused by the jealousy that a child felt when his mother became pregnant again. Judging from the symptoms and numbers of deaths, however, many cases of *chipilez* were probably due to nutritional deficiencies and/or intestinal parasites (2: NU37, 377–8).

Adaptations were made within various cultures to counter digestive difficulties and other problems associated with weaning. In Okinawa the area around the infant's navel was cauterized with nine brown dots which were believed to protect the child from digestive complications that often followed his introduction to solid foods (2: AC7, 467). The drinking of ink used in writing Koranic texts was believed to help a Hausa child grow strong and healthy after weaning (3: M212, 147). Probably much more effective were the prolonged nursing practices adopted by mothers of many of the surveyed cultures. Such nurslings were given, for a longer period of time, resistance to the effects of vitamin shortage, infections, and nutritional deficiencies suffered by older children.

In summary, although weaning was described generally as a gradual and uneventful process in many cultures, there were commonly accepted methods for hastening this transition that may have caused weaning children some emotional difficulties. Weaning was considered an important transitional period in some cultures and was marked by accompanying ceremonies. Finally, many peoples recognized that the weaned child was often more likely to become ill, although the reasons were not always the currently accepted diagnoses of Western medicine.

Beliefs Reinforcing Breastfeeding

Although many attitudes and beliefs regarding breastfeeding have already been discussed in the preceding section, there remain several which could not conveniently be described in relation to the previous categories. We feel, however, that they are important enough to be included in this final section. Most such attitudes center around the reciprocal mother's duty/child's right relationship and the "milk-relationship."

It can be generally stated on the basis of data collected in this survey that there was an awareness of the importance of breastfeeding for children in all cultures. This awareness was reflected in the various social strictures that enforced a widespread belief that it was both the child's right and the mother's duty to breastfeed. A two-year period of nursing prescribed by Islamic law is one example of a social stricture reinforcing the mother's duty/child's right belief (16: MGI, 248). The fellahin never weaned a child before one year because they believed he had the "right" to nurse (1: MR13, 100). City pediatricians in Greece, encouraging mothers to breastfeed, stated that a baby had inherited a "right" to his mother's milk (10: EHI, 98). Concomitant obligations were sometimes imposed on the child. Among the fellahin nothing was more binding in the mother-child relationship than memories of breastfeeding which were invoked to remind children to obey their mothers and to assist them in old age (1: MR 13. 107).

Social strictures enforcing sexual abstinence, hopefully to prevent pregnancy while a child was nursing, varied and were by no means universal but they still underline the recognized importance of breastfeeding in most cultures. Among the Hausa, it was believed that suckling women would spoil their milk if they had sexual relations (3: M212, 147). Although the Chagga debarred intercourse for suckling women, in fact, coitus interruptus was practiced. Social disapproval of pregnancy inside the three years prescribed by Chagga custom was so strong, however, that women were known to practice infanticide sometimes and even suicide when they conceived (2: FN4, 88). The Shilluk shamed a woman who became pregnant before her child was weaned. She was often accused of adultery (2: FJ23, 70). Among the Fanti a woman was supposed to live apart from her husband for a two-year period, or until her child was weaned (10: FE12, 406).

The "milk-relationship" was a custom found in a number of cultures whereby a child nursed by a woman other than his natural mother was thereafter considered related to her with the concomitant rights and obligations of a natural child. The reckoning of kin ties through the "milk-relationship" could also be extended to an adult who either actually or symbolically was suckled by a woman to whose kin group he wished to belong. The "milk-relationship" was especially prevalent in Islamic cultures. A foreign child was received into a Chagga family when he was offered the mother's breast (1: FN4, 9). In Senegal (1: MX3, 273–4), Turkey (7: MBI, 189), and Kerala (8: AWI1, 273), when a mother had insufficient milk and her child was nursed by another woman, that act formed a link equal to a biological one in terms of reckoning incest. The nursling was considered to be son or daughter to the nurse and thus a sibling to her children. Other kin relations were also binding between a nursling and his milk-siblings. A Nayar (India) king refused to punish the son of an attendant woman who had suckled him regardless of the son's treasonous attempts (8: AWI1, 274). In Caucasia, the "milk-relationship" was thought to predate Islamic contact because it was found among the Christian tribes of Armenia and some of the nomadic peoples from Asia as well (8: RHI, 55–6).

Related to the belief in a "milk-relationship" was the widespread belief that a mother could pass personality characteristics to her infant as she suckled him. In Iran, it was believed that the mother's milk would influence the morals, traits and habits of her child. The same belief was held of the milk of a wet-nurse (7: MAI, 28). Thus a wet-nurse in many areas was carefully chosen. In Afghanistan the nurse's character had to be above reproach; she had to be of good parentage and her husband had to be honest and brave as well (2: AUI, 40). Among the fellahin there was a slightly different twist to the belief in character influence through nursing. Men were advised to check out the maternal uncles because it was believed that their influence would be passed to the child through the milk of his mother (1: MR13, 102).

In conclusion, both the belief in the reciprocal child's right/mother's duty relationship and the "milk-relationship," along with the associated idea of passing character traits through the mother's milk, can be seen as attitudes which reinforced a more general belief in the importance of breastfeeding.

Summary Recommendations

A more thorough cross-cultural study of breastfeeding practices and beliefs might concentrate on the investigation of the following cultural characteristics. But even without further study, these customs and beliefs can generally be utilized by nutritionists. We will therefore present them as guidelines.

1. Despite changes brought about largely by Western influence, many traditional cultures have maintained some of their integrity. Most of these groups have taught that breastfeeding was both important and necessary, and it is possible that this belief may still exist in many cultures. Where it does, it should be used in programs for reinstituting the practice of breastfeeding.
2. The psychological ties of the close relationship between mother and child might also be used to promote breastfeeding.
3. Ailments resulting from or associated with weaning, particularly early weaning, might be emphasized to discourage mothers from following this practice.
4. The belief in the child's "right" to nurse might be further studied, particularly in theological law of Islam and other world religions.
5. Further investigation of the "milk-relationship" might yield ways in which this belief might be applied in programs to reinstitute breastfeeding.

Culture and the Problem of Weaning

CECIL SLOME

A T THE BEGINNING OF THE TWENTY-FIRST CENTURY, most American pediatricians recommend nursing a child for the first year of life despite its in-
compatibility with the schedules of working women. This desideratum is
more of an exigency in developing countries, however, where weaning a child before
the age of six months can contribute to early undernutrition (M. Cameron and Y.
Hofwander, *Manual of Feeding Infants and Young Children* [Oxford: Oxford University
Press, 1983]). Oddly, however, in many cultures, the colostrum, the yellowish and
sticky breast milk produced in the first week, is considered unhealthy and is dis-
carded—called useless and thought to promote diarrhea. For discussion of these and
related issues, see J. Goldsmith, *Childbirth Wisdom* (Brookline, Mass.: East West Health
Books, 1990); N. M. Scaletta, "Childbirth: A Case History from West New Britain,
Papua New Guinea," *Oceania* 57 (1986): 33–52; D. Sich, "Traditional Concepts and
Customs on Pregnancy: Birth and Post-Partum Period in Rural Korea," *Social Science
& Medicine* 15B (1981): 65–69; and M. Shostak, *The Life and Words of a !Kung Woman*
(Cambridge: Harvard University Press, 1981). See also J. Saucier, "Correlates of the
Long Postpartum Taboo: A Cross-Cultural Study," *Current Anthropology* 13 (1972):
238–249; and L. Meiser, "Child-Bearing and Child-Rearing among the Kaean of the
Northern Coast of New Guinea," *Anthropos* 54 (1959): 232–234; and A. V. Millard
and M. A. Graham, "Principles That Guide Weaning in Rural Mexico," *Ecology of Food
and Nutrition* 16 (1984): 177–188.

By reading this older essay in chapter 11 (taken from *African Child Health* 6 [1960]:
23–34) by Cecil Slome of the University of North Carolina School of Public Health,
the reader may gain some idea of the diversity in the duration of breastfeeding and
the age at which weaning is initiated. The possible significance of whether weaning is
or is not "severe" or "abrupt" was considered in a landmark study by Harvard anthropologist John W. M. Whiting and Yale psychologist Irvin L. Child. In their path-
breaking *Child Training and Personality: A Cross-Cultural Study* (New Haven: Yale University

Press, 1953), they attempted to find statistically meaningful correlations between the nature of weaning (and other aspects of infant conditioning such as toilet training) in a culture and adult fixations, in that same culture, both positive and negative. For an earlier study, see G. Devereux, "Mohave Orality: An Analysis of Nursing and Weaning Customs," *Psychoanalytic Quarterly* 16 (1947): 519–546. The psychological consequences of weaning are still being hotly debated. See T. Lubbe, "Who Lets Go First? Some Observations on the Struggles around Weaning," *Journal of Child Psychotherapy* 22 (1996): 195–213.

Culture and the Problem of Weaning　　　11

CECIL SLOME

THE COMPLEX BIOLOGICAL PROCESS OF WEANING, which all mammals have undergone since their evolution, has been receiving recognition of late, particularly in the human species, as a hazardous, rather than a natural process. The wide variations found in different societies in the time and method of weaning, the reasons for the cessation of breastfeeding, the ritual and beliefs associated with the process, and the effects of weaning on the species add enormously to the intricacy of the study. As compared with some animal species, humans set about the process consciously; it is this conscious act which seems to be changing the process from a natural milestone in life to an experience to be endured.

Recently, interest in the subject has been shown by social scientists describing the practices and customs of societies, by physicians and nutritionists faced with the necessity of introducing sufficient and adequate dietary supplements and by practitioners of psychology endeavoring to explain human emotional and psychical abnormalities.

The term "wean" is derived from the Anglo-Saxon *awenian*, to accustom (a child or young animal) to the loss of its mother's milk. It is recognized that weaning may be partial or temporary, as when a mother is ill or incapacitated, or a rural African mother is doing the seasonal ploughing, planting and weeding of the crops. In this text, however, weaning is taken as indicating the complete and permanent cessation of suckling.

Present-day knowledge about weaning revolves around varying aspects of the process, and it will be necessary to examine some facts in greater detail.

Weaning Time

Under this heading must be included the different phases of time:

a. the age of the child at which weaning occurs
b. any seasonal or ritual times of weaning, and

c. the time of weaning as determined by the developmental level reached by the child.

(a) *The age of the child at the time of weaning.* Social anthropologists, missionaries, medical practitioners and others have recorded the ages of children at weaning in many different non-literate unsophisticated societies, while some details are available about modern societies, and table 11.1 summarizes some of the recorded ages of infants at weaning in different societies.

It can be seen that in general the period of breastfeeding is much longer in non-Western societies, the earliest time of weaning being well over one year, extending even up to 15 years in the Eskimo. On the other hand, most mothers in the United Kingdom have weaned their infants by the age of 6 months, this presenting a remarkable change from the mother of the 19th and early 20th centuries. In the 18th century, the Western mother herself breastfed her child or employed a wet nurse for the purpose, whereas her modern counterpart knows the composition of cow's milk, and the supply is ready— in effect " the cow is now being used as a mother substitute" (Spence, 1938).

No study could be found which has assessed the impact of Western ideas of breast-feeding on non-Western societies; but it has been observed by the staff of the Polela Health Centre that rural mothers, when employed in towns, are weaning their babies earlier. Motivated by economic factors, they resort to the bottle and dummy of the Western mother. These apparently permit the African baby to be weaned early, and deposited in the care of the elderly grandmother in the Reserve (the rural area in South Africa inhabited by Africans), whilst the mother returned to her employment in the city.

(b) *Seasonal or ritual time of weaning.* No recorded study of the seasons of weaning could be found. While some physicians advise that weaning should occur in the cool season of the year, no assessment could be found of the response of mothers to this advice.

In many unsophisticated societies, there is a tribal ceremony attached to the weaning process, e.g. the Zulu frequently slaughter a goat or other beast to mark the occasion and to satisfy the ancestors as to its completeness, but there is no record of any ritual time for weaning in these or other groups.

(c) *Developmental stage of infant at weaning.* Some societies determine their weaning time by the level of development reached by the child. For example, among the Maori, many wean a child when it can turn over (Best, 1924); the Zulu paternal grandmother, traditionally the person to determine the time of weaning, especially of the first-born, often decides on weaning the third at a certain critical level of ability—usually when the child can walk, run, or talk well enough to request food. In fact, it is rare to find the traditional Zulu determining the time for weaning by the chronological age of the infant.

Reasons and Indications for Weaning

There are many reasons for weaning, some culturally determined, others "medically" determined, varying from modern to primitive peoples; even within each group, differences exist, but certain common features appear.

Table 11.1. Age of Children at Weaning in Different Groups

	Age of Child	Year
Non-Western Societies:		
Basuto (Ashton 1952)	Av. 2 years (1–3 years)	1952
Bareshe* (Richards 1932)	Av. 3 years 3 months (males)	1932
	Av. 4 years 4 months (females)	
Burmese (UNESCO 1953)	3–4 years	1953
Chinese (Feldman 1927)	5–6 years	1927
Caroline Islanders (Feldman 1927)	10 years	1927
Eskimo (Feldman 1927)	Up to 15 years	1927
French West Africa (Brock and Autret 1952)	18 months–2 years	1952
Greeks (UNESCO 1953)	14 months–2 years	1953
Japanese (Feldman 1927)	5–6 years	1927
Kasai (Brock and Autret 1952)	18 months–2 years	1952
Masai (Brock and Autret 1952)	3 years	1952
Navaho (Le Gros Clark 1953)	Av. 2 years 4 months	1947
Sudanese (Housden 1950)	2–4 years	1950
Western Societies:		
Irish (Health 1907)	2 years	1907
North America (Kardiner 1945)	1–7 years	"old days"
English (Craig 1946)	50% by 3 months	1943
	60% by 6 months	
English (Hughes 1948)	83% by 6 months	1945
English (Dummer 1949)	25–65% by 8 weeks	1949
N. Americans (North West) (Schlesinger 1953)	71% by time of discharge from nursery	1953
N. Americans (South, East and South West) (Schlesinger 1953)	18% by time of discharge from nursery	1953

*It appears that the Bareshe attach magic significance to the number 3 for males and 4 for females.

In tables 11.2 and 11.3, some of the reasons are summarized. It can be seen that in certain societies, some conditions or events motivate immediate cessation of breast-feeding, e.g. among the Basuto and Zulu, the onset of pregnancy leads to immediate weaning, based on the belief that the breast milk then would prove injurious to the suckling baby.

This is modified by the Masai who wean their children at the end of the 3rd month of pregnancy (Brock and Autret, 1952). This belief is not limited to unso-phisticated people, for even in Western societies it is a common belief that the milk of a pregnant lactating mother is potentially injurious to the suckling child. In fact, Bloom (1937) states that "pregnancy contraindicates breast." It is interesting that Greek mothers are encouraged to breastfeed during pregnancy, this practice being con-sidered good for the growing embryo (UNESCO, 1953).

Many other reasons for weaning exist in Western societies; their physicians advise slow weaning and argue that prolonged breastfeeding may produce an anemia in the child.

Table 11.2.   Reasons and Indications for Weaning: Western Societies

Reasons for (or Causes of) Weaning		Year
Ignorance Inability to breastfeed Reluctance to breastfeed	Spence 1938	1938
Generalized maternal illness Localized maternal illness Infant illness Economic Psychological Physiological	Dummer 1949	1949
Errors in technique Sweetened water	Craig 1946	1943
Medical Indications for Weaning: Prolonged illness of mother Pregnancy Return of menses Delicate mother Mentally ill mother Drugs used by mother Unsatisfactory nursing	Bloom 1937	1937

Prevention of anemia in baby
    (if weaned too late)
Prevention of digestive disturbances
    (if weaned too early)
Loss of weight in child
	Feldman 1927	1927

Prevention of habit	Spock 1957	1952

Table 11.3.   Reasons and Indications for Weaning: Non-Western Societies

Reasons for (or Causes of) Weaning		Year
Pregnancy: Zulu	Bryant 1949	1949
Pregnancy: Basuto	Ashton 1952	1952
Third month of pregnancy: Masai	Brock and Autret 1952	1952
For resumption of parental cohabitation (i) To appease male mate (ii) To produce further offspring (Zulu, Basuto)	Ashton 1952	1952
Economic factors (mothers having to earn) : Zulu*		1953
Discipline: Chaga	Raum 1940	1940

Medical Indications for Weaning:
  Umkhondo, a bewitchment syndrome
  manifesting with diarrhea, loss of weight,
  and a sunken fontanelle: Zulu*
		1953

*Personal observations.

Pearse and Crocker (1943) condemn any group system of indications or reasons for weaning, and suggest that each child is one unto itself, and should be weaned at its own time.

Socio-economic factors appear to enter into the determination of weaning. Dummer (1949), in a study of the relationship between housing and weaning in England (table 11.4), showed the higher proportion of children weaned by 8 weeks of age to be among the families in rooms, or living with in-laws, than among those living in other housing.

The non-Western mothers wean their children because of the onset of pregnancy, the developmental level attained by the child, or the need for resumption of parental cohabitation. Housing does not appear to enter into the process but the economic need for some African mothers to re-enter employment may cause the weaning to be effected.

Methods of Weaning

These vary widely from culture to culture (table 11.5) the Western mother depending mainly upon the early and gradual introduction of dietary supplements, with the

Table 11.4.   Correlation of Housing Distribution with Percentage of Babies Weaned by 8 Weeks (North Hertfordshire, Great Britain, 1949)

	Sharing	Detached	Semi-detached	Flat	Rooms	With in-laws
Overall (N = 545)	8.1	7.2	48.5	9.1	11.7	15.4
% weaned by 8 weeks	25.0	26.6	33.4	31.2	39.6	40.0

Source: Dummer 1949.

Table 11.5. Methods of Weaning in Some Unsophisticated Societies

Society	Applications to Breast	Other Methods
Zulu (personal observations; Bryant 1949; Albino and Thompson 1946)	Bitter aloe juice, snuff	Temporary adoption. iMfingo cycad tied around neck to make it forget. Fly around neck to stop crying.
Mundugummor, (New guinea; Mead 1948)	Bitter sap	Thrust away or slapped.
Antimelangers (Du Bois 1941)		Pushing child away or placing breast beyond reach.
Thonga (Richards 1932)		Temporary adoption.
Samoa	Lime juice	
Manus	Human hair	
Omaha (Mead, quoted in Le Gros Clark 1953)		Temporary adoption.
Zuni (Mead, quoted in Le Gros Clark 1953)		Mocking.
Greeks (UNESCO 1953)	Bitter stuff	Sweetened cow's milk offered.
Tchambuli (Mead 1948)		Stuffing infant's mouth with delicacies.
Basuto (Ashton 1952)	Tobacco, aloe juice, tight cloth	Prepared by mocking of neighbors. Temporary adoption.
Maori (Best 1924)	Bitter sap of Kawakama fern	
Comanche (Kardiner 1945)	Bitter stuff	Temporary adoption. Porcupine tail on cradle for quick weaning.
Alorese (Kardiner 1945)		Pushing away, slapping and teasing.

bottle and/or dummy available to meet the sucking demands of the infant, and then the withdrawal of the breast. It is as well to remember, however, that in England during the middle of the 15th century, other methods were used. As described in Jacob Well (about 1440) (quoted by *Oxford English Dictionary*) that " when the modyr wanyth here child sche wetyth here tetys with sum byttere thyng." The use of applications to the breasts is still frequently the practice in unsophisticated societies, but the variation among them is wide too.

Some non-sophisticated mothers introduce supplementary foods early in infancy, and ultimately, with the breast milk minimal, use the breast as a supplementary comforter. The Chaga, for example, believing that the mother's milk is insufficient, spit food into the baby's mouth from the second day of the infant's life, and with gradual introduction of foods, the breast serves just as a comforter. However, the ultimate weaning is recognized to be distasteful and is the occasion of the first disciplinary action (Raum, 1940).

Similarly amongst the Atimelangers (mountain villagers of the East Indies), pre-masticated foods and gruels are offered early in the baby's life, this feeding being increased as the baby's ability improves, but the weaning is effected by pushing the child away, or placing the breast beyond reach (Du Bois, 1941).

Among the traditional Zulu, foods are introduced even before breastfeeds, because of the belief that colostrum is injurious to the infant. The breast is withheld for the first 24–28 hours, or even longer, during which time other forms of food are given. In pre-20th-century times, *amaas* (curds of soured milk) was given to the baby immediately after birth, but now with the great shortage of milk in the reserve areas (in Polela, even in the best season, and with an equal distribution, 1/20th of a pint is available per person per day), *ncumbe*, a finely sieved pulped maize and water gruel, is used as a substitute. This is introduced a few hours after birth, any resistance by the infant being overcome by forcibly pouring the gruel from the cupped hand into the baby's mouth with the nose held closed, or more recently by the use of a feeding bottle. Breastfeeds are introduced after 1 to 3 days, and then continued, with feeds of *ncumbe*, other maize dishes and milk, when available, being gradually introduced.

The ultimate weaning, after this gradual introduction to other foods, is facilitated either through a piece of iMfingo cycad plant which is strung around the infant's neck in order to make it forget, or if the baby remembers, through the application in the presence of the baby of *umhlaba* (bitter aloe juice) to the nipples. The infant is then repeatedly offered the breast during the day. In most cases, a charm is tied around the baby's neck to encourage it to forget the breast. The charm may consist of a fly because of this insect's inability to cry, a cockroach so that its large appetite may encourage the baby to eat well, or iMfingo, breast milk or baby's tears, all of which are said to make the child forget the breast. Often, temporary adoption is imposed, the weanling being removed for a period to the maternal grandparent's home.

As can be seen in table 11.5, similar methods are employed in most unsophisticated groups, with various applications or measures being used to make the breast distasteful to the child.

However, indications for early weaning do arise, e.g. amongst the Zulu, pregnancy during early lactation is a decisive reason for immediate weaning, or the onset of a persistent diarrhea with green stools (usually diagnosed by the witch-doctor as *umkhondo*, a syndrome carried to the baby through breast milk from a bewitched mother, which is treated by immediate weaning). In these circumstances, the drastic measures are introduced for the cessation of suckling, often before the baby has been adequately established on supplementary feeds.

The Effects of Weaning

It is generally recognized that weaning may produce certain effects, but their nature, immediate or late, are not entirely agreed upon. Possible emotional disturbances are closely connected with any nutritional disorders produced.

Immediate Effects of Weaning

These, as yet, are not clearly understood and are still a matter of conjecture and argument. Richards (1932) decries the lack of anthropological contribution to the study of weaning as a change in the way of life, mentioning that the magic and ritual of the process received all the attention of the writers on the subject. Le Gros Clark (1953) reasons that some anthropologists may be forgiven on the grounds that "the mating habits and taboos of savages are doubtless more intriguing than what happens to babies, many of whom will probably be dead anyway before they are three years old." Richards (1932), Piddington (1950) and Malinowski (quoted by Richards, 1932) suggest that the savage infant, contrary to the child of well-to-do parents, is not weaned until it has developed emotionally a much more complex attitude towards the mother, and until it has reached physiologically a more or less independent stage. Richards argues that the effects of weaning are thus minimized but she does not suggest what the effects are.

Weaning does cause the first barrier between a previously indulgent mother and the child, at an age when breastfeeding is associated more with sensual pleasure for the child.

The wrench may be worsened by the non-sophisticated mother not caressing or fondling the child, who depends entirely upon the breast for providing care (Richards, 1932) and by the child understanding the punishing nature of the process (Piddington, 1950).

Psychologists and psychoanalysts generally agree that there are immediate effects on the child at weaning. Freud (1949) writes "the child will always resent weaning, even at a later period, because of its association with mother," but there are few descriptions of any prospective studies of these effects.

Friedlander (1947) mentions that the child, despite its ability to displace on to another object, e.g. a bottle, must give up instinctive pleasure by losing the close intimacy of body contact with mother, but he does not describe any actual immediate effects.

Almost all descriptions of these effects are based upon psychoanalysis. Analysts describe acts of aggression by the weanling, resulting from the unsatisfied love and desire for the breast. They maintain that the deprivation of the breast acquaints the child with reality, and he is made aware of his love (in the form of desire) and his own dependence (in the form of need). A depressive phase commences with his mourning for the breast, aggravated by guilt feelings, dependent upon the child's belief that the loss of the breast was due to his own greed and aggression (Klein, 1948; Klein and Reviere, 1953).

The only available prospective study of the changes occurring among a group of babies at weaning was made by Albino and Thompson (1956). They studied 16 Zulu babies (average age 18.9 months), and 10 controls (average age 23.6 months), performing pre-weaning assessments, and observing the process and the weanling's reactions at the time and afterwards. By providing adequate nutrients in the form of dried milk powder, they attempted to offset any nutritional disturbances resulting from the loss of breast milk. They found that the children studied were disturbed by the application of the *umhlaba* to the breast. Some even refused the breast without a prior taste of the bitter application. Later behavior disturbances were frequent, consisting of aggressiveness, particularly towards the mother, but also towards others, accompanied by bouts of fretfulness and/or apathy. This was followed by positive attempts to gain the mother's love and finally a period of increasing independence away from the mother.

The early change in behavior has been noticed by the physicians of the Polela Health Centre, who found that the previously playful, cheerful, co-operative baby, soon after weaning displayed violent tantrums, withdrawal, extreme tensing of the body, screaming, biting and gross active resistance to the same physician's advances.

An interesting finding in the study was a sudden increase in maturity of behavior from the 5th to the 13th day after the weaning. The weanlings appeared to spurt forward in their domestic activities in the homes and in their desire to assist with the family chores. Some developed an increased facility in speech, and a greater independence of the support of adults.

Clinically, physicians have noted effects of weaning, varying from death to minor digestive disturbance. As long ago as in the 14th century, weaning was recognized as a process fraught with danger, "as a childe that has nede to be on his modur kne, and fostird with hur mylke, perisch if he be wenyd, and taken fro mylke" (*Oxford English Dictionary* after Hampole, c. 1300). Similarly, high mortality rates have been observed among prematurely weaned rural Zulu babies (Polela Health Centre, 1949).

Gillman and Gillman (1951) note that in South Africa, where the price of eggs and dairy products is beyond the African's means and where even the staple diet of mealie meal (maize meal) is no longer home-grown, "it is not entirely unexpected that the weaning of African babies is attended by an extremely high mortality rate." Among Kenya Africans, Johnstone (1925) (quoted by the Gillmans, 1951), found a death rate at weaning between the ages of 9 and 18 months, of 21.7 per cent.

It is amazing that the effects of weaning have not been studied more by physiologists, for very few descriptions of this inevitable process occupy a place in physiological text books, so that we are unable to estimate any changes that must surely occur, within the range of normality and below the clinical disease level.

Even Western medical practitioners' interest in the problem is not great, probably because of the availability of a mixed diet to meet the dietary requirements of a Western society, in which cow's milk figures largely. The African baby, after weaning, passes abruptly to the diet of the family, consisting almost entirely of carbohydrate foods, because of the unavailability of other supplements, especially cow's milk (Brock and Autret, 1949).

It is thus that the acute nutritional deficiency amongst the African babies often arises. Kwashiorkor is a common disease of African babies, all too frequently following weaning. Le Gros Clarke (1953) suggests that up to then the prolonged breast-feeding had managed to supply the minimal necessary requirements to supplement the carbohydrate diet, but it is possible that non-dietary stresses of weaning play a part in the pathogenesis of kwashiorkor.

As Gillman and Gillman (1951) point out, even in the healthy, gastrointestinal upsets may follow weaning; they add a rider too, as a result of their animal experimentation, that a change from a *bad* to a *good* diet may result in morbidity or even mortality.

Most medical practitioners suggest that digestive disturbances do occur with weaning, but that these are minimized by gradual introduction to other foods. Anemia in the child is presented as a result of late weaning, especially where other adequate supplements are not introduced early on.

Despite the emphasis of study being directed towards the harmful effects of weaning on the child, the mother certainly enters into the problem. It has been noticed that the previously placid African mother frequently changes her attitude, emerging from weaning as a non-indulgent, forceful feeder, e.g. the mothers of the Tchambuli tribe stuff their infant's mouths with delicacies to stop their crying (Mead, 1948). The Basuto mother, after weaning, tends to "snap at the child and treat it harshly with no cuddling or coaxing" (Ashton, 1952).

It is recognized that weaning releases the infant from the vagaries of the mother's diet; this would appear to be important in a malnourished pellagrous African mother, whose nutritional state may permanently alter the metabolic physiological regulations of the infant (Gillman and Gillman, 1951). This has been seen in Polela, where the rearing of the infant of a pellagrous Zulu mother is frequently fraught with crises.

In addition, the temporary adoption of the African infants by the maternal grandmother makes the physical break between mother and child greater, especially in patrilocal society where the weanling might not see the mother for weeks or even months.

Changes in Family Relationships after Weaning

In many African societies, sexual intercourse is forbidden during lactation, and weaning heralds the time for resumption of cohabitation between mother and father. This does not often occur in private, so that the parental relationships are observed by the child (Richards, 1932; Piddington, 1950). This tends to increase the reactions of the weanling, especially of a male child, who is separated from his mother and his sensual (sexual) satisfaction, while he observes his father resuming sexual possession of his mother and becoming first claimant for her love and attention. This may result in infants wandering off for days, and lead to intense hatred of the mother and father (Ritchie, 1943).

This resumption of sexual relations is not only to gratify the father's urges, but also to produce further children. In fact, the Basuto mother, realizing this, may postpone weaning as long as possible "as they like suckling and do not regard child bearing as an unmixed pleasure" (Ashton, 1952).

With weaning changing his diet, the child enters into the family's social activity in relation to food making, and must compete with the fellow children for food. It is then that rivalry commences and emotional ties are formed with other children. Albino and Thompson, (1956) in fact, report a post-weaning attachment of the child to some other member of the family.

Changes in the Parents Associated with Weaning

Mother. Few physical changes in the mother in weaning have been described, but it is well recognized amongst the Zulu that the lactating mother loses her temporal hair (*ubu tete*) and regains this soon after weaning (Bryant, 1949).

Father. Apart from the satisfaction of his sexual urges, no effects on the father have been ascribed to the weaning of his child.

Remote Effects of Weaning on Infant

Almost all the remote effects of weaning are described by psychoanalysts who attribute some disturbances to the deprivation of the breast, and a maladjustment following it. Traditional Zulu do not attribute any psychopathological states to weaning and believe that the infant soon forgets the loss incurred.

However, remote biological effects are possible, so that with ever-earlier weaning becoming customary, a human race may ultimately be bred, incapable of breastfeeding at all.

The possibility, too, that premature weaning may cause the diatheses that determine the direction of future abnormalities or degenerative diseases in adulthood, has been suggested (Spence, 1938; Pearse and Crocker 1943) but no confirmatory study has been described.

It is not generally agreed that adult personality and behavior are related to weaning. The positive relationship of adult states to weaning has been measured by psychoanalysts in studies of adults, but no follow-up study from the weaning time has been recorded. Klein (1948) believes that the release of the Oedipus complex is timed by the frustration caused by weaning, which arouses feelings of guilt in the child; and that the complex in this way leads to neurotic troubles and disturbances of potency and depressive states in adulthood.

Eysenek (1952) too, agrees that there is a definite correlation between weaning and character. In a study of 115 middle-class adults, he found that the orally gratified type (late weaners) were the optimists, generous, bright, ambitious and accessible to new ideas; while the ungratified type (early weaners) were the pessimists, moody and depressive, with feelings of insecurity.

However, others deny any such correlation in studies of nursery and school-aged children, adolescents or even adults (Thurston and Mussen, 1951; Peterson and Spanot, 1941). Others suggest that the age of infants at weaning plays an important part in the determination of adult responses.

Childers and Hamil (1932) found a lower incidence of "abnormal behavior manifestations" in children who had been breastfed less than 1 month and more than 5 months, as compared with those breast fed for 1–5 months. This is supported by Maslow and Smilagyi-Kessler (1946) who found that the highest scores on a test of security were made by students breastfed little or not at all or fed for longer than one year. The method of weaning, too, appears to affect the results and as Klein and Reveire (1953) remark, "the normal psychological growth of an infant depends on the slow and gradual detachment from mother."

It would appear, therefore, that psychologists recognize the trauma associated with weaning, but disagree on the remote effects produced, and the relationship to adult behavior.

Prolonged thumb and finger sucking, which is probably a manifestation of an ungratified oral phase and all too common in Western societies, is extremely rare among the rural Zulu, or among other unsophisticated peoples (Mead, 1948). Further, among the Zulu, this habit is almost entirely confined to the prematurely weaned child.

Remote Effects of Weaning on Mothers

Mothers who have breastfed their children successfully seem to be different from those who weaned their children early, or never breastfed. Perhaps it is due to a "glowing" satisfaction at the fulfillment of the maternal role, or the realization of most mothers' desires. This has been observed by Spence (1938) who described his finding a woman who has successfully breastfed an infant "to be a saner and more sensible woman than her sister who has failed to do so."

Discussion

It has been shown how varied a process the weaning of humans is. The time and method of weaning is culturally determined, and often specific to each society, the causes of weaning differ widely, and include a physiological state of pregnancy, a pathological state such as diarrhea, or illness in the mother, while socio-economic factors including housing and the apparent necessity for mothers to work enter into the determining factors.

Our evolutionary predecessors were possessed of infants less dependent and more able to fend for themselves. The agility of the baby monkey in clinging instinctively to its mother, finding the nipple, and soon learning the mother's methods of seeking food leads to self-demand breastfeeding and ultimate self-weaning when capable of feeding itself. This permits no necessity of conscious entry of the mother into the process, so that in most lower mammal species, weaning is the resultant of the young acquiring the species-feeding habits, and thus reaching mature self-sufficiency.

But with its evolution, the human infant is now entirely dependent for feeding, with remnants such as the grasp reflex of the hands to remind us of its ancestry. Fairly early in its existence, the human infant takes everything to its mouth, but only relatively late in its existence is the child capable of obtaining the food for itself, and socialized enough for self-feeding. The conscious entry into weaning by the mother deciding the time and method, be she Westernized Briton or unsophisticated Zulu, is now constant in all humans. It is obvious that most groups, little influenced by Western societies, wean later than present day Western mothers, unless sudden contra-indications to breastfeeding arise. But with the rapid Western-style acculturating of the unsophisticated societies, weaning amongst them may occur earlier in infancy. This must raise the evolutionary possibility of the human female checking the function to such a degree as to reproduce descendants with the function lost, and procreating females incapable of breastfeeding at all.

The human race then would be entirely dependent upon the production of artificial foods, itself an unpredictable factor. Perhaps dietetically the loss of breast milk can be made up with artificial complements, especially using cow's milk, but it is recognized by most that weaning is psychologically traumatizing. If so, then it is improbable that the weanling's needs are adequately supplied without the use of the breast, despite a sufficiency of calories, proteins and other dietary constituents.

But the emphasis of medical study being on the values and constituents of breast milk, most Western medical advisers recommend weaning at a certain time, presuming that adequate foods are available. On the other hand, Zulu mothers, maintaining their prolonged breastfeeding as a form of comforting, do not realize, from the birth of the infant, the food value of breast milk, and when asked what the young infants are fed on, frequently reply, "*lutho*" (nothing). To them the breast is primarily a comforter and maintains this function until weaning, being offered to the child on all occasions of stress and crying. Weaning removes their child's comforter, so that sweetmeats and delicacies are given to appease the child for its loss, while any other available foods are given to satisfy hunger. The Zulu mother does speak of the weanling "missing" the breast, but believes it to be soon forgotten.

As westernization encourages early weaning all over the world, the problem of adequate foods arise; the plight of the recently westernized groups without access to the essential foods is becoming increasingly difficult.

But is the Western child weaned in the first year of life, on to a diet adequate in all the necessary requirements, really on the right road to health? It is always argued that even babies never breastfed do as well as others breastfed for years. The psychoanalysts contend that they can always detect a yearning for the breast in them, but this practice is not entirely accepted universally.

Even more important, perhaps, this argument merely reveals our lack of knowledge about health and its assessment. As measured by somatometric clinical and developmental tests, a baby, never breastfed, may be labeled "healthy" but modern science is incapable, as yet, of assessing the early laying down of diatheses to ill health which may be manifested only in adulthood. Only by long-term study will some progress be made; examination not only of the weanling but all concerned in the process; especially the mother who, when consciously making the weaning decision, could readily be filled with the feelings of guilt at depriving her child of the breast, and manifest them in some form of disturbance. Until such time, it would be probably best to familiarize the child with the diet of the family, slowly accustoming the child to the foods available. This would permit each child to wean itself when it reaches that stage of maturity and development.

It is possible that the Zulu mother copies this, weaning the child when it is ready for the next step towards maturity, this showing as the increased socialization effect described by Albino and Thompson (1956).

Far too many systems, timings and methods of weaning have been dogmatically ritualized. Each child is one unto itself. As Pearse and Crocker (1943) aptly put it, so capable in applying therapy are we that we have almost ceased to look for the causes that necessitate it. We seem to be forgetting "that each child is the product of its own nurture and must move forward according to its own specificity and at its own inherent tempo."

The problem of weaning is a complex one, and the need for a long-term study of all its dynamic intricacies by those concerned with the humanities should certainly prove to be of the greatest interest.

Summary

The complex intricacy of the process of human weaning is presented. The variations in time and method of weaning in different societies are shown. The immediate and remote effects of the process of weaning are discussed. In view of a possible biological species-change resulting from the curbing of the breastfeeding function, the need for a long-term study of weaning is presented.

References

Albino, R. C., and Thompson, V. J. (1956). Brit. J. Med. Psychol., 29, 177.
Ashton, H. (1952). The Basuto. London. Oxford University Press.
Best, E. (1924). The Maori. Harry H. Tombs.
Bloom, F. (1937). The Care and Feeding of Babies in Warm Climates. London. Pelican Publishing Co.

Brock, J. F., and Autret, M. (1952). Kwashiorkor in Africa. Geneva World. Health Org. Monogr. Ser. 8.

Bryant, A. T. (1949). The Zulu People. Pietermaritzburg. Shooter and Shuter.

Childers, A. T., and Hamil, B. M. (1932). Amer. J. Orthopsychiat., 2, 134.

Craig, W. S. (1946). Child and Adolescent Life in Health and Disease. Edinburgh. Livingstone Press.

Du Bois, C. (1941). Attitudes towards Food and Hunger in Alor (in Language, Culture and Personality, Editors: Spier, L., Hallowell, A. I., and Newman, S. S.) Wisconsin. Sapir Memorial Publication Fund.

Dummer, F. H. M. (1949). Brit. Med. J., 2,14

Eysenek. P. (1952). The Scientific Study of Personality, London. Routledge and Kegan Paul.

Feldman, J. (1927). Principles of Antenatal and Postnatal Child Hygiene. John Bale and Sons.

Freud, S. (1949). Outline of Psycho-analysis. New York. Norton and Co.

Friedlander, K. (1947). The Psycho-analytical Approach to Juvenile Delinquency. London. Routledge and Kegan Paul and Co.

Gillman, J., and Gillman, T. (1951). Perspectives in Human Malnutrition. New York. Grune and Stratton.

Health, H. L. (1907). The Infant, the Parent and the State. P.S. King and Son.

Housden, L. (1950).Brit. Med J., 2, 456.

Hughes, E. L. (1948). Ibid., 2, 597.

Kardiner, A. (1945). The Psychological Frontiers of Society. New York. Columbia University Press.

Klein, M. (1948). Contributions to Psycho-analysis (1921–1945). London. Hogarth Press.

Klein, M., and Reviere, J. (1953). Love, Hatred and Reparation. London. Hogarth Press.

Le Gros Clark, F. (1953). Nutrition. London. Newman Books Ltd.

Malinowski, B. Quoted by A. Richards.

Maslow, A. H., and Smilagyi, S. (1946). J. Abnorm. Psychol., 41, 83.

Mead, M. (1948). Sex and Temperament in Three Primitive Societies. London. Routledge and Kegan Paul.

Mead, M. Quoted by F. Le Gros Clark.

Pearse, I. H., and Crocker, L. H. (1943). The Peckham Experiment: A Study in the Living Structure of Society. London. George Allen and Unwin.

Peterson, C., and Spanot, T. (1941). Character and Pers., 10, 62.

Piddington, R. (1950). An introduction to Social Anthropology. Edinburgh. Oliver and Boyd.

Polela Health Centre (1949). Annual Report (Mimeograph).

Raum, O. F. (1940). Chaga Childhood. London. Oxford University Press for the International Institute of African Languages and Cultures.

Richards, A. (1932). Hunger and Work in a Savage Tribe. London. Routledge and Sons.

Ritchie, J. F. (1943). Rhodes Livingstone Papers, No. 9. Livingstone. Rhodes Livingstone Institute.

Schlesinger, E.R. (1953). Health Services for the Child. New York. McGraw-Hill Book Co.

Spence, J.C. (1938). Brit. Med. J., 2, 729.

Spock, G. (1957). Baby and Child Care. New York, Pocket Books.

Thurston, J. R., and Mussen, P. H. (1951). J. Personality, 19, 4.

UNESCO Committee (1953). Cultural Pattern and Technical Change. Paris. UNESCO Publications.

Editor's Introduction
Child Rearing in Certain European Countries

12

RUTH BENEDICT

RUTH BENEDICT (1887–1948), a professor at Columbia University, was one of the major anthropologists of the twentieth century. Her 1934 *Patterns of Culture* was a basic required textbook for generations of anthropology students. In a brilliant posthumously published essay, Benedict, influenced by Freudian theory that stressed the importance of early infantile conditioning, examined swaddling in several central and eastern European countries. In her provocative essay, reprinted in chapter 12 (taken from the *American Journal of Orthopsychiatry* 19 [1949]: 343–348), Benedict suggests that culturally specific parental attitudes can be extrapolated from observing childcare practices, in this case, swaddling. In contrast to American culture, where children are encouraged to express their interests and follow their own individual path for growth, Benedict argues that in other cultures, parents seek to exercise tight control over their children by swaddling them for varying periods of time.

For other considerations of swaddling, see M. Mead, "The Swaddling Hypothesis: Its Reception," *American Anthropologist* 56 (1954): 395–409; E. L. Lipton, A. Steinschneider, and J. B. Richmond, "Swaddling, a Child Care Practice: Historical, Cultural and Experimental Observations," *Pediatrics*, Supplement 35 (1965): 529–567; R. B. Scott, "Some Turkish Women's Attitudes towards Swaddling," *Turkish Journal of Pediatrics* 9 (1967): 71–75; C. M. Hudson and H. Phillips, "Rousseau and the Disappearance of Swaddling among Western Europeans," in *Essays in Medical Anthropology*, edited by T. Weaver (Athens: University of Georgia Press, 1968): 13–22; H. F. Stein, "The Slovak-American 'Swaddling Ethos': Homeostat for Family Dynamics and Cultural Continuity," *Family Process* 17 (1978): 31–45; and M. Bydlowski, "Childbirth Customs: A Psychoanalytic Approach," *Journal of Reproductive and Infant Psychology* 9 (1991): 35–41. For details of Benedict's career, see J. S. Modell, *Ruth Benedict: Patterns of a Life* (Philadelphia: University of Pennsylvania Press, 1983) and M. M. Caffrey, *Ruth Benedict: Stranger in This Land* (Austin: University of Texas Press, 1989).

Child Rearing in Certain European Countries   12

RUTH BENEDICT

S YSTEMATIC STUDY OF NATIONAL CHARACTER is an investigation into a special and paradoxical situation. It must identify and analyze continuities in attitudes and behaviors yet the personnel which exhibits these traits changes completely with each generation. A whole nation of babies have to be brought up to replace their elders. The situations two different generations have to meet—war or peace, prosperity or depression—may change drastically, but Americans, for instance, will handle them in one set of terms, Italians in another. Even when a nation carries through a revolution or reverses fundamental state policies, Frenchmen do not cease to be recognizable as Frenchmen or Russians as Russians.

The cultural study of certain European nations on which I am reporting[1] has taken as one of its basic problems the ways in which children are brought up to carry on in their turn their parents' manner of life. It accepts as its theoretical premise that identifications, securities, and frustrations are built up in the child by the way in which he is traditionally handled, the early disciplines he receives, and the sanctions used by his parents. The study has been carried on in New York City by a staff of interviewers who have supplemented their work with historical, literary, journalistic and economic materials. The aims of the research have been to isolate exceedingly fundamental patterns and themes that can then be tested and refined by study of local, class, and religious differences. It is believed that such preliminary hypotheses will make future field work in the home countries more rewarding, and such field work in the Old World is already being carried out under other auspices by students who have taken part in this research.

The Project has necessarily seen its work as a comparative study of cultures. It has blocked out large culture areas and their constituent subcultures. When a great area shares a generalized trait, the particular slants each sub-area has given to these customs is diagnostic of its special values and the range of variation gives insight which could not be obtained from the study of one nation in isolation. This culture area approach commits the student, moreover, when he is working outside his own cultural area, to a detailed study of behaviors which, since they are not present in his own experience, have not been incorporated into his own theoretical apparatus. It is therefore a testing ground for theoretical assumptions and often involves a rephrasing of them.

The custom of swaddling the baby during its first months of life in Central and Eastern Europe illustrates well, in the field of child rearing, the methodological value of a culture area approach. It illustrates how the comparison of attitudes and practices in different areas can illuminate the characteristics of any one region that is being intensively studied, and the kind of inquiry that is fruitful. Specifically I shall try to show that any such student of comparative cultures must press his investigation to the point where he can describe *what is communicated* by the particular variety of the widespread technique he is studying. In the case of swaddling, the object of investigation is the kind of communication that in different regions is set up between adults and the child by the procedures and sanctions used.

Because of our Western emphasis on the importance of the infant's bodily movement, students of child care who discuss swaddling in our literature often warn that it produces tics. Or with our stress on prohibition of infant genitality, it is subsumed under prevention of infant masturbation. Any assumption that swaddling produces adults with tics ignores the contradictory evidence in the great areal laboratory where swaddling occurs, and the assumption that it is simply a first technique to prevent a child from finding pleasure in its own body is an oversimplified projection of our Western concern with this taboo. Any systematic study of the dynamics of character development in the swaddling area is crippled by these assumptions. Infant swaddling has permitted a great range of communication.

Careful studies of mother-child relations in this country have abundantly shown the infant's sensitivity to the mother's tenseness or permissiveness, her pleasure or disgust, whether these are expressed in her elbows, her tone of voice or her facial expression. Communications of these sorts take place from birth on, and when a particular form of parental handling is standardized as "good" and "necessary" in any community, the infant has a greatly multiplied opportunity to learn to react to the traditional patterns. Local premises, too, about how to prepare a child for life will be expressed in modification of procedure in swaddling, and these detailed differences are means of communication to the child, no less than his mother's tone of voice. Any fruitful research in national character must base its work upon such premises and utilize them as basic principles in comparative study.

Swaddling is tightest and is kept up longest in Great Russia. The baby's arms are wrapped close to its sides and only the face emerges. After tight wrapping in the blanket, the bundle is taped with criss-cross lashings till it is, as Russians say, "like a log of wood for the fireplace." Babies are sometimes lashed so tight that they cannot breathe, and are saved from strangling only by loosening the bindings. The bundle is as rigid as if the babies were bound to a cradleboard, and this affects carrying habits and the way a baby is soothed in an adult's arms. It is not rocked in the arms in the fashion familiar to us, but is moved horizontally from right to left and left to right.

The swaddling in Russia is explicitly justified as necessary for the safety of an infant who is regarded as being in danger of destroying itself. In the words of informants, "It would tear its ears off. It would break its legs." It must be confined for its own sake and for its mother's. In the '30's the Soviet regime made a determined effort to adopt Western customs of child rearing and to do away with swaddling. Young women were trained to instruct mothers that a baby's limbs should be left free for better muscular development and exhibitions of pictures of unswaddled baby care were distributed widely. But swaddling persisted. Informants who have recently lived in Russia say constantly, "You couldn't carry an unswaddled baby." "Mothers were so busy they had to make the child secure." Several hundreds of pictures of babies available at the Sovfoto Agency show the prevalence of swaddling, photographs taken in 1946 and 1947 still show the completely bunted baby with only the face exposed. This physical restriction of the baby is traditionally continued for nine months or longer. It is not accompanied by social isolation. Babies are kept where adults are congregated, and their little sisters and grandmothers act as nurses; they are talked to and their needs are attended to.

In many ways the infant apparently learns that only its physical movement is restricted, not its emotions.[2] The Russian emphasis upon the child's inherent violence appears to preclude any belief among adults that its emotions could be curbed. The baby's one means of grasping the outside world is through its eyes, and it is significant that in all Russian speech and literature the eyes are stressed as the "mirrors of the soul." Russians greatly value "looking one in the eyes," for through the eyes, not through gestures or through words, a person's inmost feelings are shown. A person who does not look one in the eyes has something to conceal. A "look" also is regarded as being able to convey disapproval more shattering than physical punishment. Throughout life the eyes remain an organ which maintains strong and immediate contact with the outside world.

The baby's physical isolation within its bindings appears to be related to the kind of personal inviolability Russians maintain in adulthood. It is difficult for foreigners to appreciate the essential privacy accorded the individual in Russian folk life, for their pattern of "pouring out the soul" would be in most cultures a bid for intimacy, and their expressive proverb, "It is well even to tie if there are plenty of people around," seems a vivid statement of dislike of isolation. These traits, however, coexist in Russia with a great allowance for a personal world which others do not, and need not, share. "Every man," they say, "has his own anger," and the greatest respect is given to one who has taken his own private vow—either in connection with a love affair or with a mission in life. Whatever an individual must do in order to carry out this personal vow, even if the acts would in other contexts be antisocial, is accepted. He must be true to himself; it is his *pravda*.

The Russian version of swaddling can also be profitably related to the traditional Russian attitude that strong feeling has positive value. Personal outbreaks, with or without intoxication, are traditionally ascribed to the merchant class and to peasants, but they were characteristic of all classes. Official pressure at present attempts to channel this strong feeling toward foreign enemies, but the uses of violence to the individual psyche seem to be stressed in traditional fashion in this modern propaganda.

Not only is violence in itself a means to attain order, but it is also relatively divorced from aggression against a particular enemy. In Czarist days "burning up the town," breaking all the mirrors, smashing the furniture on a psychic binge were not means of "getting even" or of avenging one's honor; they were "in general." Even the peasants characteristically fired the home of a landowner other than the one on whom they were dependent. This trait is prepared for in the first years of life by the relative impersonality of the swaddling. Even in the villages of Great Russia, moreover, there is constant use of wet nurses and *nyanyas*, older women who are engaged to care for the baby; there is consequently a much more diffuse relationship during the first year of life than in societies where the child's contact is more limited to that with its own mother. It is characteristic of Russia, also, that poems and folk songs with the theme of mother love are practically nonexistent. The Great Russian mother is not specifically a maternal figure; she is quite sure of her sex without having to produce children to prove that she is female—as the man also is sure of his sex.

The Polish version of swaddling is quite different from the Russian. The infant is regarded not as violent, but as exceedingly fragile. It will break in two without the support given by the bindings. Sometimes it is emphasized that it would be otherwise too fragile to be safely entrusted to its siblings as child nurses; sometimes that the swaddling straightens its bent and fragile legs. Swaddling is conceived as a first step in a long process of "hardening" a child. "Hardening" is valued in Poland, and since one is hardened by suffering, suffering is also valued. A man does not demean himself by retelling his hardships and the impositions put upon him. Whereas an Italian, for instance, will minimize his dissatisfactions and discouragements and respect himself the more for so doing, Poles characteristically tend to prove their own worth by their sufferings. A usual peasant greeting is a list of his most recent miseries, and Polish patriots have exalted Poland as "the crucified Christ of the Nations." From infancy the importance of "hardening" is stressed. In peasant villages it is good for a baby to cry without attention, for it strengthens the lungs; beating the child is good because it is hardening; and mothers will even deny that they punish children by depriving them of dessert and tidbits, because "food is for strengthening; it would be no punishment to deprive them of any food."

Another theme in Polish swaddling has reference to the great gulf fixed between clean and dirty parts of the body. The binding prevents the infant from putting its toes into its mouth—the feet are practically as shame-ridden as the genitals in Poland—or from touching its face with its fingers which may just before have touched its crotch or its toes. When the baby is unswaddled for changing or for bathing, the mother must prevent such shameless acts. Whereas the Russian baby is quite free during the occasional half hours when it is unswaddled, the Polish baby must be only the more carefully watched and prevented. Polish decency is heavily associated with keeping apart the various zones of the body.

Although it was possible to sketch Russian infancy without describing details of nursing and toilet training, which are there warm and permissive, in Poland this is impossible. The high point of contrast is perhaps the weaning. In Russia supplementary food is given early; a very small swaddled baby has a rag filled with chewed bread tied around its neck; this is pushed down on its mouth as a "comforter" by anyone present. The baby is eating many foods long before it is weaned. In Poland, however, weaning is sudden. It is believed that a child will die if it is nursed beyond two St. John's Days of its life—or the day of some other saint—and therefore, when the child is on the average eighteen months old, the mother chooses a day for weaning. The child is not given an opportunity beforehand to accustom itself to eating solid food; the sudden transition is good because it is "hardening." It is further believed that a twice-weaned child will die and though many mothers relent because of the child's difficulties, it is necessarily with guilt.

Another contrast with Russia is a consequence of the strong feeling about the evil eye in Poland. Only the mother can touch the baby without running the danger of harming it; in the villages even the baby's aunts and cousins fall under this suspicion. Certainly no woman except the mother can feed the baby at the breast. During the spring and summer months the babies are left behind at home with three- and four-year-olds since all older children go to help their parents in the fields. In house after house neglected children are crying and women incapacitated for the fields might advantageously care for them. But this is regarded as impossible.

The Polish child gets nothing from crying. He is hurried toward adulthood, and the steps which reach it are always ones which "harden" him; they are not pleasant in themselves. As a child he has tantrums, but the word for tantrums means literally "being stuck," "deadlocked." He does not cry or throw himself about as the Jewish child in Poland does; he sits for hours with rigid body, his hands and his mouth clenched. He gets beaten but he takes it without outcry or unbending. He knows his mother will not attempt to appease him. His defense of his honor in his later life is the great approved means of unburdening himself of resentments and turning them into personal glory. There are many Polish proverbs which say idiomatically and with great affect: Defend your honor though you die. The long process of childhood "hardening" lies back of their insult contest and their spirited struggles in lost causes.

The swaddling of the Jewish baby, whether in Poland or the Ukraine, has characteristics of its own. The baby is swaddled on a soft pillow and in most areas the bindings are wrapped relatively loosely around the baby and his little featherbed. The mother sings to the baby as she swaddles it. The specific stress is upon warmth and comfort, and the incidental confinement of the baby's limbs is regarded with pity and commiseration. People say in describing swaddling, "Poor baby, he looks just like a little mummy," or, "He lies there nice and warm, but, poor baby, he can't move." Swaddling is also good, especially for boys, because it insures straight legs. There is no suggestion that it is the beginning of a process of "hardening" or that it is necessary because the baby is inherently violent. Rather, it is the baby's first experience of the warmth of life in his own home—a warmth which at three or four he will contrast with the lack of comfort, the hard benches, the long hours of immobility and the beatings at the *cheder*, the elementary Jewish school where he is taught Hebrew.[3] In strongest contrast to the experience of the Gentile child, swaddling is part of the child's induction into the closest kind of physical intimacy; within the family the mother will expect to know every physical detail of her children's lives and treats any attempts at privacy as a lack of love and gratitude. The pillowed warmth of his swaddling period apparently becomes a prototype of what home represents, an image which he will have plenty of opportunity to contrast with the world outside, the world of the *goy*.

It is profitable also to relate Jewish swaddling to another pattern of Eastern European Jewish life: its particular version of complementary interpersonal relations. I am using "complementary" in a technical sense as a designation of those interpersonal relations where the response of a person or group to its vis-à-vis is in terms of an opposite or different behavior from that of the original actors. Such paired actions as dominance-submission, nurturance-dependence, and command-obedience are complementary responses. The Jewish complementary system might be called nurturance-deference. Nurturance is the good deed—*mitzvah*—of all parents, elders, wealthy, wise and learned men toward the children, the younger generation, the poor, and the still unschooled. In interpersonal relations these latter respond to the former with deference, "respect," but not with *mitzvah*. One never is rewarded in a coin of the same currency by one's vis-à-vis, either concurrently with the act or in the future. Parents provide for all their children's needs, but the obligation of the child to the parent does not include support of his aged parents when he is grown, and the saying is: "Better to beg one's bread from door to door than to be dependent on one's son." The aged parent feels this dependence to be humiliating, and this is in strongest contrast to the non-Jews of Poland, for instance, among whom parents can publicly humiliate their children by complaining of nonsupport. Among the Jews, a child's obligation to his parents is discharged by acting toward his own children, when he is grown, as his parents acted toward him. His aged parents are cared for, not by a son in his role as a son, but in his role as a wealthy man, contributing to the poor. Such impersonal benefactions are not humiliating to either party.

The swaddling situation is easily drawn into this Jewish system of complementary relations. The personnel involved in swaddling is necessarily complementary; it includes the binder and the bound. The bound will never reciprocate by binding the binder, and the Jewish binder conceives herself as performing a necessary act of nurturance out of which she expects the child to experience primarily warmth and comfort; she is rather sorry for the accompanying confinement but she regards random mobility as a sign of the baby's being uncomfortable. She is not, like the Polish mother, "hardening," the baby or preventing indecencies, or, like the Russian mother, taking precautions against its destroying itself. She is starting the baby in a way of life where there is a lack of guilt and aggression in being the active partner in all complementary relationships and security in being the passive partner.

In swaddling situations the communication which is then established between mother and infant is continued in similar terms after swaddling is discontinued. Diapering of older babies is understood by Jewish mothers as contributing to the baby's comfort, and by Polish non-Jewish mothers as preventing indecencies by insuring that the baby's hands do not come in successive contact with "good" and "bad" parts of his body. In Rumania, where all informants from cities and towns stressed first, last and always that swaddling was necessary to prevent masturbation, the infant's hands, when he is too old to be swaddled, are tied to his crib, incased in clumsy mittens and immobilized by special clothing. His nurse or mother spies on him and punishes any slip. The different kinds of swaddling communication which are localized in Central and Eastern Europe make it clear that the practice has been revamped to conform to the values of the several cultural groups. As in any culture area study, investigation discloses the patterning of behavior in each culture. The diversities do not confuse the picture; they enrich it. And the detailed study of this one widespread trait, like any other, throws light on the individuality of each cultural group, while at the same time it emphasizes the kinship among them.

Notes

1. Research in Contemporary Cultures, government-aided Columbia University Research Project sponsored by the Psychological Branch of the Medical Sciences Division of the Office of Naval Research. The Russian material was collected and organized under the leadership of Geoffrey Gorer and Margaret Mead, and I am especially indebted to Mr. Gorer's skill and insights; Prof. Conrad M. Arensberg directed the group gathering Jewish material, and Dr. Sula Benet organized the information on Poland. Thanks are due to these leaders and to all their co-workers.

2. In this entire section I am indebted to Mr. Gorer's analysis.

3. For a fascinating, detailed account of the early school experience among Eastern European Jews, see "From the Kheyder to the Grave," a chapter in a book which grew directly out of Ruth Benedict's research project, Mark Zborowski and Elizabeth Herzog, *Life Is with People: The Jewish Little-Town of Eastern Europe* (New York, 1952), pp. 88–104.—*Editor's note.*

Editor's Introduction
Ethnic Differences in Babies

DANIEL G. FREEDMAN

I N CHAPTER 13 (taken from *Human Nature* 2 [1979]: 36–43), Freedman, a University of Chicago psychologist emeritus, ponders the role of nature and nurture in infant behavior. Freedman does not separate influences of genetics and the environment; rather he points to genetics as allowing a range of behavior dependent on culture or nurture for its expression. This fascinating area of investigation has been stymied by concerns about abuses of research findings related to fears about eugenics crusades. There have been a few attempts to disentangle biological and culture factors in the formation of human development; see, for example, T. B. Brazelton, B. Koslowski, and E. Tronick, "Neonatal Behavior among Urban Zambians and Americans," *Journal of Child Psychiatry* 15 (1976): 97–107. This remains, however, an exciting one ripe for further study.

In the age-old debate with respect to nature versus nurture, scholars tend to argue one way or the other. One such perspective is championed by so-called sociobiologists who essentially contend that "nature" takes precedence over "nurture." One of the principal advocates of "sociobiology" was Harvard entomologist Edward O. Wilson, a specialist in ants. His central thesis was expounded most fully in *Sociobiology: The New Synthesis* published by Harvard University Press in 1975. This was followed by *On Human Nature*, published by the same press in 1978. In the latter book, Wilson defined sociobiology as "the systematic study of the biological basis of all forms of social behavior, in all kinds of organisms, including man" (p. 16). For Wilson "Biology is the key to human nature" and "The genes hold culture on a leash" (*On Human Nature*, pp. 13, 167).

Not surprisingly, cultural anthropologists objected to this extreme form of biological determinism. In effect, it reduced the influence of "culture" to negligible proportions. Inasmuch as "culture" is the key concept in cultural anthropology, anthropologists quite naturally felt obliged to challenge Wilson's thesis. Samples of the ensuing debate include J. H. Barkow, "Culture and Sociobiology," *American Anthropologist* 80 (1978): 5–20; Bobby Joe Williams, "A Critical Review of Models in Sociobiology," *Annual Review of Anthropology* 10 (1981): 163–192; and F. Nielsen, "Sociobiology and Sociology," *Annual Review of Sociology* 20 (1994): 267–303. The literature is far too voluminous to survey, but suffice it to say that the debate continues. See, for example, U. Segerstrale, *Defenders of the Truth: The Battle for Science in the Sociobiology Debate and Beyond* (Oxford: Oxford University Press, 2000) and J. Alcock, *The Triumph of Sociobiology* (New York: Oxford University Press, 2001).

Psychologist Daniel G. Freedman was sympathetic to the sociobiological approach. His book, *Human Sociobiology: A Holistic Approach* (New York: Free Press, 1979), set forth his views. It is surely no accident that Freedman's research received praise from Edward O. Wilson (*On Human Nature*, pp. 48–50). Yet Freedman's position, as articulated in this final essay in the volume, seeks to find some kind of balance between the "nature" and "nurture" extremists.

Ethnic Differences in Babies

13

DANIEL G. FREEDMAN

THE HUMAN SPECIES comes in an admirable variety of shapes and colors, as a walk through any cosmopolitan city amply demonstrates. Although the speculation has become politically and socially unpopular, it is difficult not to wonder whether the major differences in physical appearances are accompanied by standard differences in temperament or behavior. Recent studies by myself and others of babies only a few hours, days, or weeks old indicate that they are, and that such differences among human beings are biological as well as cultural.

These studies of newborns from different ethnic backgrounds actually had their inception with work on puppies, when I attempted to raise dogs in either an indulged or disciplined fashion in order to test the effects of such rearing on their later behavior.

I spent all my days and evenings with these puppies, and it soon became apparent that the breed of dog would become an important factor in my results. Even as the ears and eyes opened, the breeds differed in behavior. Little beagles were irrepressibly friendly from the moment they could detect me; Shetland sheepdogs were very, very sensitive to a loud voice or the slightest punishment; wire-haired terriers were so tough and aggressive, even as clumsy three-week olds, that I had to wear gloves while playing with them; and finally, Basenjis, barkless dogs originating in Central Africa, were aloof and independent. To judge by where they spent their time, sniffing and investigating, I was no more important to them than if I were a rubber balloon.

When I later tested the dogs, the breed indeed made a difference in their behavior. I took them, when hungry, into a room with a bowl of meat. For three minutes I kept them from approaching the meat, then left each dog alone with the food. Indulged terriers and beagles waited longer before eating the meat than did disciplined dogs of the same breeds. None of the Shetlands ever ate any of the food, and all of the Basenjis ate as soon as I left.

I later studied 20 sets of identical and fraternal human twins, following them from infancy until they were 10 years old, and I became convinced that both puppies and human babies begin life along developmental pathways established by their genetic inheritance. But I still did not know whether infants of relatively inbred human groups showed differences comparable to the breed differences among puppies that had so impressed me. Clearly, the most direct way to find out was to examine very young infants, preferably newborns, of ethnic groups with widely divergent histories.

Since it was important to avoid projecting my own assumptions onto the babies' behavior, the first step was to develop some sort of objective test of newborn behavior. With T. Berry Brazelton, the Harvard pediatrician, I developed what I called the Cambridge Behavioral and Neurological Assessment Scales, a group of simple tests of basic human reactions that could be administered to any normal newborn in a hospital nursery.

In the first study, Nina Freedman and I compared Chinese and Caucasian babies. It was no accident that we chose those two groups, since my wife is Chinese, and in the course of learning about each other and our families, we came to believe that some character differences might well be related to differences in our respective gene pools and not just to individual differences.

Armed with our new baby test, Nina and I returned to San Francisco and to the hospital where she had borne our first child. We examined, alternately, 24 Chinese and 24 Caucasian newborns. To keep things neat, we made sure that all the Chinese were of Cantonese (south Chinese) background, the Caucasians of northern European origin, that the sexes in both groups were the same, that the mothers were the same age, that they had about the same number of previous children, and that both groups were administered the same drugs in the same amounts. Additionally, all of the families were members of the same health plan, all of the mothers had had approximately the same number of prenatal visits to a doctor, and all were in the same middle-income bracket.

It was almost immediately clear that we had struck pay dirt: Chinese and Caucasian babies indeed behaved like two different breeds. Caucasian babies cried more easily, and once started, they were harder to console. Chinese babies adapted to almost any position in which they were placed; for example, when placed face down in their cribs, they tended to keep their faces buried in the sheets rather than immediately turning to one side, as did the Caucasians. In a similar maneuver (called the "defense reaction" by neurologists), we briefly pressed the baby's nose with a cloth. Most Caucasian and black babies fight this maneuver by immediately turning away or swiping at the cloth with their hands, and this is reported in most Western pediatric textbooks as the normal, expected response. The average Chinese baby in our study, however, simply lay on his back and breathed through his mouth, "accepting" the cloth without a fight. This finding is most impressive on film.

Other subtle differences were equally important, but less dramatic. For example, both Chinese and Caucasian babies started to cry at about the same points in the examination, especially when they were undressed, but the Chinese stopped sooner. When picked up and cuddled, Chinese babies stopped crying immediately, as if a light switch had been flipped, whereas the crying of Caucasian babies only gradually subsided.

In another part of the test, we repeatedly shone a light in the baby's eyes and counted the number of blinks until the baby "adapted" and no longer blinked. It should be no surprise that the Caucasian babies continued to blink long after the Chinese babies had adapted and stopped.

It began to look as if Chinese babies were simply more amenable and adaptable to the machinations of the examiners, and that the Caucasian babies were registering annoyance and complaint. It was as if the old stereotypes of the calm, inscrutable Chinese and the excitable, emotionally changeable Caucasian were appearing spontaneously in the first 48 hours of life. In other words, our hypothesis about human and puppy parallels seemed to be correct.

The results of our Chinese-Caucasian study have been confirmed by a student of ethnologist Nick Blurton-Jones who worked in a Chinese community in Malaysia. At the time, however, our single study was hardly enough evidence for so general a conclusion, and we set out to look at other newborns in other places. Norbett Mintz, who was working among the Navaho in Tuba City, Arizona, arranged for us to come to the reservation in the spring of 1969. After two months we had tested 36 Navaho newborns, and the results paralleled the stereotype of the stoical, impassive American Indian. These babies outdid the Chinese, showing even more calmness and adaptability than we found among Oriental babies.

We filmed the babies as they were tested and found reactions in the film we had not noticed. For example, the Moro response was clearly different among Navaho and Caucasians. This inaction occurs in newborns when support for the head and neck suddenly disappears. Tests for the Moro response usually consist of raising and then suddenly dropping the head portion of the bassinet. In most Caucasian newborns, after a four-inch drop the baby reflexively extends both of the arms and legs, cries, and moves in an agitated manner before he calms down. Among Navajo babies, crying was rare, the limb movements were reduced, and calming was almost immediate.

I have since spent considerable time among the Navaho, and it is clear that the traditional practice of tying the wrapped infant onto a cradleboard (now practiced sporadically on the reservation) has in no way induced stoicism in the Navaho. In the halcyon days of anthropological environmentalism, this was a popular conjecture, but the other way around is more likely. Not all Navaho babies take to the cradleboard, and those who complain about it are simply taken off. But most Navaho infants calmly accept the board; in fact, many begin to demand it by showing signs of unrest when off. When they are about six months old, however, Navaho babies do start complaining at being tied, and "weaning" from the board begins, with the baby taking the lead. The Navaho are the most "in touch" group of mothers we have yet seen, and the term mother-infant unit aptly describes what we saw among them.

James Chisholm of Rutgers University, who has studied infancy among the Navaho over the past several years, reports that his observations are much like my own. In addition, he followed a group of young Caucasian mothers in Flagstaff (some 80 miles south of the reservation) who had decided to use the cradleboard. Their babies complained so persistently that they were off the board in a matter of weeks, a result that should not surprise us, given the differences observed at birth.

Assuming, then, that other investigators continue to confirm our findings, to what do we attribute the difference on the one hand, and the similarities on the other? When we first presented the findings on Chinese and Caucasians, attempts were made to explain away the genetic implications by posing differences in prenatal diets as an obvious cause. But once we had completed the Navaho study, that explanation had to be dropped, because the Navaho diet is quite different from the diet of the Chinese, yet newborn behavior was strikingly similar in the two groups.

The point is often still made that the babies had nine months of experience within the uterus before we saw them, so that cultural differences in maternal attitudes and behavior might have been transferred to the unborn offspring via some, as yet un-known, mechanism. Chisholm, for example, thinks differences in maternal blood pres-sure may be responsible for some of the differences between Navahos and Caucasians, but the evidence is as yet sparse. Certainly Cantonese American and Navaho cultures are substantially different and yet the infants are so much alike that such speculation might be dismissed on that score alone. But there is another hidden issue here, and that involves our own cultural tendency to split apart inherited and acquired charac-teristics. Americans tend to eschew the inherited and promote the acquired, in a sort of "we are exactly what we make of ourselves" optimism.

My position on this issue is simple: We are totally biological, totally environmental; the two are as inseparable as are an object and its shadow. Or as psychologist Donald O. Hebb has expressed it, we are 100 percent innate, 100 percent acquired. One might add to Hebb's formulation, 100 percent biological, 100 percent cultural. As D. T. Suzuki, the Zen scholar, once told an audience of neuropsychiatrists, "You took heredity and envi-ronment apart and now you are stuck with the problem of putting them together again."

Navaho and Chinese newborns may be so much alike because the Navaho were part of a relatively recent emigration from Asia. Their language group is called Athabaskan, after a lake in Canada. Although most of the Athabaskan immigrants from Asia set-tled along the Pacific coast of Canada, the Navaho and Apache contingents went on to their present location in about 1200 A.D. Even today, a significant number of words in Athabaskan and Chinese appear to have the same meaning, and if one looks back sev-eral thousand years into the written records of Sino-Tibetan, the number of similar words makes clear the common origin of these widely separated peoples.

When we say that some differences in human behavior may have a genetic basis, what do we mean? First of all, we are not talking about a gene for stoicism or a gene for irritability. If a behavioral trait is at all interesting, for example smiling, anger, ease of sexual arousal, or altruism, it is most probably polygenic—that is, many genes contribute to its development. Furthermore, there is no way to count the exact number of genes involved in such a polygenic system because, as geneticist James Crow has summarized, the situation biological traits are controlled by one, two, or many genes.

Standing height, a polygenic human trait, can be easily measured and is also notoriously open to the influence of the environment. For this reason height can serve as a model for behavioral traits, which are genetically influenced but are even more prone to change with changing environment.

There are, however, limits to the way that a given trait responds to the environment, and this range of constraint imposed by the genes is called a reaction range. Behavioral geneticist Irving Gottesman has drawn up a series of semihypothetical graphs illustrating how this works with regard to human height; each genotype (the combination of genes that determine a particular trait) represents a relatively inbred human group. Even the most favorable environment produces little change in height for genotype A, whereas for genotype D a vast difference is seen as nutrition improves.

When I speak of potential genetic differences in human behavior, I do so with these notions in mind: There is overlap between most populations and the overlap can become rather complete under changing conditions, as in genotypes D and C. Some genotypes, however, show no overlap and remain remote from the others over the entire reaction range, as in genotype A (actually a group of achondroplastic dwarfs; it is likely that some pygmy groups would exhibit a similarly isolated reaction range with regard to height).

At present we lack the data to construct such reaction range curves for newborn behavior, but hypothetically there is nothing to prevent us from one day doing so.

The question naturally arises whether the group differences we have found are expressions of richer and poorer environments, rather than of genetically distinguishable groups. The similar performance yet substantial difference in socioeconomic status between Navaho and San Francisco Chinese on the one hand, and the dissimilar performance yet similar socio-economic status of San Francisco Chinese and Caucasians on the other favors the genetic explanation. Try as one might, it is very difficult, conceptually and actually, to get rid of our biological constraints.

Research among newborns in other cultures shows how environment—in this case, cultural learning—affects reaction range. In Hawaii we met a Honolulu pediatrician who volunteered that he had found striking and consistent differences between Japanese and Polynesian babies in his practice. The Japanese babies consistently reacted more violently to their three-month immunizations than did the Polynesians. On subsequent visits, the Japanese gave every indication of remembering the last visit by crying violently; one mother said that her baby cried each time she drove by the clinic.

We then tested a series of Japanese newborns, and found that they were indeed more sensitive and irritable than either the Chinese or Navaho babies. In other respects, though, they were much like them, showing a similar response to consolation, and accommodating easily to a light on the eyes or a cloth over the nose. Prior to our work, social anthropologist William Caudill had made an extensive and thorough study of Japanese infants. He made careful observations of Japanese mother-infant pairs in Baltimore, from the third to the twelfth month of life. Having noted that both the Japanese infants and their mothers vocalized much less to one another than did Caucasian pairs, he assumed that the Japanese mothers were conditioning their babies toward quietude from a universal baseline at which all babies start. Caudill, of course, was in the American environmentalist tradition and, until our publication appeared, did not consider the biological alternative. We believe that the mothers and babies he studied were, in all probability, conditioning each other, that the naturally quiet Japanese babies affected their mothers' behavior as much as the mothers affected their babies'.

With this new interactive hypothesis in mind, one of my students, Joan Kuchner, studied mother-infant interactions among 10 Chinese and 10 Caucasian mother-infant pairs over the first three months of life. The study was done in Chicago, and this time the Chinese were of north Chinese rather than south Chinese (Cantonese) ancestry. Kuchner started her study with the birth of the babies and found that the two groups were different from the start, much as in our study of newborns. Further, it soon became apparent that Chinese mothers were less intent on eliciting responses from their infants. By the third month, Chinese infants and mothers rarely engaged in bouts of mutual vocalizing as did the Caucasian pairs. This was exactly what the Caudill studies of Japanese and Caucasians had shown, but we now know that it was based on a developing coalition between mothers and babies and that it was not just a one-way street in which a mother "shapes" her infant's behavior.

Following our work, Caudill and Lois Frost repeated Caudill's original work, but this time they used third-generation Japanese American mothers and their fourth-generation infants. The mothers had become "super" American and were vocalizing to their infants at almost twice the Caucasian rate of activity, and the infants were responding at an even greater rate of happy vocalization. Assuming that these are sound and repeatable results, my tendency is to reconcile these and our results in terms of the reaction-range concept. If Japanese height can change as dramatically as it has with emigration to the United States (and with post–World War II diets), it seems plausible that mother-infant behavior can do the same. On a variety of other measures, Caudill and Frost were able to discern continuing similarities to infant and mother pairs in the old country. Fourth-generation Japanese babies, like babies in Japan, sucked their fingers less and were less playful than Caucasian babies were, and the third-generation mothers lulled their babies and held them more than Caucasian American mothers did.

A student and colleague, John Callaghan, has recently completed a study comparing 15 Navaho and 19 Anglo mothers and their young infants (all under six months). Each mother was asked to "get the attention of the baby." When videotapes of the subsequent scene were analyzed, the differences in both babies and mothers were striking. The Navaho babies showed greater passivity than the Caucasian babies. Caucasian mothers "spoke" to their babies continually, using linguistic forms appropriate for someone who understands language; their babies responded by moving their arms and legs. The Navaho mothers were strikingly silent, using their eyes to attract their babies' gaze, and the relatively immobile infants responded by merely gazing back.

Despite their disparate methods, both groups were equally successful in getting their babies' attention. Besides keeping up a stream of chatter, Caucasian mothers tended to shift the baby's position radically, sometimes holding him or her close, sometimes at arm's length, as if experimenting to find the best focal distance for the baby. Most of the silent Navaho mothers used only subtle shifts on the lap, holding the baby at about the same distance throughout. As a result of the intense stimulation by the Caucasian mothers, the babies frequently turned their heads away, as if to moderate the intensity of the encounter. Consequently, eye contact among Caucasian pairs is of shorter duration (half that of the Navaho), but more frequent.

It was clear that the Caucasian mothers sought their babies' attention with verve and excitement even as their babies tended to react to the stimulation with what can be described as ambivalence: The Caucasian infants turned both toward and away from the mother with far greater frequency than did the Navaho infants. The Navaho mothers and their infants engaged in relatively stoical, quiet, and steady encounters. On viewing the films of these sequences, we had the feeling that we were watching biocultural differences in the making.

Studies of older children bear out the theme of relative unexcitability in Chinese as compared to Anglos. In an independent research project at the University of Chicago, Nova Green studied a number of nursery schools. When she reached one in Chicago's Chinatown, she reported:

> Although the majority of the Chinese-American children were in the "high arousal age," between three and five, they showed little intense emotional behavior. They ran and hopped, laughed and called to one another, rode bikes and roller skated just as the children did in the other nursery schools, but the noise level stayed remarkably low, and the emotional atmosphere projected serenity instead of bedlam. The impassive facial expression certainly gave the children an air of dignity and self-possession, but this was only one element affecting the total impression.
>
> Physical movements seemed more coordinated, no tripping, falling, bumping, or bruising was observed, nor screams, crashes or wailing was heard, not even that common sound in other nurseries, voices raised in highly indignant moralistic dispute! No property disputes were observed, and only the mildest version of "fighting behavior," some good-natured wrestling among the older boys. The adults evidently had different expectations about hostile or impulsive behavior; this was the only nursery school where it was observed that children were trusted to duel with sticks. Personal distance spacing seemed to be situational rather than compulsive or patterned, and the children appeared to make no effort to avoid physical contact.

It is ironic that many recent visitors to nursery schools in Red China have returned with ecstatic descriptions of the children, implying that the New Order knows something about child rearing that the West does not. When the *New Yorker* reported a visit to China by a group of developmental psychologists including William Kessen, Urie Bronfenbrenner, Jerome Kagan, and Eleanor Maccoby, they were described as baffled by the behavior of Chinese children:

> They were won over by the Chinese children. They speak of an attractive mixture of affective spontaneity and an accommodating posture by the children: of the "remarkable control of young Chinese children"—alert, animated, vigorous, responsive to the words of their elders, yet also unnervingly calm, even during happenings (games, classroom events, neighborhood play) that could create agitation and confusion. The children "were far less restless, less intense in their motor actions, and displayed less crying and whining than American children in similar situations. We were constantly struck by [their] quiet, gentle, and controlled manner . . . and as constantly frustrated in our desire to understand its origins."

The report is strikingly similar to Nova Green's description of the nursery school in Chicago's Chinatown. When making these comparisons with "American" nursery schools, the psychologists obviously had in mind classrooms filled with Caucasian or Afro-American children.

As they get older, Chinese and Caucasian children continue to differ in roughly the same behavior that characterizes them in nursery school. Not surprisingly, San Francisco schoolteachers consider assignments in Chinatown as plums—the children are dutiful and studious, and the classrooms are quiet.

A reader might accept these data and observations and yet still have trouble imagining how such differences might have initially come about. The easiest explanation involves a historical accident based on different, small founding populations and at least partial geographic isolation. Peking man, some 500,000 years ago, already had shovel shaped incisors, as only Orientals and American Indians have today. Modern looking skulls of about the same age, found in England, lack this grooving on the inside of their upper incisors. Given such evidence, we can surmise that there has been substantial and longstanding isolation of East and West. Further, it is likely that, in addition to just plain "genetic drift," environmental demands and biocultural adaptations differed, yielding present-day differences.

Orientals and Euro-Americans are not the only newborn groups we have examined. We have recorded newborn behavior in Nigeria, Kenya, Sweden, Italy, Bali, India, and Australia, and in each place, it is fair to say, we observed some kind of uniqueness. The Australian aborigines, for example, struggled mightily against the cloth over the nose, resembling the most objecting Caucasian babies; their necks were exceptionally strong, and some could lift their heads up and look around, much like some of the African babies we saw. (Caucasian infants cannot do this until they are about one month old.) Further, aborigine infants were easy to calm, resembling in that respect our easygoing Chinese babies. They thus comprised a unique pattern of traits.

Given these data, I think it is a reasonable conclusion that we should drop two long-cherished myths: (1) No matter what our ethnic background, we are all born alike; (2) culture and biology are separate entities. Clearly, we are biosocial creatures in everything we do and say, and it is time that anthropologists, psychologists, and population geneticists start speaking the same language. In light of what we know, only a truly holistic, multidisciplinary approach makes sense.

For Further Information

Caudill, W., and N. Frost. "A Comparison of Maternal Care and Infant Behavior in Japanese-American, American, and Japanese Families." *Influences on Human Development*, edited by Urie Bronfenbrenner and M. A. Mahoney. Dryden Press, 1972.

Chisholm, J. S., and Martin Richards. "Swaddling, Cradleboards and the Development of Children." *Early Human Development*, 2(3): 255–75.

Freedman, D. G. "Constitutional and Environmental Interaction in Rearing of Four Breeds of Dogs." *Science* 127, 1958, pp. 585–586.

Freedman, D. G. *Human Infancy: An Evolutionary Perspective*. Lawrence Erlbaum Associates, 1974.

Freedman, D. G., and B. Keller. "Inheritance of Behavior in Infants." *Science* 140, 1 1963. pp. 196–198.

Gottesman. I. I. Developmental Genetics and Ontogenetic Psychology." *Minnesota Symposia on Child Psychology*, Vol. 8, edited by A. D. Pick. Minneapolis: University of Minnesota Press, 1974.

Suggestions for Further Reading

Baines, Elizabeth. 1983. *The Birth Machine*. London: Women's Press.

Chalmers, Beverly. 1990. *African Birth: Childbirth in Cultural Transition*. River Club, South Africa: Berev Publications.

Davis-Floyd, Robbie E. 1992. *Birth As an American Rite of Passage*. Berkeley: University of California Press.

Davis-Floyd, Robbie E., and Carolyn F. Sargent, eds. 1997. *Childbirth and Authoritative Knowledge: Cross-Cultural Perspectives*. Berkeley: University of California Press.

Edonard, Lindsay. 1985. Maternal and Child Health Unit, Division of Family Health, World Health Organization. *Traditional Birth Practices: An Annotated Bibliography*.

Fraser, Gertrude. 1992. *Afro-American Midwives, Biomedicine, and the State*. Cambridge, Mass.: Harvard University Press.

Gebbie, Donald A. M. 1981. *Reproductive Anthropology—Descent through Woman*. Chicester: John Wiley and Son.

Gelis, Jacques. 1991. *History of Childbirth: Fertility, Pregnancy and Birth in Early Modern Europe*. Boston: Northeastern University Press.

Ginsburg, Faye, and Rayna Rapp, eds. 1995. *Conceiving the New World Order: The Global Politics of Reproduction*. Berkeley: University of California Press.

Goer, Henci. 1995. *Obstetric Myths versus Research Realities: A Guide to Medical Literature*. Westport, Conn.: Bergin & Garvey.

Goldsmith, Judith. 1990. *Childbirth Wisdom*. Brookline, Mass.: East West Health Books.

Granqvist, Hilma. 1947. *Birth and Childhood among the Arabs: Studies in a Muhammadan Village in Palestine*. Helsingfors: Söderström and Co. Forlagsaktiebolag.

Haire, Doris. 1973. *The Cultural Warping of Childbirth*. Environmental Child Health, Special Issue, monograph no. 27, pp. 171–191.

Hampe, Ruth. 1995. *Frau und Geburt im Kulturvergleich: eine kunst-und kulturanalytische Studie* [Woman and Birth in Cultural Comparison: An Analytical Study of Art and Culture]. New York: P. Lang.

Jeffery, Patricia, Roger Jeffery, and Andrew Lyon. 1988. *Labor Pains and Labor Power*. London: Zed Books.

Jordan, Brigitte. 1993. *Birth in Four Cultures*, 4th edition. Prospect Heights, Ill.: Waveland Press.

Kahn, Robbie Pfeufer. 1995. *Bearing Meaning: The Language of Birth*. Urbana: University of Illinois Press.

Kay, Margarita Artschwager, ed. 1982. *Anthropology of Human Birth*. Philadelphia: F. A. Davis Company.

Kitzinger, Sheila. 1984. *The Experience of Childbirth*. New York: Penguin.

Liamputtong, Pranee. 1994. *Asian Mothers, Australian Birth: Pregnancy, Childbirth, and Childrearing: The Asian Experience in an English-Speaking Country*. Melbourne: Ausmed Publications.

Lukere, Vicki, and Margaret Jolly, eds. 2002. *Birthing in the Pacific: Beyond Tradition and Modernity*. Honolulu: University of Hawaii Press.

MacCormack, Carol P., ed. 1994. *Ethnography of Fertility and Birth*, 2nd edition. Prospect Heights, Ill.: Waveland Press.

Martin, Emily. 1992. *The Woman in the Body—A Cultural Analysis of Reproduction*. Boston: Beacon Press.

McClain, Carol, ed. 1989. *Women As Healers: Cross-Cultural Perspectives*. New Brunswick: Rutgers University Press.

Michaelson, Karen L., ed. 1992. *Childbirth in America: Anthropological Perspectives*. Berkeley: University of California Press.

Mitford, Jessica. 1992. *The American Way of Birth*. London: Gallancz.

Oakley, Ann. 1980. *Women Confined: Towards a Sociology of Childbirth*. New York: Schocken Books.

Ploss, Hermann Heinrich, Max Bartels, and Paul Bartels. 1902. *Das Weib in der Natur und Völkerkunde: anthropologische Studien* [Women in Nature and Culture: Anthropological Studies]. Vol. 2. Leipzig: T. Grieben (L. Fernau).

Raphael, Dana, ed. 1975. *Being Female*. The Hague: Mouton Publishers.

Schlumbohm, Jürgen, Barbara Duden, Jacques Gelis, and Patrice Veit. 1998. *Rituale der Geburt* [Rituals of Birth]. München: Verlag C. H. Beck.

Sterk, Helen M., Krista Ratcliffe, Carla H. Hay, Leona Vande Vusse, and Alice B. Kehoe. 2002. *Who's Having This Baby?: Perspectives on Birthing*. East Lansing: Michigan State University Press

Turner, Ann Warren. 1978. *Rituals of Birth: From Prehistory to the Present*. New York: David McKay Company, Inc.

Wilson, Philip K., ed. 1996. *Childbirth: Changing Ideas and Practices in Britain and America, 1600 to the Present*. 5 vols. Hamden, Conn.: Garland Publishing.

Witkowski, Gustave J. 1887. *Histoire des Accouchements Chez Tous les Peuples* [History of Childbirth among all Peoples]. Paris: G. Steinheil.

Yamaji, Katsuhiko, ed. 1990. *Kinship, Gender and the Cosmic World: Ethnographies of Birth Customs in Taiwan, the Philippines and Indonesia*. Taipei: SMC Publishing.

Index

About the Editor

Lauren Dundes received her bachelor of arts degree in human biology from Stanford University in 1984. She then received both her master of health science and doctor of science degrees in maternal and child health from the Johns Hopkins Bloomberg School of Public Health. Dr. Dundes is an associate professor of sociology at McDaniel College in Westminster, Maryland, where she teaches medical sociology. She has published many articles in professional journals such as the *American Journal of Public Health, Academic Medicine, Journal of Clinical Epidemiology, American Journal of Infection Control, Illness, Crisis and Loss, Alternative and Complementary Therapies,* and the *Journal of Health and Social Policy.*